The Diagnosis and Treatment of Amyotrophic Lateral Sclerosis

From a Symposium Sponsored by the

Amyotrophic Lateral Sclerosis Society of America

Tucson, Arizona

February 1979

The Diagnosis and Treatment of Amyotrophic Lateral Sclerosis

Edited by

Donald W. Mulder, MD

Andersen Professor of Neurology

Mayo Medical School, Rochester, Minnesota

HMMD Houghton Mifflin Professional Publishers
Medical Division, Boston, Massachusetts

Library of Congress Cataloging in Publication Data

Main entry under title:

The Diagnosis and treatment of amyotrophic lateral
sclerosis.

Includes index.
1. Amyotrophic lateral sclerosis. [DNLM:
1. Amyotrophic lateral sclerosis. 2. Amyotrophic
lateral sclerosis—Therapy. WE550 D536]
RC406.A24D5 616.8'3 80-13398
ISBN 0-89289-403-2

ISBN 0-89289-403-2

LCCCN 80-13398

Contents

Contributors

Arnold E. Aronson, PhD, Head, Section of Speech Pathology, Department of Neurology, Mayo Clinic, Rochester, Minnesota

H. Eames Bishop, President, Amyotrophic Lateral Sclerosis Society of America, Sherman Oaks, California

Christine Cassel, MD, Fellow in Geriatric Medicine, Veterans Administration Hospital; University of Oregon Health Sciences Center, Portland, Oregon

Stanley L. Cohan, MD, PhD, Associate Professor of Neurology and Pharmacology, Department of Neurology, Georgetown University School of Medicine, Washington, DC

Nancy Jones Crigger, RN, Veterans Administration Medical Center, Kansas City, Missouri

Robert D. Currier, MD, Professor of Medicine; Chairman, Department of Neurology, University of Mississippi, Jackson, Mississippi

Arthur Dawson, MD, Head, Division of Chest Medicine, Scripps Clinic and Research Foundation, La Jolla, California

Eric H. Denys, MD, ALS Research Center, Institutes of Medical Sciences, Pacific Medical Center, San Francisco, California

Katharine M. Donohoe, RN, MS, University of Rochester School of Nursing, Rochester, New York

Janice L. Elliott, MCl Sc, Department of Speech Pathology, University Hospital, London, Ontario, Canada

W. King Engel, MD, Chief, Neuromuscular Diseases, National Institute of Neurological and Communicative Diseases and Stroke, National Institutes of Health, Bethesda, Maryland

Robert J. Fallat, MD, ALS Research Center, Institutes of Medical Sciences, Pacific Medical Center, San Francisco, California

Barry W. Festoff, MD, Chief, Neurology Service, Veterans Administration Medical Center, Kansas City, Missouri; Associate Professor, Department of Neurology, University of Kansas Medical Center, Kansas City, Kansas

Parvis Foroozan, MD, Division of Gastroenterology, Scripps Clinic and Research Foundation, La Jolla, California

David Goldblatt, MD, Professor of Neurology, University of Rochester School of Medicine and Dentistry, Rochester, New York

Brian S. Gould, MD, Medical Director, In-Patient Psychiatry; Director, Division of Biological Research, Department of Psychological and Social Medicine, Pacific Medical Center, San Francisco, California

Robert C. Griggs, MD, Professor of Neurology, Medicine, and Pathology, University of Rochester School of Medicine and Dentistry, Rochester, New York

Arthur J. Hudson, MD, Professor of Neurology and Medicine, Department of Clinical Neurological Sciences, University Hospital, London, Ontario, Canada

Steven M. Juergens, MD, Resident, Department of Medicine, Hennepin County Medical Center, Minneapolis, Minnesota

Richard T. Johnson, MD, Eisenhower Professor of Neurology and Professor of Microbiology, The Johns Hopkins University School of Medicine, Baltimore, Maryland

Claudia Kempf, RD, Department of Dietetics, University of Rochester School of Medicine and Dentistry, Rochester, New York

William R. Kennedy, MD, Professor of Neurology, University of Minnesota, Minneapolis, Minnesota

Leonard T. Kurland, MD, DPH, Chairman, Department of Medical Statistics and Epidemiology, Mayo Medical School, Rochester, Minnesota

Kathleen Landon, Patient Service Coordinator, Muscular Dystrophy Association, Rochester, New York

Edward H. Lambert, MD, PhD, Professor of Physiology and Neurology, Mayo Medical School, Rochester, Minnesota

Bahram Mokri, MD, Assistant Professor of Neurology, Mayo Medical School, Rochester, Minnesota

Richard T. Moxley III, MD, Associate Professor, Department of Neurology and Pediatrics, Center for Brain Research, University of Rochester School of Medicine and Dentistry, Rochester, New York

Donald W. Mulder, MD, Andersen Professor of Neurology, Mayo Medical School, Rochester, Minnesota

Theodore L. Munsat, MD, Professor and Chairman, Department of Neurology, Tufts University School of Medicine; Neurologist and Chief, New England Medical Center Hospital, Boston, Massachusetts

Forbes H. Norris, Jr, MD, ALS Research Center, Institutes of Medical Sciences, Pacific Medical Center, San Francisco, California

Bernard M. Patten, MD, Associate Professor of Neurology, Department of Neurology; Chief, Neuromuscular Disease Division, Baylor College of Medicine, Houston, Texas

Victor M. Rivera, MD, Neurologist, Assistant Professor, Baylor University College of Medicine, Houston, Texas

Rita A. Roelofs, RN, Section of Patient and Health Education, Mayo Clinic, Rochester, Minnesota

Lewis P. Rowland, MD, Henry and Lucy Moses Professor and Chairman, Department of Neurology, College of Physicians and Surgeons, Columbia University; Director, Neurological Service, Neurological Institute, Presbyterian Hospital; Director, H. Houston Merritt Clinical Research Center for Muscular Dystrophy and Related Diseases, New York, New York

Mehrsheed Sinaki, MD, Assistant Professor of Physical Medicine, Mayo Clinic, Rochester, Minnesota

Richard A. Smith, MD, Experimental Medicine Section, Center for Neurologic Study, La Jolla, California

H. Richard Tyler, MD, Professor of Neurology, Harvard Medical School; Director of Neurology Services, Affiliated Hospital Center, Inc., Boston, Massachusetts

Kwei Sang Ü, MD, ALS Research Center, Institutes of Medical Sciences, Pacific Medical Center, San Francisco, California

Mark J. Utell, MD, Assistant Professor of Medicine, University of Rochester School of Medicine and Dentistry, Rochester, New York

Foreword

This book is about amyotrophic lateral sclerosis (ALS). Its primary purpose is to provide physicians and paramedical personnel with practical information to aid in the diagnosis and care of the patient with ALS. It presents no "breakthrough" in our knowledge of the cause or cure of the disease. Unfortunately, ALS remains the cruel enigma it has been since it was first recognized over 100 years ago. What the book reveals and fosters is an increasing awareness that despite our ignorance of the cause and cure, something can and must be done for the patient with ALS. It reflects an increasing sensitivity of the medical and lay community to the emotional, intellectual, and physical needs of the patient and the realization that, with appropriate care, the patient with ALS may have a longer and more satisfactory life than heretofore thought possible.

Remarkable advances in medical science over the past century have conquered some diseases and have made many others manageable, but ALS is one of those that remains incurable—an invariably fatal, progressive degeneration of motor neurons that leaves the patient paralyzed, but, all the more poignant, with the intellect preserved until the end. Progress in our understanding of the disease has been documented in several medical symposia. The first on ALS was held in Paris in 1925 on the occasion of the centenary of the birth of Jean Martin Charcot (1825–1893), the French neurologist who gave us the first concise and convincing description of the syndrome. Symposia at the Mayo Clinic in 1957 and the Royal Society of Medicine in 1962 were published in the Proceedings of those institutions. Additional publications followed the first comprehensive conference on motor neuron disease in San Francisco in 1967 and a conference at The Johns Hopkins Hospital in 1972. A series of symposia on ALS were held in Japan in 1961, 1975, 1977, and 1979, and another was organized by the Council of the Medical Society of London in 1976. A symposium on recent research trends in ALS was sponsored by the Amyotrophic Lateral Sclerosis Society of America (ALSSOA) in 1975. These symposia were concerned primarily with the epidemiology and pathology of the disease, with attempts to find specific etiologic factors or specific therapeutic agents, and with studies of possible experimental models that might facilitate research on the disease.

The symposium that resulted in the publication of this book was concerned with patients and their care rather than with the disease itself. For the first time symptomatic therapies available for the ALS patient have been collated. The various medical and paramedical specialists who provide such therapy were brought together to discuss the clinical aspects of the disease and the role and importance of the family and other support systems in the treatment of the illness.

In such a devastating disease the psychologic, sociologic, and ethical implications of the disorder are of first magnitude. These factors, the interpersonal relationships, and subsequent problems of patient and family that evolve in treatment of this disorder are defined. The psychologic and psychiatric implications of the diagnosis and treatment are outlined, and the ethical implications of treatment of this relentlessly progressive disease are discussed. The formal chapters cover most of the topics of interest to those who care for patients with this disease. The discussions of the chapters by the members of the symposium, all of whom are experienced in the treatment of this disorder, serve to identify points of disagreement, to stress what is essential, and perhaps most important to point up the need for further investigation in symptomatic therapy as well as the need to press toward the final goal of finding a specific therapy. These comments add a dimension and depth that might not be obtained from a formal statement by any one individual.

The book stresses the role of the neurologic physician as a guide, not only to the patient but also to family members as they attempt to improve the quality of the patient's life while adapting to the increasing limitations of the disease. Physicians are reminded that in addition to their role as diagnostic specialists, they must also be caring. The book describes ALS in some depth. It notes what has been tested in the past and has failed as specific treatment and indicates some of the trends in continuing research. However, emphasis is placed on recounting and analyzing the clinical picture of the disease in its broadest sense. From this should come a better outlook for the patient, hopefully a fresh approach in the search for the cause and cure of ALS, but certainly renewed enthusiasm for research and support of research of the disease.

Edward H. Lambert, MD, PhD

Acknowledgments

This monograph is an outgrowth of a symposium entitled "The Care and Treatment of Amyotrophic Lateral Sclerosis," held in Tucson, Arizona, in February 1979 under the auspices of the Amyotrophic Lateral Sclerosis Society of America (ALSSOA). The organizing committee for the meeting included Drs. David Goldblatt, William R. Kennedy, Donald W. Mulder, Theodore L. Munsat, Forbes Norris, Jr, and Mr. H. Eames Bishop.

The authors and the ALSSOA are most appreciative of the significant underwriting of both the planning meetings and the conference by the ALS Foundation, Incorporated, of Milwaukee; the ALS Trust in Memory of Henry A. Wallace, Washington, DC; Mr. Aron Birmann of São Paulo, Brazil; Mr. Justin Friedman of Cincinnati; the Saint Gerard Foundation of Clearwater, Florida; and Mr. Huston Huffman of Oklahoma City.

The editor wishes to thank Mrs. Marian Dubbels, who left retirement to contribute her time as executive secretary in the preparation of this book.

1 Introduction

Donald W. Mulder

Disorders of the anterior horn cells of the spinal cord are associated with a group of diseases for which there is no known etiology and no specific therapy. The onset of these diseases is insidious and their clinical course is slowly progressive. These disorders have been classified according to age of patient at onset, prognosis, and clinical findings. In young infants, they are diagnosed as infantile muscular atrophy (Werdnig-Hoffmann syndrome); in adolescents, as juvenile muscular atrophy (Wohlfart-Kugelberg-Welander syndrome); and in adults, as amyotrophic lateral sclerosis (ALS).

Amyotrophic lateral sclerosis is the most common of these syndromes. This monograph is an outgrowth of a symposium entitled Diagnosis and Clinical Care of the Patient with ALS, held under the auspices of the Amyotrophic Lateral Sclerosis Society of America* in Tucson, Arizona, February 1979. The various chapters deal with the diagnosis of ALS and with the care that physicians and paramedical professionals can provide for patients with this disease. In addition, this is the first monograph that deals directly with symptomatic treatment of patients with ALS.

Amyotrophic lateral sclerosis was first described in the nineteenth century, and the name was first used by Charcot in 1874 (1). The syndrome is characterized by progressive, asymmetric muscular atrophy; hyperreflexia; and occasionally Babinski's signs; but there is no loss of ocular movement or bladder control. There are no other neurologic signs

*Headquarters address: P.O. Box 5951, Sherman Oaks, CA 91403.

regularly associated with the disorder. No descriptions of this clinically characteristic syndrome have been found in the medical literature published before the nineteenth century, although a privately published family history from the eighteenth century describes patients with a hereditary form of the disease (3). It is not known whether the disease was at one time confused with other paralytic disorders of the aged or whether it is a new disease that may be etiologically related to changes in the ecosystem during the past century. However, the incidence of ALS is uniform throughout most of the world and does not suggest a close etiologic relation between the disorder and the modern environment.

Two major themes to be discussed in the initial chapters are diagnosis and epidemiology of ALS. The diagnosis of ALS traditionally has been surrounded by an aura of hopelessness. In one text on neurology, the following comment is found: "Such a diagnosis means helplessness, despair, and ultimate death" (8). In the past, many physicians have felt that treatment for ALS should not be attempted because of the inability to alter the pathology of the anterior horn cell. However, some patients with ALS live productive lives long after the diagnosis has been established. Many of them continue in their occupations, and some have carried out outstanding work in spite of advanced ALS. The ability of the patient to cope with this disease has been largely overlooked in the medical literature, even though it is well documented that after the severe poliomyelitis epidemics of the early part of this century many patients with polio returned to a productive life despite severe loss of anterior horn cells.

The first few chapters of this volume highlight the observation that the diagnosis of ALS is only a clinical one and that there is no specific laboratory test for the disease. The diagnosis is made on the basis of a group of clinical findings and on the patient's history. In most cases, the examining neurologists agree on the diagnosis of ALS by the time the disease is well established. However, significant differences of opinion exist regarding patients who are atypical or in whom the disease occurs in early adult life. Occasionally, a patient with a disorder that is actually benign or treatable is improperly diagnosed as having ALS. More frequently, the diagnosis is overlooked for a long time. Clinical diagnosis, laboratory tests, and differential diagnosis for ALS are discussed in detail throughout the volume (see chapters 2, 4, and 5).

Analysis of epidemiologic data on ALS can be of considerable value in establishment of the diagnosis, prognosis, and care of patients suffering from the disorder. The incidence of ALS is approximately twice that of myasthenia gravis or muscular dystrophy and nearly that of multiple sclerosis (5). However, it is less prevalent than multiple sclerosis because it primarily affects older persons and causes death sooner than does multiple sclerosis. The disease has a predilection for three distinct groups of people. First, and most commonly, it is a disease of the elderly (see chapter 3). Second, it occurs in families as a dominant hereditary trait with good penetrance. Finally, it is prevalent in a small and distinct population in the Mariana Islands. These and other observations suggest that ALS occurs in the presence of a defect (possibly metabolic) of the anterior horn cells that renders these cells vulnerable to toxins or other noxious stimuli that are widespread in the environment (7). It is now apparent that epidemiologic data reported from clinical series studied at large medical centers are distorted by the relative mobility of their patient populations, which are younger and have less severe disease. In addition, the difficulty for older and more severely ill patients of traveling to such centers acts as a selective process and thus prevents their inclusion in such series. The data furnished in chapter 3, which are based on a specific population study, not only present a more valid description of the disorder as it is observed in the examining room of most practitioners, but also suggest that the disease is commonly overlooked in elderly patients.

Patients with ALS or other diseases of the motor system do not initially associate their disease with a feeling of illness. This is particularly true in cases where loss of motor function is very slow. In instances in which loss of movement occurs over months, it is possible for a patient to compensate so fully by using other muscles in order to carry out a function similar to that which was lost that he or she may not recognize the disability. Thus, a patient who, after many years, walks or eats with great difficulty will assure the physician that he or she is not sick. However, rapid loss of motor function may result in diminished ability of the patient to cope with the disease; such a patient is more likely to report to a physician at an early stage with a feeling of illness. A patient will also consult a physician early if loss of anterior horn cells occurs sufficiently rapidly that secondary symptoms, such as impairment of walking, writing, talking, and swallowing, begin to develop. In this situation, the patient's feeling of illness is probably related more to the response of others to his or her loss of function than to the disease itself. Many patients associate their first awareness of being ill with their physician's feeling of hopelessness toward the disease.

The primary concern of the patient and physician, and another major theme of this monograph, is how to provide the most effective and economical care for the individual suffering from ALS. The role of the neurologist in the treatment of ALS and related disorders is significant but limited. It is usually the neurologist who makes or confirms the diagnosis. However, most advice regarding care of these patients is a responsibility shared by several specialists, including physiatrists, nutritionists, internists, specialists in respiratory care, paramedical personnel, and nurses.

Specific therapy for patients with ALS includes rehabilitative measures, speech therapy, and various techniques designed to aid in nutrition and respiratory function. In addition, surgical procedures and drug therapies are available to patients with ALS. However, caution is essential in performing surgery or administering drugs; patients with ALS may be fragile, and the side effects of some treatments may be worse than the disease. Variability in the course of the disease, including variability of both initial site and maximal involvement, dictates that each patient be treated according to the character of his or her individual disease.

In the past, clinical trials of new drugs for ALS have constituted the most common form of treatment offered to patients with this disorder. At present, such trials may offer hope to both patient and physician. However, a careful review of clinical trials conducted thus far reveals that few have been competently carried out or adequately reported. New methods of performing and reporting such trials are clearly needed.

The strategy needed to supply each element of care differs for each patient and family. Patients who have been most successful in coping with ALS have themselves been instrumental in the ordering of care. Home care is regarded as an ideal arrangement for most patients with ALS. In fact, in many cases the care of a patient is primarily a family endeavor that is supplemented by the physician's advice and expertise. Such care also presupposes that the patient or family has access to medical support.

Home care of the patient with ALS is not without difficulty and can also pose problems with regard to actual implementation of supportive measures; considerable attention is given to this aspect throughout the volume. Some difficulties relate to psychologic problems of specific individuals (other than the patient) in handling the situation. Even the physician may be the source of some difficulties (see chapter 10).

Among the issues that were left unexplored at this symposium was the great cost of care, both financial and emotional, for patients with ALS, particularly for patients who are completely paralyzed. The financial cost of such home care is usually beyond the resources of the family, and the difficulty of obtaining financial support from outside sources is often insurmountable. Thus, some patients may be institutionalized against their wishes or the wishes of their families. Yet attempts to provide this care in an institutional setting or with use of paid professionals are usually only partially satisfactory and are useful only as an adjuvant to the care and understanding of family or friends. The reported scarcity of resources for meeting the general medical needs of the population (6) poses ethical problems with regard to patients suffering from ALS. Physicians and others who are interested in patients with ALS and related disorders must call attention to such problems. This topic is discussed in detail in the final chapters of the volume.

Another issue left essentially unexplored in this volume is the neuropathology of ALS, although the final chapter contains a brief discussion of the basic pathology of ALS from divergent viewpoints. Previous textbooks on ALS have focused on the anatomic pathology of diseases of the anterior horn cells in an attempt to find a cause and cure for ALS. The reader is referred to some excellent reviews of this subject (2, 4).

It is hoped that the information presented in relation to the theme of patient care will help to broaden the patient's self-determination by providing an understanding of the disease and its treatment. Such understanding will be derived in large part from open and honest interaction among patient, family, and physician. One such approach and the ethics involved in this interaction are discussed in detail in chapter 8.

The following are some questions that were raised during the symposium that need further investigation.

1. How can the physician discuss with patient and family the diagnosis and clinical implications of ALS in a manner that will help them to cope with the disorder?

2. What is the physician's response to the illness, and what impact does this response have on the care of the patient?

3. What rehabilitative measures are useful in the treatment of ALS and related disorders?

4. Is exercise of the muscles associated with severely involved anterior horn cells helpful or harmful?

5. Which surgical approach (e.g., gastrostomy, esophagostomy, cricopharyngeal myotomy) is most therapeutic for severe bulbar palsy?

6. What is the ideal respiratory aid for the patient with ALS?

7. What is the most effective kind of home care for patients with severe paralysis?

8. What is the relation of ALS to other motor neuron diseases?

9. Which tests are of most value in establishment of the initial diagnosis of ALS?

10. What tests are essential for determination of the best type of care for the patient during the course of illness?

11. What are the most important differential diagnoses that should be recognized in the diagnosis of ALS?

It is clear from the papers in this volume that we have only begun to identify the techniques that will be most helpful to patients with ALS and related disorders. It is hoped that this book will stimulate the research that is needed in order for more effective and economical treatment of such diseases to be discovered.

REFERENCES

1. Charcot JM: De la sclerose laterale amyotrophique. Progres Med 2:325, 341, 453, 1874

2. Chou SL: Pathognomy of intraneuronal inclusions in ALS. In *Proceedings of the International Symposium on ALS,* 2–3 February 1978. Edited by TT Subaki, Y Toyokura. Tokyo, University of Tokyo Press, 1979, pp 135–176

3. Hammond WA: *A Treatise on the Diseases of the Nervous System.* New York, D Appleton & Company, 1876, pp 526–530

4. Hirano A, Malamud N, Kurland LT, et al: A review of the pathologic findings in ALS. In *Motor Neuron Diseases: Research on Amyotrophic Lateral Sclerosis and Related Disorders.* Edited by FH Norris, LT Kurland. New York, Grune and Stratton, 1969, pp 51–61

5. Kurtze JF, Kurland LT: The epidemiology of neurologic disease. In *Clinical Neurology,* Vol. 3. Edited by AB Baker, LH Baker. Hagerstown, MD, Harper and Row, 1978, pp 1–80

6. Lazarus M, Gleason HP: Health care: a view from Europe. N Engl J Med 301:730–731, 1979

7. Mulder DW: The clinical syndrome of ALS. Proc Staff Meet Mayo Clin 32:427–436, 1957

8. Parker HL: *Clinical Studies in Neurology.* Springfield, IL, Charles C Thomas, 1956, p 162

2 Motor Neuron Diseases: The Clinical Syndromes

Lewis P. Rowland

The clinical characteristics of motor neuron disease have been reported in several recent comprehensive reviews (8, 10, 41, 48, 81, 94, 96, 99, 102, 118, 137). I will try to avoid redundancy by stressing points of contemporary interest.

In practice, neurologists act as though the clinical diagnosis of motor neuron disease were accurate, even though there is no pathognomonic laboratory test. It is likely that the clinical diagnosis is almost always accurate, but the precision of the diagnosis has not yet been formally assessed, and there are errors to be found. Some patients are subjected to unnecessary delay in diagnosis, thus creating emotional problems, or to cervical laminectomy or other procedures that in retrospect are inappropriate. It is probably even worse when the neurologist informs a patient or family that the most likely diagnosis is motor neuron disease and informs them of the gloomy prognosis, only to find out later that the diagnosis was wrong.

Clinical decisions about motor neuron disease are based on two general sources of information: postmortem studies and clinical analysis of series of living patients. Both sources have obvious limitations. Postmortem series reduce the margin of diagnostic error, but there are problems of classification of atypical cases that even pathologists cannot resolve. Postmortem series also are biased, because the patients died in the hospital rather than at home or in a chronic care facility; such studies are therefore weighted by cases of more rapid evolution. For instance, in the autopsy series conducted by Brownell et al., the mean duration of disease was only two years (21). On the other hand, analysis of series of living patients is limited to an unknown (but presumably small) extent because of diagnostic error. Another kind of limitation affects both postmortem and clinical analysis: it is suspected that there is more than one form of motor neuron disease, but it is not known how to separate the different types.

DEFINITION OF MOTOR NEURON DISEASES

Motor neuron diseases are manifest by weakness and wasting of skeletal muscle. Fasciculation may or may not be evident. Tendon reflexes may be either lost or increased, and signs of damage to the corticospinal tract may or may not be present. Sensory loss and cerebellar or extrapyramidal signs are not found in uncomplicated neuron disease (43). It is not certain whether dementia implies an additional diagnosis (20, 45, 100, 124, 129). The course is inexorably progressive. Nerve conduction velocities are normal or only slightly decreased, electromyographic and histologic changes in muscle are compatible with denervation, and postmortem changes are restricted to alterations of motor neurons and their axons or to secondary gliosis. In sum, all symptoms, signs, and histopathologic changes in motor neuron disease can be explained by, and are restricted to, disease of the upper or lower motor neurons, or both.

There are several problems of definition: First, clinical and pathologic problems arise when most of the characteristic features of motor neuron disease are present, but there are atypical features as well. Second, there has been a tendency in recent years to abolish the distinction between diseases of the motor neuron and purely motor syndromes attributed to dying-back peripheral neuropathies (36, 37, 85). To me, this concept is filled with ambiguity and uncertainty, especially in cases where nerve conduction velocities are normal and there is no clear evidence of peripheral nerve disease in other members of the family. Finally, some disorders of motor neuron function (e.g., myokymia, cramps, benign fasciculations) are not ordinarily included by the term *motor neuron disease* because they are not manifest by weakness and wasting. The syndrome of benign fasciculation in particular is important in relation to concepts of motor neuron disease. It would be expected that fasciculation should sometimes precede weakness in motor neuron disease, but we have never seen this, and there is no documented example of it in the literature. By the time of first examination, patients with motor neuron disease are always weak; conversely, fasciculation, with or without cramps but without weakness, does not evolve into motor neuron disease.

TERMINOLOGY

The term *motor neuron disease* encompasses several different syndromes, depending on clinical signs. *Spinal muscular atrophy* designates syndromes of limb weakness and wasting, regardless of whether cranial muscles are affected, and there are only signs of lower motor neuron disease. *Progressive bulbar palsy* is dominated by weakness of cranial muscles of the lower motor neuron type. *Amyotrophic lateral sclerosis* is characterized by both upper and lower motor neuron signs. *Primary lateral sclerosis* designates a syndrome manifest by corticospinal tract signs alone, with no evidence of disorder of lower motor neurons. Because these syndromes overlap clinically and pathologically, *ALS* and *motor neuron disease* have become equivalent terms for designating any or all of these syndromes in adults. (However, the clinical syndrome of primary lateral sclerosis can be due to diverse causes, including compressive lesions of the cervical spinal cord and multiple sclerosis, so the term should probably be reserved for autopsy-proven cases.)

There are still debates about terminology. Norris attempted to distinguish spinal muscular atrophy from ALS with the assertion that the pure lower motor neuron syndrome has the following characteristics: earlier age at onset (third to fourth decades, in contrast to the sixth decade for ALS); bulbar muscles affected late; loss of reflexes instead of hyperactive reflexes; flaccidity instead of spasticity; less frequent fasciculation and cramps; better prognosis (survival for 20 years is more common); and lack of histologic evidence of degeneration of the corticospinal tract (104). These may actually be different diseases, but the generalities do not differentiate them; even though patients may never show upper motor neuron signs clinically, the corticospinal tracts are almost always found to be affected at autopsy (21, 78). In postmortem series, cases of pure motor neuron degeneration and cases of pure corticospinal tract degeneration are equally rare (21, 78). Therefore, most students consider the several clinical forms of motor neuron disease to be manifestations of the same disorder.* This viewpoint does not exclude the likely possibility that, once we can identify the pathogenesis of some of these syndromes, we will understand that there is actually more than one disease.

---

* For purposes of this essay, the term *ALS* implies a syndrome of both upper and lower motor neuron disease; *spinal muscular atrophy*, lower motor neurons alone. The term *motor neuron disease* encompasses idiopathic forms of both of these syndromes and bulbar palsy as well. In the plural, *motor neuron diseases* includes still other diseases that affect the motor neuron. The terminology is obviously not satisfactory.

VARIETIES OF MOTOR NEURON DISEASES

There is a subtle distinction between the differential diagnosis of a syndrome and the recognition that the same clinical or pathologic disorder may result from more than one cause. For instance, cervical spondylosis may be difficult to distinguish from motor neuron disease, but it is a different condition. On the other hand, chronic lead intoxication may be a cause of motor neuron disease in the truest sense (11). Recognizing the several different kinds of motor neuron disease may help in assessing the prognosis for individual patients and may also provide clues to the pathogenesis of the most common, currently idiopathic, form of these disorders (27).

Genetic forms of motor neuron disease provide the most secure evidence that the syndrome comprises more than one disease. Different modes of genetic transmission require different biochemical abnormalities, even if the clinical syndromes are similar, and motor neuron disorders have been reported in patterns that suggest autosomal dominant, autosomal recessive (35, 42, 108), or X-linked recessive transmission (130). Horton et al. concluded that autosomal dominant transmission could account for almost all recorded cases, but they distinguished three different types: two with relatively short courses (one with degeneration of posterior columns, but with no sensory disorder in life; the other purely motor in pathology) and one with a longer course (61). Duration, however, may vary even in a single family (53). The differences between families suggest more than one genetic form of the disease; it is not known whether the pathogenesis of any of these heritable diseases is the same as that of the idiopathic form.

Other genetic diseases merge with motor neuron disease. For instance, the only differences between juvenile spinal muscular atrophy (Kugelberg-Welander syndrome) and motor neuron disease are age at onset and the predominantly proximal weakness that characterizes the juvenile disorder. However, some families could be regarded as having "late-onset Kugelberg-Welander syndrome" or "familial motor neuron disease of relatively early onset," since the age used for differentiation of these disorders is arbitrary. It is also uncertain whether there is a distinct juvenile form of motor neuron disease (10, 80, 101).

Amyotrophy may also be part of several inherited neurologic disorders that include cerebellar degeneration (14), parkinsonism (16), Pick's disease (31, 93), Huntington's disease (47), and other combinations (13, 63, 64, 108, 140). Evidence of a link with other heritable diseases of the spinal cord is found in cases that are clinically indistinguishable from ALS but that exhibit degeneration of the posterior column at autopsy (26, 40, 58). A special form on Guam was implied pathologically (17, 18, 46, 58, 75).

Acquired diseases may also cause syndromes of motor neuron disease (24, 142). For example, the clinical syndromes resulting from lead or mercury intoxication in some cases may be identical to spinal muscular atrophy or ALS (11, 19, 67), but this need not imply heavy metal intoxication in the more common forms (29, 30, 115). It is not clear whether there is a true syndrome of postpoliomyelitis progressive motor neuron disease (23, 32, 98, 141), since some patients with residual muscle weakness after paralytic poliomyelitis may function by compensatory actions that simply wear out with advancing age (4, 5, 56, 69). This observation does not explain all cases of postpolio motor neuron disease because corticospinal signs are found in some (98, 104). Amyotrophy has also been recorded after epidemic encephalitis (25, 54, 88, 116, 139) and may occur in Jakob-Creutzfeldt disease (113).

Similarly, it is not certain whether the incidence of motor neuron disease is increased in patients with malignant tumors; this paraneoplastic syndrome was suggested by Norris et al. (106) and by Brain et al. (15), but was not apparent in two autopsy series (21, 78) or in several clinical series (9, 10). Nevertheless, there have been individual cases in which the association of motor neuron disease with a malignant neoplasm seemed more than coincidental (22, 51, 114, 120), and both clinical and pathologic evidence of motor neuron disease may be part of more extensive syndromes of paraneoplastic encephalomyelitis (34, 120). Other syndromes of uncertain pathogenesis are related to hyperinsulinism (7, 57, 95, 132, 138), electric shock (60, 126), and ischemia (33, 123). Irradiation of the lower spinal cord may also cause a restricted form of motor neuron disease (55, 74, 83, 121, 128), as the following case illustrates.

Case 1

This man was well until age 32, in 1966, when he noticed a mass in the right testicle. The mass was excised and proved to be an embryonal cell carcinoma of the testis. Bilateral retroperitoneal and periaortic lymphadenectomy was performed; 11 of 12 nodes were normal. The node that contained tumor lay along the spermatic artery on the right abdominal wall. After the operation, radiotherapy was given with a six-million-volt acceleration. He received a midplane dose of 5000 rad in 32 days, covering the area between groin and diaphragm. A few months later, but so gradually that he could not be certain of the time of onset, he noticed weakness and twitching of the legs, with frequent nocturnal cramps of the gastrocnemius muscles. In 1970, weakness was pronounced, and he had lost five pounds during the preceding year. He was admitted to another hospital, where myelogram, intravenous urogram, skeletal survey, gastrointestinal series, and barium enema disclosed no evidence of metastasis. The patient had no history of toxic exposure or of similar disease in the family.

We examined him later in 1970. General examination was normal; there was no radiation dermatitis. Cranial nerve and arm functions were normal. He was barely able to walk without assistance, but moved rapidly with canes. Psoas and hamstrings were weak against firm resistance; quadriceps muscles were normal. The anterior tibials, peroneals, and extensors of the toes were virtually paralyzed. The posterior tibials and gastrocnemii had slight function, with more on the left. He could not stand on his toes. Knee and ankle jerks were absent. There was spontaneous fasciculation of both gastrocnemii, and twitching was elicited by percussion of the hamstrings. Reflexes in the arms were normal, and there was no Hoffmann's sign. Plantar responses, cremasteric and abdominal reflexes, and sensation were normal.

Routine laboratory studies gave normal results, except that the cerebrospinal fluid protein content was 62 mg/dl. An intravenous venocavogram was normal, and chorionic gonadotropin hormone was not present in the urine. Serum creatine kinase activity was normal. There was no spontaneous activity on the electromyogram (EMG) (performed by Dr. P. V. DeJesus) in the vastus lateralis; mean duration of motor unit potentials was normal (15.3 msec), but there was a mixed-to-single oscillation pattern with increased amplitude (7.5–10.5 mV) and 25% polyphasia. The loss of motor units and the high amplitude of the remaining units were compatible with denervation. The pattern in the left flexor digitorum profundus was normal, and motor conduction velocities were normal in the left peroneal and medial nerves. The patient was examined annually for the next three years and there was essentially no change.

Finally, there are syndromes of motor neuron disease that differ so much from the usual form, which implies progression with no remission, that a separate disease is implied (86, 87). Perhaps the best documented example of this is the syndrome of wasting of the arms at about age 20, which is often unilateral (though sometimes bilateral), and is always of such slow progression that it seems to be static (77, 109, 127). A similar disease may affect the legs (37, 89, 85). Even more striking aberrations of clinical course are provided by the few documented examples of significant improvement (39) or complete recovery (97, 105). We have seen one case of complete recovery in a patient with spinal muscular atrophy that was typical except for the age of the patient.

Case 2

In December 1968, an 18-year-old man first noted weakness of his arms and occasional twitching of the deltoids and biceps. By March 1969, he had difficulty playing tennis and later had difficulty raising his arms; he also noted weakness of his legs at this time. Frequent cramps affected the biceps and gastrocnemius muscles, and he lost 13 pounds within two months. While he was traveling in July 1969, he had so much trouble that he was admitted to a university hospital in Ireland. Cervical myelogram and laboratory studies conducted there were normal except for signs of denervation in the EMG. We examined him in August 1969. Cranial nerve functions were normal. There was weakness against gravity of the deltoids, and weakness against resistance of parascapular muscles, biceps, and triceps, with only slightly less weakness of the hand muscles. Wasting corresponded to the weakness. His gait was normal, and his leg muscles were strong except for slight weakness of the psoas against resistance. Fasciculations were seen in deltoid, triceps, and scapular muscles. Myotatic reflexes were absent in the arms, elicited with reinforcement at the knees, and active at the ankles. Plantar responses were normal, and there was no clonus or Hoffmann's sign. Sensation was normal.

Laboratory data were normal except for a cerebrospinal fluid protein content of 76 mg/dl, and signs of denervation on EMG (fasciculations, polyphasic motor unit potentials, and decreased interference patterns were seen in arm muscles, but were normal in leg muscles) and muscle biopsy (many angular fibers, mostly type 2; few targetoid fibers). Nerve conduction velocities were normal.

One year later, he reported that the weakness had progressed for about six months, affecting the legs as well as the arms, but that he was still able to walk. In the spring of 1970, he began to improve, and by September 1970 he was essentially asymptomatic. He never had had paresthesias. There were no abnormalities on examination at that time. Two years later, he was still well.

IDIOPATHIC MOTOR NEURON DISEASE

Antecedent Events

Although the effects of traumatic injury may sometimes merge with the initial symptoms of motor neuron disease, this phenomenon is rare and not easily explained (2, 52, 65, 90, 133). The most skeptical view is that the patient was injured in an accident caused by weakness that he or she had not yet recognized; in such cases the injury could bring the weakness to the patient's attention. Alternatively, the injury might have activated the disease in some nonspecific way, as general surgery or antecedent viral infection sometimes precipitates Guillain-Barré syndrome. No other event seems to occur with inordinate frequency in a population of patients with motor neuron disease. Ask-Upmark (5) and Kniffen and Quick (70) were impressed with the frequency of history of gastric surgery in patients who presented with signs of motor neuron disease, and implied that nutritional deficiency might have been a cause. Jokelainen found that 10 of 255 patients with motor neuron disease had previously undergone gastrectomy (66); however, this was not true of patients in other series (10, 71, 131). Felmus et al. noted syndromes resembling motor neuron disease in patients with hyperparathyroidism (44), but disorders of calcium metabolism are exceptional in patients with motor neuron disease and have not been recorded in the analysis of clinical series. There is no clear indication that paralytic poliomyelitis occurred significantly more often in patients with motor neuron disease (117), and serum antibody titers to poliovirus in patients with motor neuron disease did not differ from those in controls (79). In addition, there is no indication that the incidence of motor neuron disease has declined with the disappearance of poliomyelitis. Greater occupational exposure to lead, participation in athletics, and consumption of milk were reported by patients with motor neuron disease than by controls (44), but the significance of these data has been disputed (68).

Clinical Forms of Motor Neuron Disease

In most series, ALS is the most common form of motor neuron disease, followed by spinal atrophy and bulbar palsy (Table 1). Some of the patients identified in Table 1 as having bulbar palsy probably also had spinal signs, and the frequency of "pure" cranial nerve syndromes is probably much lower than 26%.

Sexual and Racial Distribution

In most series, men were affected more frequently than women, in a ratio of 1.5:1.0 or greater. In some series, however, men and women were affected equally and without apparent reason for the discrepancy

Table 1 Clinical Forms of Idiopathic Motor Neuron Disease[a]

Form of Disease	Percentage of Total (N = 466)
Upper and lower motor neurons together (ALS)	66.3
Progressive bulbar palsy	26.3
Lower motor neuron only	7.3

[a] Data taken from Bonduelle M: Amyotrophic lateral sclerosis. In *Handbook of Clinical Neurology*, vol. 22. Edited by PJ Vinken, GW Bruyn. New York, American Elsevier; Amsterdam, North-Holland, 1975, pp 281–338.

(9, 10, 82). The disease occurs everywhere and in all races; Japanese people living in the United States and Filipinos living in Hawaii may be more susceptible, and Mexicans may be less susceptible (8).

Age at Onset

The most common age of onset as calculated from living patients was 50 to 55 years, whereas analysis of patients who died from the disease showed a mean age of onset of 62 years, with a mean duration of 3 to 4 years (10, 96). However, death certificates may fail to list ALS as a cause of death (59), and Aimard et al. found a rising incidence in recent years of cases beginning before age 40 (1). Approximately 80% of cases begin between 40 to 70 years of age, with about 10% of patients younger and about 10% older than these limits (10).

Clinical Manifestations

The major symptoms of motor neuron disease are due to weakness, but cramps and weight loss are also common. Cramps have been recorded infrequently in some series (10), but when specific inquiry is made, our experience coincides with that of Mulder and Espinosa, who noted cramps in 40% of patients questioned (96). Cramps seem to be more prominent early in the disease and may occur during the day when limbs are stretched or twisted, or during sleep. As weakness progresses, cramps occur less frequently. Weight loss is presumably a manifestation of muscle wasting, alone or with dysphagia, and it is rarely the presenting manifestation.

Limb weakness may first be evident in the arms, the legs, or in all limbs simultaneously. Although weakness may be asymmetric at first, all limbs are ultimately involved. There seems to be no difference in prognosis if symptoms start in the arms rather than in the legs. Cranial symptoms are essentially restricted to dysphagia and dysarthria; facial weakness may be present but is rarely symptomatic; mastication is affected late; the eyelids and ocular muscles are always spared, and no convincing case of oculomotor weakness has been documented (62, 136). Respiratory muscles are usually affected late in the disease, although pulmonary function tests may be abnormal before onset of dyspnea (72), and, in rare instances, ventilatory insufficiency may be prominent early (91, 92, 111).

The signs of the disease conform to its pathology. Wasting is almost always evident in weak muscles. Fasciculation may not be seen clinically or may be very active; these differences are not understood. Fasciculation is occasionally noted by the patient, but more commonly patients become aware of twitching only after it is pointed out by the physician. As the disease progresses, fasciculation usually becomes less prominent, but it may persist. Upper motor neuron signs are present in most cases, but even when they are not evident, the combination of brisk reflexes and weak, wasted, and twitching muscles in the same limb is virtually pathognomonic of the disease.

Dysphagia and dysarthria may be attended by lower motor neuron signs of cranial nerves IX, X, and XII but may also be due to pseudobulbar palsy because of supranuclear corticobulbar lesions. In some cases, there is evidence of both nuclear and supranuclear disorders; that is, there may be wasting and fibrillation of the tongue, which implicate lower motor neuron pathology, but there also may be emotional incontinence and "release" signs (e.g., snout reflexes, jaw jerks), which implicate supranuclear disorder. The vocal cords are virtually never involved alone, but may be paralyzed in advanced cases (28).

Autonomic functions are generally spared (112). Special tests may reveal distorted esophageal motility (12, 28, 125), but overt disorders are exceptional. Urinary symptoms are usually attributed to weakness of muscles of the abdominal wall, and preservation of sacral neurons subserving bladder function may be apparent histologically (84). The anal sphincter is also spared (122). Furukawa and Toyokura (50) and Jokelainen (66) noted the absence of bedsores in patients with motor neuron disease; it is not clear whether this implies involvement of cutaneous circulation or other cutaneous functions (49, 135). Although some observers have been impressed with the frequency of sensory symptoms (38, 110), others have found a singular lack of persistent paresthesias. There have been no well-documented cases of sensory loss, although it has been recorded in familial cases (3).

Course and Prognosis

Duration of motor neuron disease has most commonly been calculated from data on patients who have died. On this basis, the mean duration of symptoms usually is found to be 1.7 years in progressive bulbar palsy and about 3 years in ALS or spinal atrophy (10). In some series, however, there has not been much difference in length of survival of patients with different clinical forms (9, 21, 66). There is no clear difference in mean survival of those with both upper and lower motor neuron signs and those with only lower motor neuron signs, but the individual cases of longest duration seem to be those with only spinal muscular atrophy. Another measure of severity was employed by Boman and Meurman (9), who found that 90% of their patients were unable to work within five years after onset of illness.

Because calculations based only on fatal cases automatically exclude living cases of longer duration, an actuarial approach was made by Kristensen and Melgaard, who found that 7.6% of 118 patients they studied were living 10 years after onset of illness and that 18.7% survived longer than 5 years after onset (73). In a prospective study, Mulder and Howard found that 50% of patients studied died within 3 years, but that 20% were alive after 5 years (97). Rosen reported a 5-year survival rate of 39.4%, but diagnoses were not ascertained (119). Among the longest survivals reported are 27 years (6), 35 years (78), and 38 years (76). Prolonged observation is the only way to detect cases of longer duration.

Age at onset does not seem to have a major effect on survival for patients whose illness begins in middle age, and life expectancy generally is shorter for patients whose symptoms start after age 60 (10). However, onset before age 40 seems more likely to be associated with longer survival (66).

In our experience, the disease is inexorably progressive, although the rate of progression varies from case to case. We have not been impressed with overt changes in rate of progression or with so-called plateaus of clinical state, although once patients lose the ability to walk, it may become difficult to discern clinical changes over a long time (103, 107). This question has not been studied formally because there is no precise way to measure rate of progression, and apparent plateaus may create false impressions of benefit from different therapies. Similarly, we have not seen clear-cut reversal of weakness, but Tyler has reported that some minor changes, such as movement of a finger that had seemed to be paralyzed, may take place (134).

Death is almost always due to weakness, directly or indirectly, through aspiration, pulmonary infection, atelectasis, or asphyxiation; however, intercurrent illness of any type can supervene.

CONCLUSIONS

The clinical diagnosis of motor neuron disease is usually accurate but has not been tested formally. Although the prognosis is grim, clinical variations suggest that more than one disease is subsumed by the term *motor neuron disease*. In individual cases, it is prudent for the physician to be circumspect about prognosis, and no therapeutic trials should be conducted without appropriate controls.

Acknowledgments

The work described in this chapter was supported by Center Grants from NINCDS [#NS-117660(04)] and the Muscular Dystrophy Association.

REFERENCES

1. Aimard G, Bady B, Boisson D, et al: Sclérose latérale amyotrophique survenue avant 40 ans. Remarques à propos de 25 observations. Rev Neurol (Paris) 132:563–566, 1976

2. Alpers BJ, Farmer RA: Role of repeated trauma by pneumatic drill in production of amyotrophic lateral sclerosis. Arch Neurol Psychiatry 62: 178–182, 1949

3. Alter M, Schaumann B: Hereditary amyotrophic lateral sclerosis. Eur Neurol 14:250–265, 1976

4. Anderson AD, Levine SA, Gellert H: Loss of ambulatory ability in patients with old anterior poliomyelitis. Lancet 2:1061–1063, 1972

5. Ask-Upmark E: Precipitating factors in the pathogenesis of amyotrophic lateral sclerosis. Acta Med Scand 170:717–723, 1961

6. Assmus H, Thiele RM: Gibt es extrem chronische Verläufe bei der myatrophischen Lateralsklerose? Nervenarzt 44:609–610, 1973

7. Barris RW: Pancreatic adenoma (hyperinsulinism) associated with neuromuscular disorder. Ann Intern Med 38:124–129, 1953

8. Bobowick AR, Brody JA: Epidemiology of motor-neuron diseases. N Engl J Med 288:1047–1055, 1973

9. Boman K, Meurman T: Prognosis of amyotrophic lateral sclerosis. Acta Neurol Scand 43:489–498, 1967

10. Bonduelle M: Amyotrophic lateral sclerosis. In *Handbook of Clinical Neurology*, vol. 22. Edited by PJ Vinken, GW Bruyn. New York, American Elsevier; Amsterdam, North-Holland, 1975, pp 281–338

11. Boothby JA, DeJesus PV, Rowland LP: Reversible forms of motor neuron disease; lead "neuritis." Arch Neurol 31:18–23, 1974

12. Bosma JF, Brodie DR: Disabilities of the pharynx in amyotrophic lateral sclerosis as demonstrated by cineradiography. Radiology 92:97–103, 1969

13. Bots GTAM, Staal A: Amyotrophic lateral sclerosis dementia complex, neuroaxonal dystrophy, and Hallervorden-Spatz disease. Neurology 23:35–39, 1973

14. Boudouresques J, Toga M, Khalil R, et al: Forme amyotrophique d'une dégénérescence spino-cérébelleuse. Rev Neurol (Paris) 125:25–38, 1971

15. Brain R, Croft PB, Wilkinson M: Motor neuron disease as a manifestation of neoplasm (with a note on the course of classical motor neuron disease). Brain 88:475–498, 1965

16. Brait K, Fahn S, Schwarz GA: Sporadic and familial parkinsonism and motor neuron disease. Neurology 23:990–1002, 1973

17. Brody JA, Edgar AN, Gillespie MM: Amyotrophic lateral sclerosis. No increase among U. S. construction workers in Guam. JAMA 240: 551–552, 1978

18. Brody JA, Hirano A, Scott RM: Recent neuropathologic observations in amyotrophic lateral sclerosis and parkinsonism-dementia of Guam. Neurology 21:528–537, 1971

19. Brown IA: Chronic mercurialism. Arch Neurol Psychiatry 72:674–681, 1954

20. Brown WA, Mueller PS: Psychological function in individuals with amyotrophic lateral sclerosis (ALS). Psychosom Med 32:141–152, 1970

21. Brownell B, Oppenheimer DR, Hughes JT: The central nervous system in motor neuron disease. J Neurol Neurosurg Psychiatry 33:338–357, 1970

22. Buchanan DS, Malamud N: Motor neuron disease with renal cell carcinoma and postoperative neurologic remission. Neurology 23:891–894, 1972

23. Campbell AMG, Williams ER, Pearce J: Late motor neuron degeneration following poliomyelitis. Neurology 19:1101–1106, 1969

24. Capasso G, Glorino A, Facciolla D, et al: Sindrome amiotrofico spastica progressiva (SLA?) insorta dopo vaccinazione anticolerica. Ospedale Psichiatrico 44:300–309, 1976

25. Capitani E, Meola G, Spinnler H: Amyotrophy and Kluever-Bucy syndrome. Eur Neurol 16:99–105, 1977

26. Castaigne P, Cambier J, Escourolle R, et al: Dégénérescence subaiguë des neurones moteurs périphériques avec inclusions neuronales et lésions des cordons postérieurs. Les limites de la sclérose latérale amyotrophique. Rev Neurol (Paris) 122:313–320, 1970

27. Castaigne P, Lhermitte F, Cambier J, et al: Etude neuropathologique de 61 observations de sclérose latérale amyotrophique. Discussion nosologique. Rev Neurol (Paris) 127:401–414, 1972

28. Colmant H: Progressive bulbar palsy in adults. In *Handbook of Clinical Neurology*, vol. 22. Edited by PJ Vinken, GW Bruyn. New York, American Elsevier; Amsterdam, North-Holland, 1975, pp 111–156

29. Conradi S, Ronnevi LO, Stibler H: Serum protein binding of lead in vitro in amyotrophic lateral sclerosis patients and controls. J Neurol Sci 37:95–105, 1978

30. Conradi S, Ronnevi LO, Vesterberg O: Increased plasma levels of lead in patients with amyotrophic lateral sclerosis compared with control subjects as determined by flameless atomic absorption spectrophotometry. J Neurol Neurosurg Psychiatry 41:389–393, 1978

31. De Morsier G: Un cas de maladie de Pick avec sclérose latérale amyotrophique. Rev Neurol (Paris) 116:373–382, 1967

32. Dereux J, Choteau P, Bedague JP: Discussion de la situation nosologique d'un cas d'amyotrophie musculaire neurogène, séquelle tardivement évolutive d'une poliomyélite antérieure aiguë de l'enfance. J Sci Med Lille 88:155–163, 1970

33. Dodson WE, Landau WM: Motor neuron loss due to aortic clamping in repair of coarctation. Neurology 23:539–542, 1973

34. Dorfman LJ, Forno LS: Paraneoplastic encephalomyelitis. Acta Neurol Scand 48:556–574, 1972

35. Dumon J, Macken J, DeBarsy T: Concordance for amyotrophic lateral sclerosis in a pair of dizygous twins of consanguineous parents. J Med Genet 8:113–115, 1971

36. Dyck PJ: Pathological alterations of the peripheral nervous system of man. In *Peripheral Neuropathy.* Edited by PJ Dyck, PK Thomas, EH Lambert. Philadelphia, WB Saunders, 1975, pp 296–336

37. Dyck PJ, Lambert EH: Lower motor and primary sensory neuron diseases with peroneal muscular atrophy. Arch Neurol 18:603–618, 1968

38. Dyck PJ, Stevens JC, Mulder DW, et al: Frequency of nerve fiber degeneration of peripheral motor and sensory neurons in amyotrophic lateral sclerosis. Morphometry of deep and superficial peroneal nerves. Neurology 25:781–785, 1975

39. Engel WK, Hogenhuis LAH, Collis WJ, et al: Metabolic studies and therapeutic trials in amyotrophic lateral sclerosis. In *Motor Neuron Diseases. Research on Amyotrophic Lateral Sclerosis and Related Disorders.* Edited by FH Norris Jr, LT Kurland. New York, Grune & Stratton, 1969, pp 199–208

40. Engel WK, Kurland LT, Klatzo I: An inherited disease similar to amyotrophic lateral sclerosis with a pattern of posterior column involvement. An intermediate form? Brain 82:203–220, 1959

41. Erbsloh F, Kunze K, Recke B, et al: Die myatrophische Lateralsklerose. Dtsch Med Wochenschr 23:1131–1141, 1968

42. Estrin WJ: Amyotrophic lateral sclerosis in dizygotic twins. Neurology 27:692–694, 1977

43. Feller T, Jones RE, Netsky M: Amyotrophic lateral sclerosis and sensory changes. Virginia Medical Monthly 93:325–335, 1966

44. Felmus MT, Patten BM, Swanke L: Antecedent events in amyotrophic lateral sclerosis. Neurology 26:167–172, 1976

45. Finlayson MH, Guberman A, Martin JB: Cerebral lesions in familial amyotrophic lateral sclerosis and dementia. Acta Neuropathol (Berl) 26:237–246, 1973

46. Forno LS, O'Flannagan FJ: Amyotrophic lateral sclerosis of the Guam type in a U. S. veteran. Neurology 23:876–880, 1973

47. Frank G, Vuia O: Chorea Huntington-ALS-spastische Spinalparalyse. Z Neurol 205:207–220, 1973

48. Friedman AP, Freedman D: Amyotrophic lateral sclerosis. J Nerv Ment Dis 111:1, 1950

49. Fullmer HM, Lazarus GS, Stam AC Jr., et al: Collagenase in neuromuscular diseases. In *Motor Neuron Diseases. Research on Amyotrophic Lateral Sclerosis and Related Disorders.* Edited by FH Norris Jr, LT Kurland. New York, Grune & Stratton, 1969, pp 242–244

50. Furukawa T, Toyokura Y: Amyotrophic lateral sclerosis and bedsores. Lancet 1:862, 1976

51. Gerling GM, Woolsey RM: Paraneoplastic motor neuron disease. Missouri Med 64:503–506, 1967

52. Geyer H: Über posttraumatische Muskelatrophien und progressive spinale Muskelatrophie. Dtsch Z Nervenheilk 134:14–29, 1974

53. Giminez-Roddan S, Esteban A: Prognosis in hereditary amyotrophic lateral sclerosis. Arch Neurol 34:706–708, 1977

54. Greenfield JG, Matthews WB: Post-encephalitic parkinsonism and amyotrophy. J Neurol Neurosurg Psychiatr 17:50–56, 1954

55. Greenfield MM, Stark PM: Post-irradiation neuropathy. Am J Roentgenol 60:617–622, 1948

56. Hallen O, Brusis T, Pfisterer H: Die Myatrophia postpoliomyelitica chronica. Ein Beitrag zum Problem der sog. Poliomyelitis anterior chronica. Dtsch Z Nervenheilk 195:333–343, 1969

57. Harrison MJG: Muscle wasting after prolonged hypoglycaemic coma: case report with electrophysiological data. J Neurol Neurosurg Psychiatry 39:465–470, 1976

58. Hirano A, Arumgasamy N, Zimmerman HM: Amyotrophic lateral sclerosis: a comparison of Guam and classical cases. Arch Neurol 16:357–363, 1967

59. Hoffman PM, Brody JA: The reliability of death certificate reporting for amyotrophic lateral sclerosis. J Chronic Dis 24:5–8, 1971

60. Holbrook LA: Delayed myelopathy: a rare complication of severe electrical burns. Br Med J 4:659–660, 1970

61. Horton WA, Eldridge R, Brody JA: Familial motor neuron disease. Evidence for at least three different types. Neurology 26:460–465, 1976

62. Hotz G: Über das Vorkommen des Parinaud-Syndroms bei amyotrophischer Lateralsklerose. Confinia Neurologica 16:25–37, 1956

63. Ishino H: Motor nuclear involvement in progressive supranuclear palsy. J Neurol Sci 22:235–244, 1974

64. Iwashita H, Inoue N, Araki S, et al: Optic atrophy, neural deafness and distal neurogenic amyotrophy. Arch Neurol 22:357–364, 1970

65. Jelliffe SE: The amyotrophic lateral sclerosis syndrome and trauma. J Nerv Ment Dis 82:415–435, 1935

66. Jokelainen M: Amyotrophic lateral sclerosis in Finland. Acta Neurol Scand 56:185–204, 1977

67. Kantarjian AA: A syndrome clinically resembling amyotrophic lateral sclerosis following chronic mercurialism. Neurology 11:639–644, 1961

68. Karis R: Statistical data questioned in amyotrophic lateral sclerosis. Neurology 27:100, 1977

69. Kayser-Gatchalian MC: Late muscular atrophy after poliomyelitis. Eur Neurol 10:371–380, 1973

70. Kniffen JC, Quick DT: Neuromuscular disorder following gastric resection. Arch Intern Med 124:315–321, 1969

71. Koch MJ, Hoffman P, Brody JA, et al: Neurologic disorder following surgery for peptic ulcer disease. Arch Neurol 32:206–207, 1975

72. Kreitzer SM, Saunders NA, Tyler HR, et al: Respiratory muscle function in amyotrophic lateral sclerosis. Am Rev Resp Dis 117:437–447, 1978

73. Kristensen O, Melgaard B: Motor neuron disease. Prognosis and epidemiology. Acta Neurol Scand 56:299–308, 1977

74. Kristensen O, Melgaard B, Schiodt AV: Radiation myelopathy of the lumbosacral spinal cord. Acta Neurol Scand 56:217–222, 1977

75. Kurland LT, Brody JA: Amyotrophic lateral sclerosis Guam type. In *Handbook of Clinical Neurology*, vol. 22. Edited by PJ Vinken, GW Bruyn. New York, American Elsevier; Amsterdam, North-Holland, 1975, pp 339–348

76. Lance JW, Enis J, Duckworth JW: Motor neuron disease in Australia. Proc Aust Assoc Neurol 14:42–50, 1977

77. Lander M, Eadie MJ, Tyrer JH: Hereditary motor peripheral neuropathy predominantly affecting the arms. J Neurol Sci 28:389–394, 1976

78. Lawyer T Jr, Netsky M: Amyotrophic lateral sclerosis: clinicoanatomic study of 53 cases. Arch Neurol Psychiatry 69:171–192, 1953

79. Lehrich JR, Oger J, Arnason BGW: Neutralizing antibodies to poliovirus and mumps virus in amyotrophic lateral sclerosis. J Neurol Sci 23:537–540, 1974

80. LeLong M, Lerboullet J, Merklen PP: Sclérose latérale amyotrophique chez une jeune fille de 16 ans. Bull Soc Franc Pediatr 30:88–95, 1932

81. Leri A: Atrophie généralisée de la musculature de tous les visceres dans une amyotrophie progressive du type Aran-Duchenne. Rev Neurol (Paris) 10:394–401, 1902

82. Mackay RP: Course and prognosis of amyotrophic lateral sclerosis. Arch Neurol 8:117–127, 1963

83. Maier JG, Perry RH, Saylor W, et al: Radiation myelitis of the dorsolumbar spinal cord. Radiology 93:153–160, 1969

84. Mannen T, Iwata M, Toyokura Y, et al: Preservation of a certain motor neuron group in the sacral cord in amyotrophic lateral sclerosis; its clinical significance. J Neurol Neurosurg Psychiatry 40:464–469, 1977

85. Marsden CD: Inherited neuronal atrophy and degeneration predominantly of lower motor neurons. In *Peripheral Neuropathy*. Edited by PJ Dyck, PK Thomas, EH Lambert. Philadelphia, WB Saunders, 1975, pp 771–790

86. Matsunaga M, Inokushi T, Ohinishi A, et al: Oculopharyngeal involvement in familial neurogenic muscular atrophy. J Neurol Neurosurg Psychiatry 36:104–111, 1973

87. McLeod JG, Prineas JW: Distal type of chronic spinal muscular atrophy. Brain 94:703–714, 1971

88. McMenemy WH, Barnard RO, Jellinek EH: A late sequel of epidemic encephalitis (von Economo). Rev Roum Neurol 4:251–256, 1967

89. Meadows, JC, Marsden CD: A distal form of chronic spinal muscular atrophy. Neurology 19:53–59, 1969

90. Milanese C, Martin L: Amyotrophic lateral sclerosis and trauma. Acta Neurol Belg 70:482–491, 1970

91. Miller RD: Pulmonary disability as a symptom of amyotrophic lateral sclerosis. Mayo Clin Proc 32:436–437, 1957

92. Miller RD, Mulder DM, Fowler WS, et al: Exertional dyspnea: a primary complaint in unusual cases in progressive muscular atrophy and amyotrophic lateral sclerosis. Ann Intern Med 46:119–125, 1957

93. Minauf M, Jellinger K: Kombination von amyotrophischer Lateralsklerose mit Pickscher Krankheit. Arch Psychiatr Nervenkr 212:279–288, 1969

94. Mulder DW: The clinical syndrome of amyotrophic lateral sclerosis. Proc Staff Meet Mayo Clin 32:427–436, 1957

95. Mulder DW, Bastron JA, Lambert EH: Hyperinsulin neuropathy. Neurology 6:627–635, 1956

96. Mulder DW, Espinosa RE: Amyotrophic lateral sclerosis: comparison of the clinical syndrome in Guam and the United States. In *Motor Neuron Diseases. Research on Amyotrophic Lateral Sclerosis and Related Disorders.* Edited by FH Norris Jr, LT Kurland. New York, Grune & Stratton, 1969, pp 12–19

97. Mulder DW, Howard FM: Patient resistance and prognosis in amyotrophic lateral sclerosis. Mayo Clin Proc 51:537–541, 1976

98. Mulder DW, Rosenbaum RA, Layton DD Jr: Late progression of poliomyelitis or forme fruste amyotrophic lateral sclerosis? Mayo Clin Proc 47:756–761, 1972

99. Muller R: Progressive motor neuron disease in adults. A clinical study with special reference to the course of the disease. Acta Psychiatr Scand 27:137–156, 1952

100. Myrianthopoulos NC, Smith JK: Amyotrophic lateral sclerosis with progressive dementia. Neurology 12:603–610, 1962

101. Nelson JS, Prensky AL: Sporadic juvenile amyotrophic lateral sclerosis: a clinicopathologic study of a case with neuronal cytoplasmic inclusions containing RNA. Arch Neurol 27:300–306, 1972

102. Nishigaki S: Zur Klinik und Pathologie verschiedener Formen der myatrophischen Lateralsklerose. Arch Psychiatr Nervenkr 213:121–138, 1970

103. Nishigaki S: Krankheitsverlauf und Prognose der amyotrophischen Lateralsklerose. Arzt Forsch 26:402–407, 1972

104. Norris FH Jr: Adult spinal motor neuron disease. In *Handbook of Clinical Neurology*, vol. 22. Edited by PJ Vinken, GW Bruyn. New York, American Elsevier; Amsterdam, North-Holland, 1975, pp 1–56

105. Norris FH Jr: Benign post-traumatic amyotrophy. Arch Neurol 27: 269–270, 1972

106. Norris FH Jr, McMenemey WH, Barnard RO: Anterior horn pathology in carcinomatous neuromyopathy compared with other forms of motor neuron disease. In *Motor Neuron Diseases. Research on Amyotrophic Lateral Sclerosis and Related Disorders.* Edited by FH Norris Jr, LT Kurland. New York, Grune & Stratton, 1969, pp 100–111

107. Norris FH Jr, Ü KS, Denys EH, et al: Amyotrophic lateral sclerosis. Mayo Clin Proc 53:544, 1978

108. Orthner H, Becker PE, Muller D: Recessiv erbliche amyotrophische Lateralsklerose mit 'Lafora-Korpern.' Arch Psychiatr Nervenkr 217:287–342, 1973

109. O'Sullivan DJ, McLeod JG: Distal chronic spinal muscular atrophy involving the hands. J Neurol Neurosurg Psychiatry 41:653–658, 1978

110. Pallis CA: Motor neuron disease: two awkward questions. In *Motor Neuron Diseases*. Edited by FC Rose. New York, Grune & Stratton, 1977, pp 60–72

111. Parhad IM, Clark AW, Barron KD, et al: Diaphragmatic paralysis in motor neuron disease. Neurology 28:18–22, 1978

112. Patten JT: Decreased lacrimation and amyotrophic lateral sclerosis. JAMA 231:24, 1975

113. Perret J, Chatelain R: Amyotrophie distale lente des quatre membres avec évolution démentielle (forme amyotrophique du syndrome de Creutzfeldt-Jakob). Etude anatomoclinique. Rev Neurol (Paris) 115:955–964, 1966

114. Peters HA, Clatanoff DV: Spinal muscular atrophy secondary to macroglobulinemia. Neurology 18:101–108, 1968

115. Petkau A, Sawatzky A, Hillier CR, et al: Lead content of neuromuscular tissue in amyotrophic lateral sclerosis; case report and other considerations. Br J Ind Med 31:275–287, 1974

116. Petrov PA: V. Vilyuisk encephalitis in Yakut Republic (USSR). Am J Trop Med Hyg 19:146–150, 1970

117. Poskanzer DC, Cantor HC, Kaplan GS: The frequency of preceding poliomyelitis in amyotrophic lateral sclerosis. In *Motor Neuron Diseases. Research on Amyotrophic Lateral Sclerosis and Related Disorders.* Edited by FH Norris Jr, LT Kurland. New York, Grune & Stratton, 1969, pp 286–290

118. Ral B, Jolly SS: Motor neuron disease: a clinical study. J Indian Med Assoc 57:315–318, 1971

119. Rosen AD: Amyotrophic lateral sclerosis. Clinical features and prognosis. Arch Neurol 35:638–642, 1978

120. Rowland LP, Schneck S: Neuromuscular disorders associated with malignant neoplastic disease. J Chronic Dis 16:777–795, 1963

121. Sadowsky CH, Sachs E Jr, Ochoa J: Post-radiation motor neuron syndrome. Arch Neurol 33:786–787, 1976

122. Sakuta M, Nakanishi T, Toyokura Y: Anal muscle electromyogram in amyotrophic lateral sclerosis and Shy-Drager syndrome. Neurology 28:1289–1293, 1978

123. Schott B, Bourrat L, Duquesnel J, et al: Syndrome de pseudosclérose latérale amyotrophique par ischémie artérielle vertébrale. J Med (Lyon) 50:581–589, 1969

124. Sherratt RM, Gibberd FB: Motor neurone disease and dementia: probably Creutzfeldt-Jakob disease. Proc Roy Soc Med 67:1063–1064, 1974

125. Smith AW, Mulder DW, Code CF: Esophageal motility in amyotrophic lateral sclerosis. Mayo Clin Proc 32:438–441, 1957

126. So SC, Lee MLK: Spastic quadriplegia due to electric shock. Br Med J 2:590, 1973

127. Sobue I, Saito N, Iida M, et al: Juvenile type of distal and segmental muscular atrophy of upper extremities. Ann Neurol 3:429–432, 1978

128. Somasundaram M, Cho ES, Posner JB: Anterior horn cell degeneration as a remote effect of lymphoma. Trans Am Neurol Assoc 100:144–148, 1975

129. Staal A: A case of hereditary juvenile amyotrophic lateral sclerosis complicated with dementia. Psychiatr Neurol Neurochir 72:129–135, 1969

130. Stefanis C, Papapetropoulos T, Scarpalezos S, et al: X-linked spinal and bulbar muscular atrophy of late onset. A separate type of motor neuron disease? J Neurol Sci 24:393–403, 1975

131. Stiehl J: The incidence of gastrectomy and gastric secretion in motor neuron disease. Aust Ann Med 16:176–177, 1967

132. Tom MI, Richardson JC: Hypoglycaemia from islet cell tumor of pancreas with amyotrophy and cerebrospinal nerve cell changes. J Neuropathol Exp Neurol 10:57–66, 1951

133. Turner JWA: Trauma and progressive muscular atrophy. Lancet 2:549–551, 1939

134. Tyler HR: Double-blind study of modified neurotoxin in motor neuron disease. Neurology 29:77–81, 1979

135. Urbánek K, Jansa P: Amyotrophic lateral sclerosis; abnormal cellular inflammatory response. Arch Neurol 30:186–187, 1974

136. Van Bogaert L: Contribution à la connaissance des troubles oculaires et vestibularies dans la S.L.A. Rev Otoneuroophthal 4:263–274, 1925

137. Vejjajiva A, Foster JB, Miller H: Motor neuron disease. A clinical study. J Neurol Sci 4:299–314, 1967

138. Williams CJ: Amytrophy due to hypoglycaemia. Br Med J 1:707–708, 1955

139. Wimmer A, Neel AV: Les amyotrophies systématisées dans l'encéphalite épidémique chronique. Acta Psychiatr Neurol 3:319–365, 1928

140. Yase Y, Matsumoto N, Azuma K, et al: Amyotrophic lateral sclerosis. Association with schizophrenic symptoms and showing Alzheimer tangles. Arch Neurol 27:118–128, 1972

141. Zilka KJ: Discussion on motor neuron disease. Proc Roy Soc Med 55:1028–1029, 1962

142. Zukerman E, Zatz S: Esclerose lateral amiotrofica e neurossifilis. Arq Neuropsiaquiatr 31:214–219, 1973

Commentary

H. Richard Tyler

The role of the clinician is to establish an accurate diagnosis and prognosis. It is critical that the neurologist-physician does this in a manner that allows him or her to treat the patient appropriately and to offer some hope. Specifically, one can stress that well cared for patients with ALS have normal mental status and no pain. Pain may result from complications such as frozen shoulders or immobilized joints, but with good care it should not be part of the disease. I think that it is important that patients realize that sexual function can be normal; this is a subject that patients with ALS are rarely able to discuss spontaneously.*

It is equally essential not to misdiagnose treatable disease. The physician must make sure that lead poisoning and mercury poisoning have been ruled out. It is easier to deal with an elevated level of lead or mercury by discovering and treating it while the patient is in the hospital than to have to make a legal defense of the oversight later.

The chief purpose of trying to separate the various clinical syndromes is to make an effective prognosis. In the case of a disease for which there is no definitive test, I think it is clear that the diagnosis must be established by the clinician. If I am to tell the patient the truth, I can make a more intelligent judgment if I assess the various clinical syndromes present in that patient than if I repeat the generalizations we make from large studies of patients with ALS in which we make no attempt to differentiate the clinical presentations, findings, and courses of illness. As Dr. Rowland has stressed, it is more useful to separate these syndromes and to avoid referring to all of them as ALS.

The form of motor neuron disease referred to as primary muscle atrophy is clearly correlated with much greater longevity than are the other syndromes, and many patients who present with that form live 5, 10, 15, or 20 years. Patients who present with typical ALS have rapid course and a poor prognosis. Any patient who comes in with a history of a disease that is progressing every six months has a poor prognosis. Conversely, patients who present with some of the aberrant syndromes, such as wasting of the hands (especially of the extensors and muscles supplied by the posterior interosseous nerve) have a good prognosis. I have attended patients 15 to 20 years with this particular kind of finding. It is clearly a motor neuron disease, will certainly spread, and will be more severe in 10 years; however, it causes

---

* Similarly, patients with ALS who become pregnant generally will deliver normal infants. The progressive nature of ALS is not altered by pregnancy (1).

much less loss of function in terms of general physical performance. One may find motor neuron disease concentrated in specific groups of neurons before the illness disseminates. For example, a form of the disease that occurs in elderly women results in complete loss of ability to use the tongue but gives no evidence of progression to other muscles for 3 to 4 years. There is a respiratory form in which the patient presents with pure loss of respiratory function but virtually no evidence of involvement in other areas of the body. Such a patient can die with respiratory involvement, and postmortem confirmation will show that the number of anterior horn cells is greatly decreased in the midthoracic area.

Most clinicians diagnose ALS reasonably well. Mistakes are still made, even by neurologists. One cannot speak of 100% accuracy of diagnosis. In general, I would say 5% of the patients referred to me with a diagnosis of ALS may have been misdiagnosed. I have also observed a fair number of patients with ALS who have undergone surgery for cervical spondylosis or who have been told they have multiple sclerosis. Five of my patients had been diagnosed as having myasthenia gravis; they had been treated appropriately and obtained symptomatic relief, yet within a year each one developed ALS. I have seen one patient who had Guillain-Barré syndrome with high protein and severe paralysis. He did not recover and went on to develop ALS. I have seen sensory loss in a patient with ALS who was originally thought to have atypical syringomyelia. Examination revealed that the patient reported sensory loss and that he had fasciculations and weakness; repeat examination a year later revealed no sensory loss but progression of weakness.

The familial motor neuron disorders are atypical. In such cases, observation of previously affected members of the family may give some prognostic indications. The fasciculations have definite characteristics in this illness, and the distribution of muscle weakness is almost unique. The clinician who is experienced in the diagnosis of ALS frequently will be able to diagnose the disease by observing the combination of muscles involved in a foot or hand.

In terms of prognosis, the question often arises of whether there is any hope of arresting the course of ALS or whether the disease is steadily progressive. I think it is desirable to give a patient hope; for example, the physician can inform the patient that some individuals reach a plateau that lasts for a few months or years. The physician can also tell the patient of therapies being tested. If treatment with a drug is tried, the patient often will not be sure for three months or longer that the condition is getting worse; hopeful patients often note minor variations with optimism. On the other hand, the physician who does not try various treatments tends to find ALS to be a steadily progressive disease. Patients often deceive themselves, even if they do not deceive the doctor. I am not sure there are real plateaus, but there certainly are minor variations in the course of illness. It is terribly important for the clinician to be cautious rather than wrong. The patient will be distressed if he or she is told mistakenly that the disease will take a particular turn at a particular time, and the patient may interpret such a mistake as an indication that the physician does not know enough about the illness. As Dr. Rowland has pointed out, it is important that the clinician pay attention to the rare cases of lead or mercury poisoning, syphilis, or combined-systems disease; routine determination of lead and mercury levels in ALS patients has become an important consideration.

The clinician also must pay a great deal of attention to clues that may give his or her laboratory colleagues some idea of the nature of the illness. I would favor breaking down the motor neuron diseases into syndromes. We must be very careful in choosing the patient populations we study to be sure we are talking about the same things, and we must be sure to communicate accurately with one another.

REFERENCE

1. Huston JW, Lingenfelder J, Mulder DW, et al: Pregnancy complicated by amyotrophic lateral sclerosis. Am J Obst Gynecol 72:93–99, 1956

Forbes H. Norris, Jr

I would like to report three observations. First, I do not think we can prognosticate early in cases of ALS. Second, I do not believe there are patterns of involvement; that is, in its capriciousness, ALS is very much like acute poliomyelitis. Third, the clinical course of ALS is also capricious: the disease usually progresses by "fits and starts" rather than by steady progression. Some patients do remain stable over many years, and there are even cases in which improvement does occur. Such improvement can be verified by objective criteria, not just by the patient's belief that he or she is better.

David Goldblatt

It is a well recognized characteristic of ALS that muscles in a weak, atrophic, fasciculating limb may have brisk stretch reflexes that are more active than would be expected in uncomplicated lower motor neuron disease. What I have observed is that, when involvement of the limbs is asymmetric, abnormalities of the upper and lower motor neuron types develop pari passu in the same limb; thus, reflexes are more active and atrophy is more pronounced in one limb than in the corresponding limb on the opposite side of the body.

In a series of 13 patients with ALS who had relatively early involvement and were ambulatory when we first examined them, the onset of weakness had been asymmetric in all, and the first limb to be affected remained weaker than its corresponding limb until late in the course of the disease. In 10 of the 13 patients, the weaker limb had more active reflexes. In two patients, these reflexes were symmetric, and in only one patient (whose reflexes were otherwise symmetrically hyperactive) was the radial pronator reflex absent on the more affected side.

In 7 of the 13 patients, plantar reflexes were asymmetric. In 6 of the 7, the abnormal response was present on the side that showed the more prominent lower motor neuron signs. The exception was a patient with a claw hand on the right side, an increase in all reflexes in the right upper limb, but with an equivocal plantar response on the left side and a flexor response on the right. Two patients showed an asymmetric palmomental reflex that was more prominent on the side of the more severely affected limb.

More than a century ago, Charcot suggested that the pathologic process of ALS may spread from the white to the gray matter or (less likely, he thought) from the gray matter to the white (1). Wilson offered the somewhat different suggestion that "outgoing root fibres might be injured, by some diffuse noxa radiating among ventral columns, only where they traverse the latter," so that a process confined to the white matter could account for both the upper and lower motor neuron signs (2). It is also worth considering that some so-called upper motor neuron signs, such as hyperactive stretch reflexes, could in fact be caused by a pathologic process confined to the gray matter, which contains gamma motor neurons, various interneurons (including Renshaw cells), and the synaptic terminals of descending motor pathways in addition to alpha motor neurons. An example of this situation might be found in the rigidity that accompanies progressive encephalomyelitis (3), which may be due to impaired inhibition (or destruction) of Renshaw cells with the release of tonic myotatic reflexes. The presence of a Babinski sign on the side of greater atrophy can only be the result of involvement of white matter.

The pathogenesis just described is compatible with a focal process, possibly an infectious one, and does not seem compatible with a degenerative disorder to which the term *abiotrophy* could be applied, or with a general toxic or dysmetabolic process.

REFERENCES

1. Goldblatt D: Motor neuron disease: Historical introduction. In *Motor Neuron Diseases. Research on Amyotrophic Lateral Sclerosis and Related Disorders.* Edited by FH Norris, LT Kurland. New York, Grune and Stratton, 1969, p 9

2. Wilson SAK: *Neurology,* Vol 2. Edited by AN Bruce. Baltimore, Williams & Wilkins, 1940, p 1028

3. Whitely AM, Swash M, Urich H: Progressive encephalomyelitis with rigidity. Its relation to subacute myoclonic spinal neuronitis and to the 'stiff man syndrome.' Brain 99:27–42, 1976

Lewis P. Rowland

I appreciate Dr. Goldblatt's emphasis on a point that I have made repeatedly in textbook articles. The combination of weak, wasted, twitching muscles in a limb with hyperactive reflexes occurs exclusively in ALS. Once, however, I said this on rounds to some residents and they immediately showed me a patient with syringomyelia who had the same combination. Nevertheless, it generally is a reliable sign of ALS. I would like to stress, however, that no formal evaluations have yet been conducted to ascertain the accuracy of clinical diagnoses of ALS. Although we depend on the accuracy of the clinical diagnosis, we do not always know for sure that it is reliable.

Of the three points made by Dr. Norris, two are basically in accord with my statements. However, I would urge all physicians to be careful in making statements about ALS patients who seem to improve. The cases I have cited from the literature (i.e., those described by Drs. Norris, Engel, and Mulder) are, like the case I discuss here, striking and unequivocal. Because these patients improved so dramatically, it is even possible that their diseases were different from "ordinary" motor neuron disease. Vague and undocumented statements about the "possibly beneficial" effects of various agents, such as snake venom or guanidine, may play havoc with the emotions of patients with motor neuron disease. Some may go from one end of the country to the other in search of a miracle, especially if a healthy-looking person who had an (unverified) condition with similar symptoms appears on television and says, "Look at me now." We must be careful about giving undue credence to anecdotes. We also must recognize that our accuracy in measuring the rate of progression of illness is limited; the best guideline is probably the Norris scale, but this is still crude in reference to "plateaus," and, once the patient is unable to walk, changes can be hard to detect. There is another reason to regard apparent plateaus with caution: the rate of progression is not the same for all patients and may not be consistent in a single patient, with or without therapy. This inconsistency is one of the reasons why controlled trials are necessary. What we need, I suppose, is an assessment that encompasses the pathogenesis of at least one of these syndromes so that we can follow the results of a laboratory test, rather than having to rely solely on clinical changes. In the end, however, if we ever do find an effective treatment for motor neuron disease, it will be the clinical effect that is important, not the laboratory test results.

Stanley L. Cohan

I think it should be stressed that clinicians must maintain a circumspect point of view regarding the possibility of cervical spondylosis in patients with ALS. These patients are in an age group in which degenerative changes in the cervical spine are prominent and common. Some patients who are diagnosed as having ALS start with an asymmetric lower motor neuron syndrome in the hands, which can be due to cervical spondylosis. In addition, some patients have degenerative disease in both the cervical and the lumbosacral spine, so that evidence of denervation on EMG in the upper and lower extremities does not unequivocally differentiate between patients with degenerative disease in the neck and those with ALS.

An additional problem in differentiating some patients with ALS from those with cervical-lumbar spondylosis is that patients with ALS may also have well established degenerative disease of the spine; thus, the demonstration of degenerative changes on x-ray does not exclude the diagnosis of ALS.

3 Epidemiology

Steven M. Juergens

Leonard T. Kurland

Amyotrophic lateral sclerosis has been the subject of a wide range of epidemiologic studies that may help to provide a better understanding of its natural history and etiology and ultimately lead to its prevention. The disease is more common in men than in women. It is a disease of adulthood, generally occurring in people who are older than 40 years. The average duration of ALS is between 2 and 5 years. There is a hereditary component in a small proportion of cases.

BACKGROUND

Except in a very few areas (e.g., Guam and the Kii Peninsula of Japan), discrete populations with a relatively high incidence of ALS have not been located. In most countries, the annual incidence of ALS is less than 2 cases per 100,000 population; this low incidence and its related problems of diagnosis, record keeping, and record retrieval can adversely affect case ascertainment in population surveys.

Several population studies have defined specific populations as the denominators with numerators consisting of the number of cases of ALS. These numerators have been determined with varying degrees of completeness and accuracy. Other sources of information are mortality reports from the United States and other countries, as described in two monographs (18, 24). Since many earlier studies are based on selected data from specialty centers, hospital records, or death certificates, one must interpret the findings with caution.

INCIDENCE

A review of population studies from the United States, Europe, Israel, Iceland, and Mexico reveals a range in incidence rates of ALS from 0.4 to approximately 1.8 per 100,000 population (Table 1). Juergens et al. (14), updating a previous study (17), examined the epidemiology of ALS in Rochester, Minnesota, with use of the central medical index of the community (based at the Mayo Clinic), which affords a high level of case ascertainment. They found an incidence of 1.76 per 100,000 population, 35 cases being identified during the period 1925 to 1977. A slight but statistically insignificant increase in the incidence rate was observed for this 52-year period. On the basis of data from 89 patients during 1951 to 1967 in northwestern Switzerland, Lorez reported an average annual incidence of 1.4 per 100,000 (20). Zack et al. identified 31 patients with ALS and reported an incidence of 1.32 per 100,000 population for Lehigh County, Pennsylvania, between 1968 and 1975 (30). Matsumoto et al. reported an incidence of 1.04 per 100,000 population and identified 118 patients with ALS in Hawaii between 1952 and 1969 (22). In a study in Carlisle, England, between 1955 and 1961, Brewis et al. found an average annual incidence of 1.0 per 100,000 population and identified 5 cases of ALS for that period (3). In Israel between 1960 and 1970, Kahana et al. identified 185 cases of ALS and reported an average annual incidence of approximately 0.8 per 100,000 population (15). Gudmundsson reported 24 cases of the disease in Iceland from 1954 to 1963, with an annual incidence of 0.76 per 100,000 population (10). In Sardinia, Rosati et al. found an average annual incidence of 0.64 per 100,000 inhabitants on the basis of data from 96 cases of ALS for the period 1965 to 1974 (26). With information from a government health plan study in Mexico City that dealt with approximately 500,000 people, Olivares et al. reported an annual incidence of 0.4 per 100,000 population during 1964 to 1969 (25). Cendrowski et al. reviewed case reports of 56 patients in Poznan, Poland, between 1955 and 1965 and estimated the incidence there to be 0.22 per 100,000 population (5).

The lower incidence figures that are generally reported in the European and Mexican studies as compared with those for the United States may reflect incomplete case ascertainment. However, these studies are in marked contrast to the much higher incidence of ALS reported on Guam (6, 19) and to comparably high rates reported on the Kii Peninsula of Japan (6, 29).

Data on mortality provide broad geographic comparisons at relatively low cost. These data are derived from death certificates, which

Table 1 Population Surveys of ALS

Investigator	*Years of Study*	*Location*	*Base Population*	*Total Cases*	*Annual Incidence per 100,000*
Juergens et al. (14)	1925–1977	Rochester, MN	36,665	35	1.76
Lorez (20)	1951–1967	Northwest Switzerland	300,000	89	1.40
Zack et al. (30)	1968–1975	Lehigh County, PA	255,304	31	1.32
Kurland et al. (17)	1925–1964	Rochester, MN	30,000	17	1.30
Matsumoto et al. (27)	1952–1969	Hawaii	632,772	118	1.04
Brewis et al. (3)	1955–1961	Carlisle, England	71,000	5	1.00
Kahana et al. (15)	1960–1970	Israel	2,360,066	185	0.78
Gudmundsson (10)	1954–1963	Iceland	187,200	24	0.76
Rosati et al. (26)	1965–1974	Sardinia	1,494,084	96	0.64
Olivares et al. (25)	1962–1969	Mexico City (ISSTE[a] population)	494,059	16	0.40
Cendrowski et al. (5)	1955–1965	Poznan, Poland	2,547,736	56	0.22

[a]ISSTE = Instituto de Seguridad y Servicios Sociales de los Trabajadores del Estado.

are often prepared by physicians who do not have expertise in neurology. Although they are not always reliable, they can serve as a general source of information and as a guide for future population surveys. Such records also are subject to errors in certification and to nonuniformity in handling and coding.

The reliability of death certification for ALS in North Carolina was investigated in 1971 by Hoffman and Brody (12). They collected data on 72 patients who were clinically diagnosed at several referral centers as having ALS. In 72% of these cases, ALS was certified as the cause of death; in 11%, multiple sclerosis was erroneously reported; and in 17%, some other cause was listed. The authors suggest that ALS is most commonly misdiagnosed as multiple sclerosis.

Of 33 patients in Rochester, Minnesota, who died of ALS, 30 (91%) had ALS listed as the cause of death, 1 (3%) had ascending paralysis of the lower extremities listed as a contributory cause, and 2 (6%) had no mention of neurologic abnormality (14). Twenty-six of the 30 (87%) had ALS listed as the primary cause of death. The accuracy of reporting is due to the fact that most of these death certificates were prepared by pathologists at the Mayo Clinic who had access to the patients' clinical history.

Amyotrophic lateral sclerosis occurs in all countries for which mortality statistics can be obtained; in the well developed countries of the West and the Pacific, the illness accounts for about 1 per 1000 adult deaths. Kurland compared statistics on mortality from ALS in 10 selected well developed countries during the early 1950s and found that the age-adjusted rates were between 0.7 and 1.0 per 100,000 population (16). Goldberg and Kurland later analyzed mortality figures for other countries during 1951 to 1958 and found that the age-adjusted rates per 100,000 population varied from 0.1 in Mexico to 1.2 in the Netherlands (9). Mortality generally was higher than 0.5 per 100,000 population. For the United States between 1949 and 1964, the crude rate varied between 0.6 and 0.7 per 100,000 population, revealing no trend in mortality from ALS in the United States during those years.

AGE, MORTALITY, AND SURVIVORSHIP

The data concerning age at onset of ALS are frequently in conflict (Table 2). Several clinical series and many population studies report a mean age at onset between the late 40s and mid-50s. However, population studies in the United States show a median age at onset of more than 60 years. Juergens et al. reported a median age at onset of 66 years in Rochester, Minn., with no demonstrable difference between ages of men and women (14). Zack et al. reported an overall median age at onset of

Table 2 Median or Mean Age at Onset or Diagnosis of ALS for Various Clinical and Population Studies

Investigator	Source of Data	Total Cases	Median or Mean Age		
			Total	*Male*	*Female*
Clinical series					
Rosen (27)	National ALS Foundation questionnaire	668	56.1[a,b]	54.9[a,b]	57.9[a,b]
Mackay (21)	Private clinical files	91	52.0	52.0[a]	52.9[a]
Friedman and Freedman (19)	Montefiore Hospital (NY) records	111	52.0[a]		
Mulder (23)	Mayo Clinic cases	100	51.5		
Boman and Meurman (1)	University of Helsinki and City of Helsinki neurologic clinic files	140	50.0		
Population studies					
Juergens et al. (14)	Central medical index (Rochester, MN)	35	66.0	65.5	68.0
Kurland et al. (17)	Central medical index (Rochester, MN)	17	64.0[a]	63.0[a]	66.0[a]
Zack et al. (30)	Hospital and clinical records (Lehigh County, PA)	31	61.0	52.5	66.0
Rosati et al. (26)	Hospital and practitioner records (Sardinia)	96	56.5[a]		
Kahana et al. (15)	Hospital and clinical records and death certificates (Israel)	122		55.4[a]	52.4[a]
Jokelainen (13)	Hospital records (Finland)	168	51.9[a]	50.8[a]	53.5[a]
Olivares et al. (25)	ISSTE[c] government health plan (Mexico City)	16	50.6[a]	52.0[a]	49.9[a]
Gudmundsson (10)	Hospital and clinical records (Iceland)	24	49.8[a]		

[a]At onset.
[b]At diagnosis.
[c]Instituto de Seguridad y Servicios Sociales de los Trabajadores del Estado.

61 years for Lehigh County, with a median age at onset of 52.5 years for men and 66 years for women (30).

Surveys of death certificates in the United States between 1959 and 1961 reveal a median age at death from ALS of approximately 62.0 years and a mean age at death of 64.4 years. If we assume a 2- to 4-year survival after diagnosis of ALS, the average age at onset would be approximately 60 years. Of the 3149 patients whose death certificate listed ALS as a primary cause of death, 8% died before the age of 45, and 73% died after the age of 54. Ninety-eight percent of these patients died between the ages of 35 and 84.

Data concerning the survivorship of patients with ALS also varied. Most of the data are from clinical series, which generally report an average survival of approximately 3 years after onset (8, 21, 23). On the basis of questionnaires from 596 patients with ALS who belonged to the National ALS Foundation registry, Rosen reported a 5-year survival for 39.4% of these patients (27). However, the study of patients in Rochester demonstrated a slightly shorter median survival of less than 2 years (22.5 months) (14). One factor that may have contributed to the shorter survival is that the patients in the Rochester series were older than both those in the clinical series and those who responded to the National ALS Foundation questionnaire. The usual range of survival reported in such studies has been 1 to 10 years.

The differences in results between series concerning age at onset and those concerning survivorship of patients with ALS may be due to several factors. If the rate of progression of disease does not vary with age, then a younger person, who generally is stronger at the onset of the disease, might be expected to live longer. A relation between younger age at onset and a longer course of ALS has been noted by some investigators (1, 14, 15, 26, 27). It is also possible that early diagnosis of ALS is more likely in younger patients than in older ones (14). That is, relatively young patients, their family, and physician may be more motivated to obtain the opinion of a specialist for diagnosis. An elderly patient may have more difficulty in traveling to a specialty center because of physical limitations associated with both age and debilitation caused by ALS. In addition, the family, physician, or patient may assume that his or her symptoms are simply part of the aging process and thus may not seek the opinion of an expert. It is also possible that the longer the interval between onset and diagnosis, the more likely that the patient will associate the time of onset with more recent milestones of the illness. Also, patients who have been referred for diagnosis must have lived long enough to obtain appointments and been able to travel far enough to have been included in the series; for this reason, elderly patients or patients with rapidly advancing disease may be excluded. Finally, studies based on patients who answer questionnaires distributed by health agencies necessarily exclude individuals who did not participate in the questionnaire, possibly because they did not live long enough to learn of its existence. Therefore, because most studies are based on data from patients who have been examined either at a specialty center or by a neurologist or who have joined a specialty organization, the younger patient with a more indolent course is more likely to be studied than the older patient.

Studies based on death certificates may be less selective than clinical series and thus may give evidence of a disease process that begins later in life, a fact that is borne out by the United States mortality figures. The ALS patients studied in Rochester were older at onset of disease than patients studied in other series. They also manifested a shorter average survival as compared with that of patients in most clinical series. These observations may reflect not only differences in the selection of the patient population, but other factors as well, such as differences in health care facilities. It is believed that the results of the Rochester study offer an accurate picture of the course of ALS, at least as it has affected that population.

The question of the age at which the incidence of ALS is highest is still unresolved. Most clinical series have shown a decline in the number of patients with ALS whose age is beyond the mid-50s. However, these series do not take into consideration the population at risk in each age group. The United States mortality figures for 1959 to 1961 show that the age-specific rates for ALS increased with age and reached a peak of approximately 70 years for white men and women and then declined. In Rochester, the observed incidence increased with age and reached a maximum in the oldest age group (≥70 years); however, because the number of cases studied was small, the age-specific rates for age groups older than 55 years did not differ significantly from one another (3).

SEX OF PATIENTS

Sporadic and Guam-type ALS have consistently been shown to occur in a greater proportion of men than women. International mortality statistics show a ratio of between 1.5:1 and 1.8:1; the ratio for the United States is 1.7:1. The ratio of men to women with ALS in Rochester is 1.6:1. The reason for this difference is unclear, but the greater number of men with ALS is consistent in nearly all mortality and morbidity studies.

HEREDITARY ALS

Many studies of ALS report that the disease occurs as an autosomal dominant inherited disorder in 5%–10% of patients (19, 21, 28). In contrast to sporadic and Guam-type ALS, the mortality ratio of men to women for this form is 1:1. The clinical pattern and course of hereditary ALS in the individual patient seem to be indistinguishable from that of sporadic ALS, but the hereditary form pathologically exhibits some clinically silent changes, such as demyelination of the posterior columns (11).

THE MARIANA (WESTERN PACIFIC) FORM

The high incidence of ALS among the Chamorro people of the Mariana Islands has been noted by investigators since the mid-1940s. Clinically, Mariana-type ALS is indistinguishable from the sporadic form (20). Although the range of age of onset is similar, the mean age at onset—46 to 48 years—is lower than that of the classic form. The mean age at death is approximately 52 years for women and 50 years for men, with a male-to-female mortality ratio of about 2.5:1. The mean duration of illness is approximately 3 to 4 years. The major pathologic features of degeneration of the anterior horn cells and demyelination of the pyramidal tract do not differ from those of the classic form; however, neurofibrillary changes and granulovacuolar bodies are common in Guam-type ALS but occur infrequently in other types (4).

GEOGRAPHY AND RACE

Amyotrophic lateral sclerosis seems to have a uniform incidence throughout the world. The increased incidence of the disease on Guam, the Kii Peninsula of Japan, and possibly western New Guinea (West Irian) are the only well documented geographic isolates. Although there is some disparity in incidence of ALS among the various population studies mentioned previously, the uncertainty of the accuracy of these studies makes it difficult to know whether the reported differences are accurate representations. Kurland et al. reviewed the mortality per 100,000 population for certain countries and for the United States by state and found that, although some differences existed (Mexico 0.1; the Netherlands, 1.2; United States, 0.3–1.0, with all but five states having death rates between 0.4 and 0.7), the variability of medical care and training, certification, and coding may have accounted for the observed differences. There was no clear-cut difference according to hemisphere, nor was there a north–south gradient. The age-adjusted rates for foreign-born and native Americans were similar (17).

Edgar et al. found that the age-adjusted death rates from ALS for native and nonnative residents of California and Washington did not vary significantly (7). Kahana et al. found a narrow range of incidence rates among both the subpopulations from different parts of the world living in Israel and the native-born in Israel; these findings are in contrast to the geographic differential reported for multiple sclerosis (15).

There is no firm evidence of racial selectivity in patients with ALS. Mortality statistics for the United States during 1959 to 1961 reveal a ratio of white to nonwhite deaths from ALS of 1.7:1; however, this difference may have been due to reporting artifacts or to differences in diagnostic services. Also, during that period, mortality from ALS among Japanese living in the United States surpassed that among whites, although the number of cases was small. It also has been suggested that there is an elevated death rate from ALS among Filipino men living in Hawaii (7). As mentioned previously, Olivares et al. reported a lower incidence of ALS in Mexico (25). It is unclear whether the data showing a lower mortality from ALS in Mexico are an artifact of underreporting or the result of decreased incidence of the disease in that country.

OCCUPATION

There have been reports in Europe (5, 26) and America (2) of a seemingly higher incidence of ALS in persons regularly engaged in physical labor. Many individuals affected are reported to have primarily agricultural occupational backgrounds, and investigators have suggested an etiologic relation between ALS and labor, toxins, or animal-transmitted infections. Data concerning this point are inconclusive at present.

SUMMARY

Amyotrophic lateral sclerosis is a disease that occurs in all countries for which mortality statistics are available. It accounts for about 1 in every 1000 deaths. The incidence of ALS varies from approximately 0.4–1.8 per 100,000 population, except in selected areas of the Kii Peninsula of Japan, Guam, and possibly western New Guinea, where the incidence is much higher.

The average age of onset and the duration of ALS have been subject to controversy. Many clinical series report that the average age of onset is between the late 40s and mid-50s. However, two recent population studies in Lehigh County, Pennsylvania, and Rochester, Minnesota, reported ages of onset of 61 and 66 years, respectively. United States mortality statistics reveal that the mean age at death is about 64 years, which would reflect an average age of onset of about 60 years.

The survivorship of ALS is reported to average approximately 3 to 5 years, although the Rochester study, in which older patients predominated, revealed a median survivorship of slightly under 2 years.

It is our opinion that the variability in reported survivorship lies in the differences in the populations studied. Studies that are based on specialty center records or on questionnaires from voluntary health agencies tend to select younger patients. Younger patients have been noted to live somewhat longer with the disease than older persons and thus would have more time and strength both to make and keep appointments with specialists as well as to learn of and join voluntary ALS organizations. Therefore, unless a study evaluates survivorship thoroughly in a well delineated population of patients, as was done in Rochester, one would expect the group to consist of younger patients and, therefore, show a more prolonged course. We believe the average age of onset to be greater than 60 years, with survival after onset varying widely but averaging under 3 years.

The question of the age at which the incidence of ALS is highest is still unresolved. It is an important point because, if the incidence of ALS increases with age, it may point toward a different etiology of ALS than if the incidence peaked and then declined. Clinical series indicate a peak incidence in the mid-50s, but the problems with population selection have been discussed above. The United States mortality figures for 1959 to 1961 reveal a peak incidence at approximately 70 years of age. In Rochester, the observed incidence rates increased with increasing age, but the age-specific rates did not vary significantly in the groups older than age 55 because of the small number of cases studied. It remains to be clarified by further population-based studies whether age-specific rates increase with age or peak between the sixth and eighth decades of life.

REFERENCES

1. Boman K, Meurman T: Prognosis of amyotrophic lateral sclerosis. Acta Neurol Scand 43:489–498, 1967

2. Breland AE Jr, Currier RD: Multiple sclerosis and amyotrophic lateral sclerosis in Mississippi. Neurology (Minneap) 17:1011–1016, 1967

3. Brewis M, Poskanzer DC, Rolland C, et al: Neurological disease in an English city. Acta Neurol Scand [Suppl] 42(Suppl 24):1–89, 1966

4. Brody JA, Stanhope JM, Kurland LT: Patterns of amyotrophic lateral sclerosis and parkinsonism-dementia on Guam. In *Topics on Tropical Neurology*. Edited by RW Hornabrook. Philadelphia, FA Davis, 1975, pp 45–70

5. Cendrowski W, Wender M, Owsianowski M: Analyse epidemiologique de la sclerose laterale amyotrophique sur le territoire de la grande-pologne. Acta Neurol Scand 46:609–617, 1970

6. Chen K-M, Brody JA, Kurland LT: Patterns of neurologic diseases on Guam. I. Epidemiologic aspects. Arch Neurol 19:573–578, 1968

7. Edgar AH, Brody JA, Detels R: Amyotrophic lateral sclerosis mortality among native-born and migrant residents of California and Washington. Neurology (Minneap) 23:48–51, 1973

8. Friedman AP, Freedman D: Amyotrophic lateral sclerosis. J Nerv Ment Dis 111:1–18, 1950

9. Goldberg ID, Kurland LT: Mortality in 33 countries from diseases of the nervous system. World Neurol 3:444–465, 1962

10. Gudmundsson KR: The prevalence of some neurological diseases in Iceland. Acta Neurol Scand 44:57–69, 1968

11. Hirano A, Kurland LT, Sayre GP: Familial amyotrophic lateral sclerosis: a subgroup characterized by posterior and spinocerebellar tract involvement and hyaline inclusions in the anterior horn cells. Arch Neurol 16:232–243, 1967

12. Hoffman PM, Brody JA: The reliability of death certificate reporting for amyotrophic lateral sclerosis. J Chronic Dis 24:5–8, 1971

13. Jokelainen M: Amyotrophic lateral sclerosis in Finland. I. An epidemiologic study. Acta Neurol Scand 56:185–193, 1977

14. Juergens SM, Kurland LT, Okazaki H, et al: ALS in Rochester, Minnesota, 1925–1977. Neurology (Minneap), in press

15. Kahana E, Alter M, Feldman S: Amyotrophic lateral sclerosis: a population study. J Neurol 212:205–213, 1976

16. Kurland, LT: Epidemiologic investigations of amyotrophic lateral sclerosis. III. Proc Staff Meet Mayo Clin 32:449–462, 1957

17. Kurland LT, Choi NW, Sayre GP: Implications of incidence and geographic patterns on the classification of amyotrophic lateral sclerosis. In *Motor Neuron Diseases. Research on Amyotrophic Lateral Sclerosis and Related Disorders.* Edited by FH Norris Jr, LT Kurland. New York, Grune and Stratton, 1969, pp 28–50

18. Kurland LT, Kurtzke JF, Goldberg ID (Editors): *Epidemiology of Neurologic and Sense Organ Disorders.* Cambridge, Mass., Harvard University Press, 1973

19. Kurland LT, Mulder DW: Epidemiologic investigations of amyotrophic lateral sclerosis. 2. Familial aggregations indicative of dominant inheritance: Part I and Part II. Neurology (Minneap) 5:182–196, 249–268, 1955

20. Lorez A: Ein Beitrag zu Klinik und Vorkommen der amyotrophischen Lateralsklerose (isolierte und familiäre Fälle). Schweiz Med Wochenschr 99:51–57, 1969

21. Mackay RP: Course and prognosis in amyotrophic lateral sclerosis. Arch Neurol 8:117–127, 1963

22. Matsumoto N, Worth RM, Kurland LT, et al: Epidemiologic study of amyotrophic lateral sclerosis in Hawaii: identification of high incidence among Filipino men. Neurology (Minneap) 22:934–940, 1972

23. Mulder DW: The clinical syndrome of amyotrophic lateral sclerosis. Proc Staff Meet Mayo Clin 32:427–436, 1957

24. Norris FH Jr, Kurland LT (Editors): *Motor Neuron Diseases. Research on Amyotrophic Lateral Sclerosis and Related Disorders.* New York, Grune and Stratton, 1969

25. Olivares L, San Estéban E, Alter M: Mexican 'resistance' to amyotrophic lateral sclerosis. Arch Neurol 27:397–402, 1972

26. Rosati G, Pinna L, Granieri E, et al: Studies on epidemiological, clinical and etiological aspects of ALS disease in Sardinia, Southern Italy. Acta Neurol Scand 55:231–244, 1977

27. Rosen AD: Amyotrophic lateral sclerosis: clinical features and prognosis. Arch Neurol 35:638–642, 1978

28. Thomson AF, Alvarez F: Hereditary amyotrophic lateral sclerosis. J Neurol Sci 8:101–110, 1969

29. Yase Y, Matsumoto N, Yoshimasu F, et al: Motor neuron disease in the Kii Peninsula, Japan. Proc Aust Assoc Neurol 5:335–339, 1968

30. Zack MM, Levitt LP, Schoenberg B: Motor neuron disease in Lehigh County, Pennsylvania: an epidemiologic study. J Chronic Dis 30:813–818, 1977

Commentary

Leonard T. Kurland

Dr. Juergens's data bring up the question of the age at which ALS has the highest incidence. The figures he presents point toward an increase in incidence with age. The study of ALS conducted in Rochester, Minnesota, was based on 35 cases and extended over a 50-year period; this is a small number of cases. However, I should point out that many other Rochester studies are based on a relatively small number of cases, and most of them have proved to be reliable when other, larger population studies have become available for comparison. Twenty years ago, I presented a descriptive epidemiologic study on primary brain tumors and reported that the incidence in the Rochester population increased with age; in contrast, all other studies showed a peak incidence at about 55 to 60 years of age (2). Recently, Dr. Bruce Schoenberg of the National Institutes of Health confirmed this observation, which reflects the level of diagnosis and the importance of our high autopsy rate (8).

Another example is the striking difference between the age distribution of patients with parkinsonism studied in Rochester over several decades and that of patients studied by Poskanzer et al. through the referral practice of the Massachusetts General Hospital in Boston (7). Poskanzer et al. concluded that there existed a cohort phenomenon that resulted from exposure of the United States population to the virus(es) responsible for the encephalitis epidemics that occurred around 1920. In Rochester during the past 40 years, there has been no change in the mean age of onset of parkinsonism, which has been about 65 years (4). Thus, I would like to stress that, although only small numbers of cases of ALS have been identified and studied, our study may be of great value and perhaps shows a more accurate picture of the true age-specific incidence for ALS and many other serious diseases.

In 1978, Wylie reported on data from the Professional Activity Study (PAS) (Commission on Professional and Hospital Activities) for hundreds of hospitals around the country. This study included a review of almost 3000 patients with ALS who had been discharged from the hospital (9). The average age of these patients was 61 years; 42% of the patients were between 50 and 64 years old, and 44% were 65 years and older.

Another feature of Dr. Juergens's report concerns the age of his patients, which is much greater than that reported in clinical studies but similar to the age distribution of deaths from motor neuron disease reported in the United States as a whole. In spite of the small number of cases studied, the Rochester data may reflect age distribution better than clinical studies

Third Symposium on Parkinsonism. Edinburgh, E and S Livingstone, 1969, pp 12–16

5. Kurland LT, Mulder DW: Epidemiologic investigations of amyotrophic lateral sclerosis: preliminary report on geographic distribution, with special reference to the Mariana Islands, including clinical and pathological observations. Neurology 4:355–378, 1954

6. Mulder DW: The clinical syndrome of amyotrophic lateral sclerosis. Mayo Clin Proc 32:427–436, 1957

7. Poskanzer DC, Schwab RS: Cohort analysis of Parkinson's syndrome: evidence for a single etiology related to subclinical infection about 1920. J Chronic Dis 16:961–973, 1963

8. Schoenberg BS, Christine BW, Whisnant JP: The resolution of discrepancies in the reported incidence of primary brain tumors. Neurology 28:817–823, 1978

9. Wylie CM (Editor): Variations of ALS incidence. PAS Reporter 16(12):1, 1978

Steven M. Juergens

In the Rochester study, autopsy was performed on 18 of the 35 patients who died from ALS. Fourteen were examined at the Mayo Clinic, and we were able to review slides on 2 others. All 16 revealed anterior horn cell degeneration; 10 also showed definite demyelination of the pyramidal tract. Neither a neuropathology report nor tissue sections were available for 1 of the remaining 2 patients; the report on the second of the 2 described changes of ALS. In none of the 16 autopsies reviewed were there findings in the posterior columns, Clark's column, or the spinocerebellar tracts; neurofibrillary tangles or hyaline inclusions were not observed in spinal cord sections.

The patients, both men and women, seemed to be reasonably representative of the Rochester community. Among the women who died were seven housewives; three nurses; two other hospital workers; and one teacher, seamstress, milliner, cashier, and elevator operator. Among the men were four unskilled laborers, two semiskilled laborers; two salesmen; two restaurant workers; and one hospital laundry worker, dogcatcher, horse trainer, grain buyer, engineer, bookkeeper, minister, and physician.

Of the 35 patients, 3 had suffered injuries to the neck or shoulder from three months to three years before onset of ALS in the same extremity that was affected by the injury.

Two patients had a history of exposure to toxin. One was a laboratory worker who was exposed to numerous solvents, and the other was a dogcatcher who worked with cyanide gas. Six patients had received various degrees of exogenous irradiation before onset of the ALS. The actual rates of these exposures are not known for the general population, so at best we are left with only an impression. The injuries, toxin exposure, irradiation, and other exogenous factors that were reported did not exceed those that might be expected in the Rochester population.

4 Differential Diagnosis of Adult Motor Neuron Diseases

Forbes H. Norris, Jr

Eric H. Denys

Kwei Sang Ü

To clinicians experienced with adult motor neuron disease, the well-established case, particularly of amyotrophic lateral sclerosis, is distinctive. However, puzzling atypical cases do exist, and almost always in very early cases, the physician may hesitate to make a firm diagnosis because it carries such a grave prognosis. These diagnostic problems are compounded by the capricious onset and course of ALS, by our ignorance of its exact etiology, and by our reliance in large part on empirical therapeutic efforts.

What we present here includes partly impressionistic clinical conclusions based on personal experience with approximately 1500 ALS patients. Our emphasis is on other conditions that are likely to confuse the diagnosis rather than on excessively rare disorders that have greater academic than practical importance. We shall also emphasize areas that need further clinical investigation.

First, it is important to recognize the capriciousness of motor neuron disease; in some cases this characteristic can create major diagnostic problems, and in our opinion it has not been given due weight in the literature. Let us consider ALS, in which onset of symptoms can occur in any part of the body below the eyes and may affect emotional reflexes in one patient, toe muscles in another, or cause almost simultaneous generalized involvement in another. The course of ALS is equally erratic and may be characterized by "fits and starts" rather than by steady downhill progression, although the latter course afflicts a small number of patients. Periods of improvement do occur, and sometimes persist for many months or even years.

We have suggested, particularly in cases where maximum disability is relatively mild or returns to a mild level through partial recovery, that the term *benign ALS* be used to distinguish this form from *rapidly progressive ALS*, which manifests a malignant disease process (26). Subtyping of motor neuron disease is almost another topic, however, and will be discussed briefly at the end of this chapter.

The major point to be made now is that motor neuron disease exhibits a capricious onset and course more frequently than the literature suggests, and this tendency can create major diagnostic problems, particularly in early or atypical cases or for inexperienced physicians. If we seem to deemphasize the usual clinical courses noted in most texts, such as those of steady progression, rapid progression, or generalized symptoms, it is because we find these "typical" aspects to be inconstant and therefore of less diagnostic value than others have taught.

DIFFERENTIAL DIAGNOSIS AT THE BEDSIDE

One well known typical finding in ALS is Babinski's sign. It is probably true that most patients with far-advanced ALS show this sign, but it is often absent in early cases and never appears in others. There may be hyperactive reflexes, even clonus, but normal (flexor) plantar responses. A patient with such signs usually will (but may not) manifest spastic gait. In these patients, there seems to be a discrepancy between the extent of upper motor dysfunction manifested by muscle-stretch reflex activity and that manifested by the plantar response.

This lack of consistent upper motor neuron findings stands in sharp contrast to the pattern that is usually seen in other disorders prominent in the differential diagnosis, particularly multiple sclerosis (MS) in younger patients and spinal cord compression syndromes (especially cervical spondylosis) in older patients. In these disorders, involvement of the long tracts typically produces Babinski's sign before the development of muscle-stretch clonus.

Another point concerns the precise Babinski sign. We find most useful the sign of toe extension in response to slightly nociceptive lateral plantar stimulation, as originally utilized by Babinski for detection of significant corticospinal tract pathology (3). Babinski later described a less frequent response to plantar stimulation, "the sign of the fan" of the small toes (4). A combination of Babinski's toe sign with fanning was later termed the "complete Babinski sign." The abnormal response to plantar stimulation in ALS is frequently either extension of the great toe with no fanning of the small toes or fanning of the small toes with no clear extension of the great toe. In other conditions, such as MS and spinal cord compression due to neoplasm or cervical spondylosis, the two Babinski components often occur together, although the experienced clinician certainly is aware of exceptions to this general rule. On the other hand, the superficial abdominal reflexes, which are often reduced or absent in MS and cord compression, usually are quite active in ALS.

To the clinician, the pathophysiology of ALS appears to affect upper motor neuron pathways to the same fine extent as it does the lower motor neurons. Although the exact mechanism is not known, this peculiar tendency to spare immediately adjacent neurons or fiber pathways is a valuable hallmark of ALS with respect to the differential diagnosis. The following examples illustrate this point.

An older man with a long history of multiple neck injuries has, over many years, slowly developed increasing rigidity of the neck and occasional neck pain, sometimes with radicular components in the shoulders and sometimes with radiation to the occiput, resulting in headache. Some weakness of the small hand muscles then appeared, accompanied later by mild atrophy but with only rare fasciculations. Although the patient had no subjective change in leg strength, examination revealed a slightly spastic gait with subclonic knee jerks and ankle jerks. Plantar responses were flexor. A reasonable diagnostic consideration would be cervical osteoarthritis and spondylosis, but the absence of Babinski's sign makes ALS more likely, even though Babinski's sign is often regarded as typical of ALS.

Another example is the young woman with slowly progressive paraparesis but with no impairment either of sensation or of bowel and bladder control. Examination revealed clonic knee jerks and significant hyperactivity of ankle jerks; however, there was flexion on plantar stimulation. A common diagnostic consideration would be MS, but again, the absence of a Babinski sign points to ALS as the correct diagnosis.

Needless to say, in neither case should the relevant diagnostic tests be neglected merely because of the absence of Babinski's sign. Conversely, the presence of Babinski's sign in these patients would not point away from a diagnosis of motor neuron disease, and the appropriate diagnostic tests for these disorders should not be ignored.

Fasciculation

Fascicular twitching of the muscles, which is characteristic of motor neuron diseases and especially of ALS, probably has intrigued physicians since the time of Aran's original description in 1850 (1). Swank and Putnam attempted to use the extent and frequency of fasciculation as a guideline for diagnosis of the specific disorder (33); for example, ALS is notable for causing the greatest amount of fasciculation. Norris's review confirmed the value of this guideline (24), though in exceptional or atypical cases, ALS-like fasciculation can be seen in benign ALS and progressive muscular atrophy, whereas fasciculation may be minimal or absent in rapidly progressive, or malignant, ALS.

Early development of prominent fasciculation in some patients with ALS also raises other, more benign considerations with regard to differential diagnosis. For example, paralytic poliomyelitis causes fasciculations that sometimes persist for many years. A 64-year-old man described having suffered an acute febrile illness with paralysis of the right leg during a poliomyelitis epidemic when he was 4 years old. Examination at age 64 revealed continued muscular weakness and atrophy with areflexia throughout the right leg, plus frequent coarse fascicular twitching in the muscles of that leg. He also experienced occasional fasciculation in the left leg. He reported being aware of the fasciculation for many years but noting little change in its activity. Follow-up examinations during the following 2 years revealed stability of these neuromuscular findings, which presumably originated with paralytic poliomyelitis some 60 years before.

Another concern in the differential diagnosis is fasciculation after fatiguing exercise, a response to which many healthy individuals are subject. Such *benign fasciculation* is frequently a result of anxiety, as, for example, in the neurology trainee who notices his own fasciculation while caring for a patient with advanced ALS.

In *benign myokymia*, many authors have described frequent or even constant undulating or rhythmic fasciculation, which is unlike the fasciculation associated with motor neuron disease. This differentiation would be strengthened by a long history of similar muscular activity and by evidence of other family members being so affected.

Diagnostic difficulties arise with all these disorders because the history may be incomplete or inaccurate or because the fasciculations are atypical (e.g., intermittent and jerky in a case of myokymia rather than constant and undulating). It is remarkable that, even so long after Aran's description (1) and the great attention given to the diagnosis and classification of motor neuron diseases in the late nineteenth century, physicians remain ignorant of the pathophysiology of fasciculations, even in healthy individuals, and frequently are unable to firmly differentiate benign from malignant fasciculations, despite the aid of sophisticated electromyographic analyses (35). Table 1 presents various characteristics of fasciculations that are valuable for clinical differentiation.

Cramps

Differentiation of frequent, painful cramps in motor neuron diseases is subject to the same problems as those encountered in differentiation of fasciculations. Cramps are so well known in the general population that they have received various specific appellations—for example, pregnancy

Table 1 Differentiation of Fasciculations According to Clinical Characteristics

Characteristic	Type of Fasciculation		
	Benign	*Myokymic*	*ALS-Related*
Extent of fasciculation	More focal	Generalized	Focal to generalized
Frequency	Slow	Fast to constant	Fast
Appearance	Fine	Coarse to undulating	Fine to coarse
Occurrence in tongue	Rare	Occasional	Common
Subsequent functional disability	None	Mild	Mild to moderate[a]

[a] Depending on the extent of the ALS before examination.

cramps, night cramps, swimmer's cramps, writer's cramp, salt-loss cramp, heat cramp, and so forth. Although the frequency of painful cramps is greater in patients with motor neuron disease, particularly in those with ALS, some patients with malignant ALS never experience painful cramps. On the other hand, there are many healthy individuals whose physical activity is restricted by the frequent occurrence of such cramps.

Again, unless the motor unit participation in the cramp includes units with grossly abnormal action potentials, there is no adequate differentiation on electromyogram (EMG) between cramps experienced by healthy individuals and those experienced by individuals with motor neuron disease (24).

In some cases of motor neuron disease, particularly in ALS, the initial symptom is frequent cramping or fasciculation, which sometimes lasts many months or even years before other symptoms appear; it is in these cases that great diagnostic difficulties arise. Extensive study with electromyography, even in the best laboratories, may yield few additional clues to the presence of early motor neuron disease.

In a series of several hundred patients with ALS, who underwent biopsy of an apparently unaffected muscle, the characteristic small, angulated fibers, occurring singly or in small groups, were invariably found. More recently, in more than 100 patients with histochemically based fiber differentiation, moderate and sometimes marked type grouping also was seen, regardless of clinical involvement. However, this result is obtained from large amounts of material removed during open biopsy and probably should not be considered an early diagnostic test, especially since there is no specific preventive or curative treatment for the motor neuron diseases.

Correct differentiation sometimes is possible after multiple evaluations of the patient's neuromuscular status over time, as exemplified by the case of the patient whose fasciculation was present 60 years after he had poliomyelitis. However, in some cases such watchful waiting is easier to recommend than to carry out, particularly when the patient's anxiety is heightened by appreciation of the ominous associations of frequent cramps and fasciculation. The following is a case in point.

A patient (male) has had prominent fasciculations and cramps for at least 10 years, but these symptoms are not associated with muscular weakness, atrophy, or alteration of reflexes. No clinical change has occurred during 2 years of observation. The symptoms were of little concern to the patient until 4 years ago, when his best friend also developed cramps and fasciculation, then weakness with atrophy, and was diagnosed as having ALS. Our patient's anxiety and complaints about the symptoms seem to have progressed in direct proportion to his friend's advancing paralysis, although from an objective viewpoint he has no cause for such concern. The working diagnoses for this patient are benign fasciculation and anxiety, or possibly the "muscular pain–fasciculation syndrome" described by Hudson and colleagues (13).

It is clear that a major advance in the care of such patients, as well as early diagnosis of ALS in other patients, would result from development of a firm means of differentiating benign forms of cramps and fasciculation from those attributable to ALS. Another consideration is that perhaps some, if not all, cases of apparently benign fasciculation or cramping do represent early and limited ALS or an ALS-like process to which the patient is resistant (20, 26). We are following such patients carefully and accumulating relevant information for comparison with data on patients with ALS in the hope of detecting some clue to the existence and perhaps the character of this hypothetical resistance factor.

Myasthenic Symptoms

Abnormal fatigability is a typical symptom in patients with ALS. There may be dramatic recovery of strength after rest, and, as in myasthenia gravis, the patient may benefit from standard anticholinesterase preparations (21). Four patients in our series had such prominent fatigability early in the illness and derived so much benefit from anticholinesterase medication that the initial diagnosis by other neurologists was myasthenia gravis. Moreover, careful nerve–muscle transmission testing during EMG examination frequently reveals a minor disturbance in synaptic transmission in ALS (7).

Except in very rare cases, the differentiation of this myasthenic state from true myasthenia gravis usually is possible at the bedside because (*a*) the orbital muscles, which are spared in motor neuron disease, frequently are affected in myasthenia gravis; (*b*) the muscle-stretch reflexes are usually pathologic in motor neuron disease; and (*c*) the patient's response to medication for myasthenia gravis usually is considerably less in motor neuron disease than in myasthenia gravis (Table 2).

Other criteria are less reliable. The presence of fasciculation on examination can be misleading if the patient has been previously diagnosed as having myasthenia gravis and has received anticholinesterase medication. Such a patient also may experience painful muscle cramps. Judicious reduction or even cessation of the medication clarifies the significance of such findings. Palatal paresis in motor neuron disease, particularly in ALS and progressive bulbar palsy, may mimic typical symptoms of myasthenia gravis (e.g., nasal speech; regurgitation of food, and especially drink, through the nose). These symptoms also can be caused by a variety of neuropathies, but since poliomyelitis and diphtheritic polyneuropathy have virtually disappeared, they are seen today almost exclusively in motor neuron disease and myasthenia gravis. Like myasthenia gravis, motor neuron disease can have acute onset, and, in the absence of other signs, differentiation between these two syndromes can rarely be quite difficult.

The Lambert-Eaton syndrome manifests more proximal involvement, usually sparing the cranial nerve–supplied muscles, with normal reflexes or hyporeflexia; these signs are strong criteria for differentiation of this syndrome from both early ALS and myasthenia gravis (Table 2). Confusion is more likely to occur between the Lambert-Eaton syndrome and early progressive muscular atrophy.

Table 2 Criteria for Differentiation of Abnormal Fatigue at Bedside Evaluation

Criterion	*ALS*	*Myasthenia Gravis*	*Lambert-Eaton Syndrome*
Muscle atrophy	++++	+	++
Spasticity	++++	0[a]	0
Babinski's sign	+++	0	0
Abnormal muscle-stretch reflexes	++++	±	++
Orbital muscle involvement	±	++++	+
Response to			
Edrophonium (iv)	+	++++	+
Oral anticholinesterase	+	++++	++

[a] 0 = not present.

Mental Symptoms

Problems in differential diagnosis also arise from the capricious effect of ALS on the emotional reflexes, with pseudobulbar emotional swings as an early manifestation. The intact mentation in ALS points against the possibility of dementing brain disease. Tongue fasciculation with hyperactivity of the jaw jerk are common findings in ALS and eliminate diagnoses of neurotic, psychosomatic, or psychiatric disorder. However, physicians in either general or community practice may examine the patient at an earlier stage of illness, when clinical differentiation is less clear and the principal concern is for major brain and psychiatric disorders. Under such circumstances one or more of the following studies is often conducted: electroencephalogram (EEG), isotope brain scan, and computed brain tomogram. These tests are safe and noninvasive.

Greater care should be exercised with respect to more extensive testing, such as arteriography, which rarely reveals a remedial lesion and which carries the risk of some morbidity. In an older individual or in a younger person with known occlusive arterial disease, the most likely cause of acute impairment of emotional control is the compounding of a previously subclinical lesion of an internal capsule with an acute infarct of the other internal capsule. The diagnosis will be more certain if paresis or sensory (including visual-field) deficits occur on either side of the body. Bilateral frontal lobe disease also may present as acute loss of emotional control but usually is accompanied by prominent alteration of mental status and by other signs of frontal lobe dysfunction, such as forced grasping. In the absence of headache and nuchal rigidity, a leaking aneurysm of the anterior communicating artery is a rare finding; the patient's ability to accept or withstand surgery should be weighed against possible morbidity from arteriography.

SENSORY INVOLVEMENT

One reason for the widespread preference for the term *motor neuron disease* to the term *ALS* is that the syndrome is clinically characterized by sparing of sensory function despite extensive sensory pathology in the nervous system. Even patients with the characteristic additional lesion of the dorsal column in familial ALS (10) show no clinical sensory loss. Thus, the absence of sensory symptoms and findings is generally considered to be an important diagnostic clue.

It must be noted, however, that some patients with ALS do have sensory symptoms and findings, albeit usually minor and sometimes transitory. Many patients with onset of weakness in the distal arm and hand muscles experienced "pins-and-needles" paresthesia in the fingertips immediately before onset of weakness. Most of these patients also noted remission of the sensory symptom before their first neurologic evaluation, but in some cases, patchy areas of diminished pin and temperature sensitivity or of altered light-touch persisted. In at least two of these rare instances, larger patches of altered sensation occurred on the hand and forearm; these patches migrated slightly on serial examination and contracted or expanded in size from time to time. Necropsy study in one case confirmed the diagnosis of ALS.

More often, slight blunting of vibratory perception in the toes has been encountered; there is rarely absence of vibratory perception. It seems safe to attribute this sensory finding to the aging process, since it is consonant with the fact that patients with ALS generally are older.

Minor autonomic involvement occurs frequently as ALS progresses, causing cold or clammy, cyanotic, swollen hands and fingers or feet and toes. Edema is increased by physical dependency, and in such cases the patient may complain of distal paresthesia in the affected parts. The examiner may find reduction in pin and temperature perception and sometimes reduction or alteration of light-touch sensation. In many cases, it seems probable that tissue edema has affected either peripheral sensory receptors or fiber conduction, although in occasional cases, vibratory sensation is also reduced. Such sensory alterations are rare early in ALS and thus are more likely to confuse the differential diagnosis in a more advanced case.

Rarely, patients with ALS also experience neuralgic pain, and in these cases the differential diagnosis may include a variety of disorders, such as neurofibroma or prolapsed intervertebral disk, depending on the part of the body that is affected. In another rare type of ALS, patients complain of generalized hypersensitivity to sensory stimuli, particularly early in the illness; this hypersensitivity sometimes affects taste and smell. The symptom rarely persists into the amyotrophic stage of illness. The relationship between such irritative sensory symptoms and ALS is obscure.

Some patients with ALS experience bone or joint pain. This discomfort can originate in the neck and radiate into the shoulders as a result of cervical instability from muscle weakness; it also may be pain secondary to osteoarthritis in this group of older patients. Similarly, both vertebral instability from paraspinal muscular weakness and coincidental osteoarthritis can cause low backache in a patient with ALS.

Occasionally these pains are quite severe and may be present early in the illness. Distal radiation of pain may simulate nerve-root pain and stimulate more intensive investigation than might otherwise be indicated.

As ALS progresses, many patients develop a kind of periarthritis known as "frozen shoulder" due to weakened shoulder muscles. On occasion, severe weakness of shoulder muscles, followed by reduced motion, occurs very early in the illness, and severe shoulder pain is prominent as a presenting symptom. The weakness and atrophy may be mistaken for secondary changes from primary joint disease, and the diagnosis may be misdirected toward rheumatic rather than neurologic disorders.

As ALS progresses further, the evolving motor signs and symptoms invariably outweigh sensory disturbances. Therefore, the latter usually cause diagnostic confusion early in the illness.

DIFFERENTIATION IN THE LABORATORY

Many sources have described the findings of electrographic studies in the motor neuron diseases and in other disorders that are likely to be confused with them (7, 17, 24). Moreover, as noted above, we have seen patients for whom neurologists mistakenly diagnose early stages of motor neuron disease as myasthenia gravis because electrographic testing was inadequate. In one patient, we overlooked a significant Lambert-Eaton syndrome during bedside evaluation. Other considerations for differentiation may also rely heavily on accurate laboratory studies.

Polymyositis

Confusion of polymyositis with motor neuron disease, particularly with progressive muscular atrophy or an early stage of ALS, has been described elsewhere (24). There are several reasons for this confusion in atypical cases. First, in polymyositis the reflexes are normal and not hyperactive, as they are in ALS; however, the range of normal muscle-stretch activity is variable, and the examining neurologist is usually not aware of the state of the patient's reflexes before the onset of illness.

Second, the pattern of weakness in motor neuron disease can be atypical and may be accompanied by prominent myalgia that is not readily explainable by muscle cramps; in fact, muscle cramps may be completely absent. The pattern of onset in polymyositis may be distal rather than proximal; in addition, the typical aching muscle pain and tenderness on palpation may be either absent or only intermittent, and thus the patient may not mention such pain.

Third, the skeletal muscle lesion in polymyositis affects the intramuscular neurovascular bundles; thus, unless the muscles subjected to EMG and biopsy are carefully selected and evaluated, the results may be misleading, depending on the sampling error involved in the test. The chance of such an error can be reduced with increased caution both in performing and evaluating the EMG and in obtaining an appropriately sized muscle biopsy specimen. In the latter, evaluation of numerous longitudinal sections, particularly those containing neurovascular bundles, is essential, since the inflammatory lesion may be segmental and thus overlooked in cross-sections. In suspected cases, it is desirable to biopsy two or three muscles.

Fourth, standard blood tests, which are usually useful in the diagnosis of polymyositis, may be positive only intermittently. This circumstance can lead to misleading negative or borderline results at some stages of illness. Conversely, the level of creatine phosphokinase (CPK) may be elevated in motor neuron disease, particularly in progressive muscular atrophy and ALS. We have had considerably less experience with determination of serum aldolase in patients with polymyositis because of the relative rarity of that condition. However, we have observed moderate elevation of serum aldolase in 4 patients with polymyositis as compared with normal levels of aldolase in more than 600 patients with motor neuron disease; the highest level of CPK observed thus far in a patient with motor neuron disease is 800 IU (normal, $\leq$ 46). Thus greater elevations of CPK can probably be used as reliable indicators of myopathy; lesser elevations are not so useful as a guideline. As reviewed elsewhere, elevated levels of CPK have been observed in a variety of brain and spinal cord diseases, and even EMG studies can cause transient increases in CPK (24).

Heavy-Metal Toxicity

Since the time of Aran's report (1), occasional cases of exposure to heavy metals have been reported to produce disorders that resemble motor neuron disease. In the past, lead and mercury were primarily associated with these disorders; more recently, exposure to selenium has been associated with ALS (15).

Kilness and Hochberg reported that some ranchers with ALS had elevated excretions of Se in 24-hour urine collections (15). We undertook to measure the level of urinary Se in a series of what is now more than 100 consecutive patients, including 2 who were born and raised in the same locale as the patients of Kilness and Hochberg. None of the 100 patients showed elevation of urinary Se. In a preliminary report early in this study, Norris and Ü suggested that the exposure to Se documented by Kilness and Hochberg represented a coincidence rather than a significant factor in the etiology or pathophysiology of the motor neuron disease (27). We have subsequently found no evidence to contradict that opinion.

For patients with both clear histories of exposure to a heavy metal and signs and symptoms of motor neuron disease, we recommend an open bone biopsy to permit spectrographic quantitation of the particular element in a dehydrated specimen of cortical bone. The biopsy is best done by an orthopedic surgeon using extensive local anesthesia to obtain a piece of cortical bone from the iliac crest. In appropriate cases, we also have obtained a segment of external-rib cortex during a muscle biopsy of the chest wall (conducted for other purposes), as described elsewhere (25).

Patients with elevated levels of metal in the cortical bone should be treated with standard chelation therapy, with intravenous calcium disodium edetate (EDTA) followed by long-term oral administration of EDTA on an outpatient basis. In each such case, we obtain 24-hour urine collections for measurement of other heavy metals as well as the one in question. The urine should be collected at least once before EDTA is administered and then every 24 hours during intravenous treatment. Excretion of the metal that is elevated more than threefold above the control level on three or more days during the five days of intravenous treatment is considered to indicate possibly significant mobilization of metal. Our review suggests, however, that the optimal schedule for administration of EDTA and the criteria for abnormality of metal excretion in urine have never been fully determined.

We rely on periodic follow-up evaluations for major diagnostic assistance in determination of abnormal levels of metal in the body. Some degree of sustained recovery may be viewed as evidence that the amount of metal in the body was elevated and that the administration of EDTA was of benefit. The development of prolonged neuromuscular stability may be gratifying but is not convincing evidence of recovery from heavy-metal toxicity as opposed to spontaneous stabilization of idiopathic motor neuron disease.

Such apparent cases of metal toxicity are extremely rare in comparison with cases of idiopathic motor neuron disease. During the last five years, of approximately 750 consecutive patients with motor neuron disease, only 3 patients had clear histories of exposure to heavy metal (lead in each case), with elevated levels of lead in cortical bone, elevated excretion of lead in urine during the period of intravenous treatment with EDTA, and subsequent sustained improvement but incomplete recovery. None of these patients showed other signs of lead toxicity; even the excretion of lead during the 24 hours before treatment was within the normal range.

Despite the rarity of exposure to heavy metals and the difficulty of establishing the diagnosis, we continue to test patients routinely for this condition. Experience to date indicates that screening of urine should perhaps be abandoned in favor of bone biopsy when the history clearly reveals exposure to a heavy metal.

Diabetic Amyotrophy

It is important to differentiate idiopathic motor neuron disease from diabetic amyotrophy because the latter condition offers chances for substantial recovery after appropriate treatment of the diabetes. Nearly all the patients described thus far have had severe, poorly regulated diabetes or were undiagnosed and thus untreated. Diabetic amyotrophy is notable for its predilection for the proximal leg muscles and is accompanied by pain and reduction or absence of muscle-stretch reflexes. Thus, these symptoms are more likely to represent a case of early but atypical progressive muscular atrophy or a case of polymyositis rather than ALS. The clinical picture of diabetic amyotrophy was originally described by Garland (11) and was reemphasized more recently by Bruyn and Garland (5). Asbury has suggested that both the clinical and pathologic spectrum of diabetic amyotrophy is broader than suspected (2).

In our experience, this complication of diabetes is rare and, in their recent review, Bruyn and Garland (5) found only about 200 cases of diabetic amyotrophy in the world literature. Although we have suspected this diagnosis in several cases, we have not been able to substantiate it in any of them. During the past five years, a diagnosis of diabetic amyotrophy was made for four patients; a vigorous diabetic treatment program was administered, and a correspondingly benign prognosis was made because each patient exhibited predominant weakness and atrophy of the proximal leg muscles of the lower motor type, absence of Babinski's sign, and severe diabetes mellitus. Two of these patients also had heavy aortofemoral calcification. Each patient progressed steadily downhill to death, and necropsy studies (done elsewhere and made available for our review) showed ALS only, in addition to generalized atherosclerosis.

Hypoglycemic neuropathy/neuronopathy may also mimic motor neuron disease (18, 30), particularly progressive muscular atrophy, but in our experience this condition has been even more rare than diabetic amyotrophy. Nevertheless, in the absence of a specific cure for ALS, each patient's glucose tolerance should be tested carefully and appropriate treatment should be prescribed whenever indicated. Swank and Putnam noticed that ALS patients seem to do better when their general state of health is good (33), an additional reason for administering appropriate diabetic treatment. As with many aspects of practical treatment of ALS patients, these efforts often seem fruitless and may contribute to the patient's despondency or depression when no definite improvement results.

DIFFERENTIATION FROM TRAUMATIC MYELORADICULOPATHY

The various syndromes of acute and chronic spinal cord and root pressure are usually clinically distinct from motor neuron disease; in fact, some readers may be surprised that we discuss the differentiation. However, about 40% of the patients with motor neuron disease whom we observed had undergone myelography earlier in the illness, and about 15% had undergone spinal surgery.

The main problems of differentiation occur early in motor neuron disease, before the extent of the illness is apparent. It is reasonable to investigate focal symptoms by means of a myelogram, and it is predictable that any incidental lesions found at or near the involved segment might be considered for surgery. While the risks of spinal surgery are not zero and the results are not always satisfactory, this approach is appropriate for some patients for two reasons. First, mass lesions of the spinal canal and foramina, particularly at two or more levels, can mimic motor neuron disease. With rapid progression of severity, surgical removal of mass lesions or decompression followed by continued neurologic observation is the only way to ensure accurate differentiation.

Second, clinicians experienced in the care of patients with motor neuron disease recognize that maintenance of a good general state of health is an important aspect of treatment (24, 33). In this context, the presence of acute or chronic neural trauma or pressure (or vascular compression) cannot be regarded as optimal health. Surgical removal of a prolapsed disk or surgical decompression of a spondylotic canal removes this additional source of neural pathophysiology. None of our patients with benign ALS has suffered from other untreated health problems, significant spinal cord or root compression in particular. These data are based on a relatively small number of cases, and it cannot be determined that these patients would not have had benign courses in the absence of spinal surgery; thus, we suggest that surgical intervention for treatment of significant compressive lesions be carefully tailored to the specific patient.

Amyotrophic Spondylotic Myeloradiculopathy

The typical case of neurologically symptomatic cervical/lumbar spondylosis can be distinguished from motor neuron disease by the presence of sensory findings and by absence on examination of the usual extensive findings that typify ALS, even in the relatively asymptomatic patient. In other words, the patient with ALS usually has more extensive findings than the initial symptoms may indicate; with rare exception, these are entirely motor findings.

Difficulties arise in atypical cases, particularly cases of spondylosis with long-standing neural encroachment at multiple levels but with minimal or no sensory changes. In more advanced cases of motor neuron disease, specifically in those referred to us by other neurologists who diagnosed this syndrome, approximately 1% of patients are found to have substantial evidence of spondylotic myeloradiculopathy, particularly neurologic stabilization or improvement after decompressive surgery.

However, differentiation can be remarkably difficult, and the physician should stress to the patient before surgery that the diagnosis depends partly on the postoperative course. Needless to say, this point will not increase the patient's enthusiasm for surgery, and the consulting neurosurgeon may also lose interest.

The presence of clearly positive bulbar and pseudobulbar motor neuron lesions strongly suggests that problems related to spondylosis are coincidental and that the postoperative course most likely will be downhill. This problem in differentiation usually arises in cases with neurologic involvement at lower levels of the neuraxis. The problem that is best known in this regard is related to cervical spondylosis, but lumbar spondylosis also can be a problem, and sometimes both conditions afflict the same patient (36).

The most satisfactory diagnostic test for amyotrophic spondylotic myeloradiculopathy is the myelogram. In one case, even though the patient refused lumbar puncture, a computerized tomogram of the cervical canal demonstrated significant narrowing in the anteroposterior diameter at several levels that corresponded to disk spaces; at one point in the saggital plane the diameter was 5.0 mm. There were extensive changes seen on plain x-rays, suggesting a process of long duration, with heavy calcification of the lesions. The computerized tomogram may be less reliable than the myelogram for patients with softer lesions and shorter courses.

All cases of compressive myeloradiculopathy that we have detected thus far showed marked encroachment that was visible at the time of decompressive surgery. We have no explanation for the sparing of sensory fibers in these patients. Thus far, we have had no autopsies in cases of this type; the lesions seen at surgery corresponded to those described previously by other authors (36).

The small number of patients in this group who had symptomatic spondylotic myeloradiculopathy showed no consistent abnormalities in spinal fluid that were not also seen in patients with idiopathic motor neuron disease. Because simple lumbar puncture sometimes produces alterations in spinal fluid that make subsequent myelography difficult or temporarily impossible, we recommend that the lumbar puncture be deferred until a complete set of spinal x-rays has been obtained and the decision for or against myelography has been made. As discussed later in this chapter, spinal fluid should be examined in every patient with motor neuron disease, but this analysis usually is not significant and thus can be deferred safely in most patients until plain x-rays of the spine are available.

Benign Posttraumatic Amyotrophy

The presence of benign amyotrophy after trauma was noted in two patients by Norris (23). Since we have not seen any other patients with this syndrome, its occurrence must be extremely rare. In a series of cases described by Sobue et al. as having benign segmental atrophy of the upper extremities (31), some patients had unilateral atrophy after trauma and thus may have represented additional instances of benign posttraumatic amyotrophy.

Etiologic Role of Acute Trauma

Some patients with motor neuron disease notice the onset of symptoms after they experience trauma. Several case reports in the literature indicate that some physicians believe in a traumatic etiology (24). The worst trauma to the spinal structures probably occurs in cases of vertebral fracture–dislocation with maceration of the spinal cord, causing permanent paraplegia. Many persons have suffered this injury as a result of war wounds, automobile accidents, falls, and the like, but we have not observed such a patient who also has developed motor neuron disease. Thus, it is difficult to ascribe any significance to lesser trauma for this syndrome, since the incidence of motor neuron disease in patients with traumatic paraplegia is so low.

DIFFERENTIATION FROM OTHER CONDITIONS

Neoplasms

Several types of spinal neoplasm can be considered in the differential diagnosis, but for practical purposes the two most likely to mimic motor neuron disease are high thoracic meningioma and multiple neurofibromata. The former, which occurs more frequently in older women than in men, causes diagnostic difficulties only early in the course, although atypical meningioma with lower cervical involvement may create more of a diagnostic problem. A major problem might occur with neurofibromata if the patient atypically lacks other signs of von Recklinghausen's disease and the family history is negative or incomplete. We know of one such case in which the attending neurologist felt the diagnosis of ALS to be so certain that neither lumbar puncture nor adequate plain x-rays of the patient's spine were done. The autopsy surgeon later diagnosed lower cervical and midthoracic neurofibromata.

Symptoms of some intracranial neoplasms are also likely to mimic motor neuron disease. Parasaggital and foramen magnum meningioma, brain stem astrocytoma, and ependymoma should be noted specifically in this regard. Perhaps a dozen of our patients had undergone vertebrobasilar arteriography after relatively acute bulbar onset, but no pontine or medullary vascular tumors (including hamartoma, arteriovenous malformation, or angioma) were detected; generalized findings subsequently indicated ALS.

Arteriosclerotic Myelopathy

Only brief attention will be given here to arteriosclerotic myelopathy, chiefly because of its rarity. As described above, two patients thought to have had the complication of arteriosclerosis in association with severe diabetes mellitus suffered steadily progressive disability, died, and at necropsy were found to have had lesions typical of ALS.

Postpoliomyelitic Amyotrophy

Several surveys show an increased incidence of a history of paralytic poliomyelitis in patients who develop ALS (24). Some of these patients seem to have symptoms typical of ALS, including rapid deterioration with a fatal outcome. In others, however, a less malignant course has been observed.

Mulder et al. drew our attention to this subgroup of patients with motor neuron disease in their description of 34 patients seen over many years at the Mayo Clinic (22). We also have encountered several patients with a similar history: focal paralysis resulted from a febrile illness (presumably poliomyelitis) many years before; relative stability followed recovery from the illness; in later years, further weakness developed, with a corresponding increase in atrophy in the part of the body that previously was paretic; the illness subsequently extended to other parts of the body but ran a much slower course than that typical of ALS, with milder corticospinal signs and symptoms, if any.

The etiology and the pathophysiology of this second neuromuscular illness remain obscure. Serum antibody titers to known polioviruses are not elevated (6, 22), and the renal glomerular immune complexes found in some patients with ALS were not found in the kidney biopsy of the one patient with postpoliomyelitic amyotrophy whom we studied (28).

The patients in our series who had motor neuron disease that developed after paralytic poliomyelitis seem to have approximately a 50–50 chance of having a relatively benign course. The benign illness may be a different subtype of motor neuron disease. Patients who eventually develop ALS, the malignant form of motor neuron disease, may have a genetically determined susceptibility to disorders of the motor neuron;

hence the high incidence of a prior history of poliomyelitis. Zamir et al. have provided some evidence from HL-A typing to support this hypothesis (37); however, these observations need further study and analysis in larger series of patients.

Chronic Inflammatory Polyradiculopathy

Dyck and associates described a series of patients at the Mayo Clinic in whom chronic inflammatory disease had greatest impact on the spinal nerve roots and the peripheral nerves (8). Administration of corticosteroids appeared to be of benefit in some of these cases. Many cases in that series are readily distinguishable from idiopathic motor neuron disease in that patients exhibited sensory loss; some had involvement of the special senses, impotence, or impaired bowel or bladder control. Motor involvement, usually the lower motor neuron type, could be the predominant feature, thus raising progressive muscular atrophy as a differential diagnosis.

Among new patients with motor neuron disease referred to us for evaluation, fewer than 1% displayed spinal fluid findings consistent with inflammatory disease. All such patients in our series had been investigated previously by experienced neurologists, who diagnosed motor neuron disease—either progressive muscular atrophy or ALS—by discounting abnormal spinal fluid findings or failing to obtain a lumbar puncture for examination of CSF. While our series so far contains no definite example of luetic amyotrophy, the possibility of its occurrence mandates that the spinal fluid be examined at least once in every patient diagnosed as having motor neuron disease and that any abnormalities be given due consideration.

We have found that the total protein in CSF of patients with motor neuron disease frequently is slightly elevated, usually less than 75 and rarely more than 100 mg/dl. The rare patients we have seen who were thought to have chronic inflammatory disease have had total protein in CSF greater than 150 mg/dl and cell counts of approximately 10–30 cells/mm^3 (predominantly lymphocytes). Protein fractionation for determination of gamma globulin has not been helpful; as reported previously, one of our patients with idiopathic ALS had elevation of gamma globulin in CSF comparable to that seen in patients with acute MS (29). An additional criterion, though one that is of little value early in the investigation, is the patient's response to a trial of corticosteroid therapy. However, such a trial in patients with idiopathic motor neuron disease is always complicated by the possibility of spontaneous improvement, so repeated trials over several months, punctuated by periods of no corticosteroid administration, provide more convincing evidence of benefit from corticosteroids than does a single brief trial.

DIFFERENTIATION FROM HEREDOFAMILIAL DISORDERS

Motor neuron degeneration occurs in a variety of hereditary disorders and, in atypical cases, may be part of the differential diagnosis, particularly when the family history is inadequate. Complete family histories are not always easy to obtain from patients with these disorders, perhaps because of a psychologic coping mechanism or because of ignorance. Sometimes the physician mistakenly assumes that lack of clear indications of these disorders in the history of a small family means that there is no genetic component. The opportunity to inspect family records, to look through photograph albums, or to interview older family members frequently is of great help in identification of hereditary motor disorders.

The major problems for clinical differentiation relate to amyotrophy early in atypical Friedreich's ataxia, unusually late onset in Wohlfart-Kugelberg-Welander disease, and adult onset and predominance of distal symptoms in muscular dystrophy. Table 3 compares the features of these disorders with those of ALS.

Rare problems in differentiation may arise in connection with either segmental distal atrophy of the upper extremities, particularly in patients of Japanese ancestry (31); the development of mild permanent weakness with atrophy in a patient who has suffered many episodes of familial periodic paralysis; the occurrence of only amyotrophy in a

Table 3 Comparison of Features of ALS and Some Heredofamilial Disorders

Feature	*ALS*	*Friedreich's Ataxia*	*Wohlfart-Kugelberg-Welander Disease*	*Muscular Dystrophy*
Usual age of onset	Adult	Child	Child	Child or adult
Relatives affected	Rare[a]	Common	Common	Common
Early proximal vs. distal involvement	Distal	Distal	Proximal	Proximal or distal
Early atrophy	Common	Rare	Common	Rare
Fasciculation	Common	Rare	Rare	0
Impaired emotional control	Common	Rare	0[b]	0
Babinski's sign	Common	Occasional	0	0
Ataxia	0	Common	0	0
Nystagmus	0	Common	0	0
Pes cavus	Rare	Common	0	0

[a] Except in familial ALS.
[b] 0 = not present.

member of a family whose other members are reported to have had only ataxia or dementia (32); or onset of amyotrophy before onset of other symptoms in a patient with familial amyotrophic dystonic paraplegia (12).

Neuronal Charcot-Marie-Tooth Disease

During investigation of a large series of patients with apparent Charcot-Marie-Tooth disease, Dyck and Lambert found that approximately 2% of these patients had normal or near normal nerve conduction velocities (9). Slow nerve conduction is a hallmark of classic Charcot-Marie-Tooth disease and is demonstrable in unaffected parts of the body and in clinically unaffected but genetically positive relatives. Additional characteristics of this subgroup of patients are relatively late onset of atrophy and weakness and even later onset of sensory loss; thus, in early cases little or no sensory abnormality is evident. This new subtype of (presumably) neuronal Charcot-Marie-Tooth–like disease also may be characterized by a more slowly progressive clinical course. We are observing four such patients at present, one of whom is in her sixties and does her own housework and shopping, despite many years of this illness.

Familial Progressive Bulbospinal Amyotrophy

Magee (19) and others (14, 34) have described a familial neurogenic disease that begins clinically in adult life and causes slowly progressive disability from mainly bulbar and proximal limb muscle weakness, accompanied by prominent fasciculation. The main difference between this disease and ALS is its relatively slow course. Familial progressive bulbospinal amyotrophy is a rare consideration in the differential diagnosis of adult motor neuron disease but merits special attention because of the prominent bulbar involvement and the coarseness and frequency of fasciculations. We have observed two patients with this disorder. Since the disease has a relatively benign course, both patients, who are in their sixties, are still ambulatory. In fact, one works every day as groundskeeper for a golf course. This patient minimizes his symptoms and has not appeared for objective reevaluation in more than three years. The other patient continually needs reassurance, having been told earlier that he was suffering from ALS because of bulbar involvement and marked fasciculation in the muscles. The familial nature of this disease should also be emphasized: these two patients are identical twins. The disease appears to be a sex-linked recessive genetic disorder, on the basis of data from families investigated by Magee (19) and by Kennedy and associates (14).

ALS CACHEXIA

We have recently drawn attention to the occurrence of undue cachexia in ALS patients (26). Many clinicians and autopsy surgeons have probably seen advanced muscular wasting that causes a cachectic appearance in patients with ALS. The concomitant loss of fatty tissue has probably also been noted but has usually been attributed either to complications of the illness, such as anorexia and dysphagia secondary to bulbar palsy, or to nonspecific toxic effects of repeated pulmonary infections from aspiration, hypoventilation, and so on. In a small percentage of cases, however, cachexia is not explainable by such factors and may even be the presenting symptom. Our series contains three patients who presented with unexplained weight loss exceeding 33% of body weight weeks to months before development of weakness or muscular atrophy, well before development of difficulty in chewing and swallowing.

One of these patients was admitted to a university hospital and was investigated extensively (including cardiac catheterization) for thyrotoxicosis and heart disease; another patient was studied exhaustively in another hospital for the possibility of occult carcinoma. Less severe unexplained weight loss has been seen in a larger number of patients with ALS as the first symptom or as part of the earliest stage of illness.

When such cachexia appears early in the illness, several possible diagnoses other than motor neuron disease seem much more important. These possibilities include thyroid/parathyroid dysfunction, occult carcinoma, heavy-metal intoxication, lung abscess and other chronic occult infections, and multiple small pulmonary emboli. In the presence of diarrhea, a malabsorption problem would be an important consideration; in countries with extensive parasitism, such diseases would rank high on the list of differential diagnoses.

Even if unexplained cachexia appears later in the disease, when signs of ALS or other motor neuron disease are prominent, reassessment should be made, with special attention to thyroid/parathyroid function, exposure to heavy metals, and inapparent lung disease. At this later stage, the appearance of cachexia does not warrant investigation for occult carcinoma. Some patients with ALS have or develop neoplasms, but none in our series presented with cachexia not readily explainable by one of the complications of ALS; nor were any of the neoplasms detected during investigation for occult carcinoma. Conversely, neoplasms were not found in any patients with ALS cachexia who underwent necropsy. Thus, it seems unnecessary to investigate the possibility of occult carcinoma in patients with established ALS.

Careful investigation should be conducted in patients with ALS whose neuromuscular disease is preceded or accompanied by ALS cachexia, with particular attention to studies of metabolic balance and neuroendocrine function in search of a systemic factor. Thus far, our preliminary studies have not yielded a clue to the cause of ALS cachexia, nor has hyperalimentation, by either nasogastric intubation or intravenous routes, been successful in reversing what has become a grave prognostic sign.

CONCLUDING DISCUSSION

The emphasis of this chapter has been on the differential diagnosis of motor neuron disease, with particular attention to other disorders. It is important to investigate all possibilities before arriving at a diagnosis of idiopathic motor neuron disease. It is particularly important not to overlook a possibly remediable disorder. Even if the diagnosis is an untreatable heredofamilial disorder, the prognosis is often quite different from that for idiopathic motor neuron disease, and the family may benefit from genetic counseling.

We have not emphasized the distinctions among the various subtypes of idiopathic motor neuron disease, such as those between progressive muscular atrophy and ALS. Many neurologists see little point in making these distinctions. On the basis of official statistics, Kurland and associates found a decline in the death rate from progressive muscular atrophy that corresponded to a rise in the death rate from ALS (16); the most likely explanation for this occurrence is that physicians do not make a diagnostic distinction between these two disorders. It is a paradox in modern medicine (in an age of organ transplantation, sophisticated biochemical probes, and pharmaceutical tools for therapy) that this basic problem of differentiation of motor neuron disorders remains unsolved nearly 130 years after Aran's original description (1).

In order to establish an accurate prognosis, the physician should attempt to specify correctly the particular idiopathic motor neuron disease syndrome in each case, despite difficulty in differentiation, especially early in the illness. Typical progressive muscular atrophy has in common with typical ALS the characteristic of lower motor neuron impairment; if this common denominator is an indication of the same disease process (i.e., identical etiology and pathophysiology), then the patient with progressive muscular atrophy should possess some resistance to the bulbar and corticospinal pathway lesions typical of ALS. Perhaps further study of patients with progressive muscular atrophy would reveal clues to the nature of this hypothetical resistance and thus lead to advances in therapy for ALS patients.

An alternative explanation is that the etiology, pathophysiology, or both differ between progressive muscular atrophy and ALS. If this is so, it is even more important to differentiate the clinical disorders so that diagnostic clues such as biochemical analyses do not become confused and misleading.

Another major problem of even greater importance to patients and their families is the differentiation between sporadic and familial ALS. Despite the prominent lesions of the dorsal column that typify most cases of familial ALS, we have yet to see one such patient with sensory loss. Clinical preservation of sensation is a puzzling feature of ALS because of prominent disturbance of myelin in the tracts of the anterior two-thirds of the spinal cord in most cases of ALS. The additional lesion of the sensory pathway in familial cases also fails to produce diagnostic clinical findings (10). Affliction of numerous family members has been a clear indication of familial ALS in a few families subject to an apparently dominant genetic trait with high penetrance. However, it is more common to encounter an ambiguous family history. For example, an aunt may be reported to have died from "bulbar palsy" several decades ago, or a cousin may be said to have recently developed leg weakness and, at the age of 65 years, is now confined to a wheelchair with a diagnosis of "multiple sclerosis." In such a case, familial ALS is a reasonable concern, but it may be difficult to establish that the affected relative actually suffered from motor neuron disease. If motor neuron disease can be established in the relative, it still is not clear whether its occurrence was an unfortunate coincidence or a case of familial ALS. A means of clinical differentiation of sporadic ALS from familial ALS is urgently needed.

We have neglected several considerations in this discussion, such as thyrotoxic myopathy, luetic amyotrophy, and atypical vitamin B_{12} deficiency with subacute combined degeneration of the nervous system, for which standard diagnostic tests are available. These disorders still may be seen by family doctors and primary-care consultants but are now rare in Western neurology clinics as causes of motor neuron disease. The weakness/wasting syndromes that accompany chronic renal disease and cancer treatment (especially antimetabolite neuropathy and radiation myelopathy) are clear diagnostic considerations in appropriate circumstances. However, most patients referred to neurologists with syndromes resembling motor neuron disease usually are found to have this disorder, the most common of which is ALS.

Acknowledgment

The work described in this paper was supported in part by an award from the Muscular Dystrophy Association (MDA), New York, New York.

REFERENCES

1. Aran FA: Récherches sur une maladie non encore décrite du système musculaire (atrophie musculaire progressive). Arch Gen Med 24:15–35, 172–214, 1850

2. Asbury AK: Proximal diabetic neuropathy (editorial). Ann Neurol 2:179–180, 1977

3. Babinski J: Sur le réflexe cutané plantaire dans certaines affections organiques du système nerveux central. CR Soc Biol (Paris) 3:207, 1896

4. Babinski J: De l'abduction des orteils. Rev Neurol (Paris) 11:728–729, 1903

5. Bruyn GW, Garland H: Neuropathies of endocrine origin. In *Handbook of Clinical Neurology*, Vol. 8. Edited by PJ Vinken, GW Bruyn. New York, American Elsevier, 1970, pp 29–71

6. Cremer NE, Oshiro L, Norris FH Jr, et al: Culture of tissues from patients with amyotrophic lateral sclerosis. Arch Neurol 29:331–333, 1973

7. Denys EH, Norris FH, Jr: Neuromuscular transmission in amyotrophic lateral sclerosis. Arch Neurol 36:202–205, 1979

8. Dyck PJ, Lais AC, Ohta M, et al: Chronic inflammatory polyradiculoneuropathy. Mayo Clin Proc 50:621–637, 1975

9. Dyck PJ, Lambert EH: Lower motor and primary sensory neuron diseases with peroneal muscular atrophy. II. Arch Neurol 18:619–625, 1968

10. Engel WK, Kurland LT, Klatzo I: An inherited disease similar to amyotrophic lateral sclerosis with a pattern of posterior column involvement. Brain 83:203–220, 1959

11. Garland H: Neurological complications of diabetes mellitus: clinical aspects. Proc Soc Med 53:137–146, 1961

12. Gilman S, Horenstein S: Familial amyotrophic dystonic paraplegia. Brain 87:51–66, 1964

13. Hudson AH, Brown WF, Gilbert JJ: The muscular pain–fasciculation syndrome. Neurology (Minneap) 28:1105–1109, 1978

14. Kennedy WH, Alter M, Sung JH: Progressive proximal spinal and bulbar muscular atrophy of late onset. Neurology (Minneap) 18:671–680, 1968

15. Kilness AW, Hochberg FH: Amyotrophic lateral sclerosis in a high selenium environment. JAMA 237:2843–2844, 1977

16. Kurland LT, Choi NW, Sayre GP: Implications of incidence and geographic patterns on the classification of amyotrophic lateral sclerosis. In *Motor Neuron Diseases. Research on Amyotrophic Lateral Sclerosis and Other Disorders.* Edited by FH Norris, LT Kurland. New York, Grune and Stratton, 1969, pp 28–50

17. Lambert EH: Electromyography in amyotrophic lateral sclerosis. In *Motor Neuron Diseases. Research on Amyotrophic Lateral Sclerosis and Related Disorders.* Edited by FH Norris, LT Kurland. New York, Grune and Stratton, 1969, pp 135–153

18. Lambert EH, Mulder DW, Bastron JA: Regeneration of peripheral nerves with hyperinsulin neuronopathy. Neurology (Minneap) 10:851–854, 1960

19. Magee KR: Familial progressive bulbar-spinal muscular atrophy. Neurology (Minneap) 10:295–305, 1960

20. Mulder DW, Howard FM: Patient resistance and prognosis in amyotrophic lateral sclerosis. Mayo Clin Proc 51:537–541, 1976

21. Mulder DW, Lambert EH, Eaton LM: Myasthenic syndrome in patients with amyotrophic lateral sclerosis. Neurology (Minneap) 9:627–631, 1959

22. Mulder DW, Rosenbaum RA, Layton DD: Late progression of poliomyelitis or 'forme fruste' amyotrophic lateral sclerosis? Mayo Clin Proc 47:756–761, 1972

23. Norris FH: Benign post-traumatic amyotrophy. Arch Neurol 27: 269–270, 1972

24. Norris FH: Adult spinal motor neuron disease. In *Handbook of Clinical Neurology,* Vol. 22. Edited by PJ Vinken, GW Bruyn. New York, American Elsevier, 1975, pp 1–56

25. Norris FH: Moving axon particles of intercostal nerve terminals in benign and malignant ALS. In *Amyotrophic Lateral Sclerosis.* Edited by T Tsubaki, Y Toyokura. Tokyo, University of Tokyo Press, 1979, pp 359–369

26. Norris FH, Denys EH, Ü KS: Old and new clinical problems in amyotrophic lateral sclerosis. In *Amyotrophic Lateral Sclerosis.* Edited by T Tsubaki, Y Toyokura. Tokyo, University of Tokyo Press, 1979, pp 3–24

27. Norris FH, Ü KS: Amyotrophic lateral sclerosis and low urinary selenium levels (letter). JAMA 239:404, 1978

28. Oldstone MBA, Perrin LH, Wilson CB, et al: Evidence for immune-

complex formation in patients with amyotrophic lateral sclerosis. Lancet 2:169–172, 1976

29. Roboz-Einstein E, Macrae D: Spinal fluid analysis in amyotrophic lateral sclerosis. In *Motor Neuron Diseases. Research on Amyotrophic Lateral Sclerosis and Related Disorders.* Edited by FH Norris, LT Kurland. New York, Grune and Stratton, 1969, pp 175–178

30. Rosner L, Elstad R: The neuropathy of hypoglycemia. Neurology (Minneap) 14:1–6, 1964

31. Sobue I, Saito N, Iida M, et al: Juvenile type of distal and segmental muscular atrophy of upper extremities. Ann Neurol 3:429–432, 1978

32. Staal A, Went LN: Juvenile amyotrophic lateral sclerosis–dementia complex in a Dutch family. Neurology (Minneap) 18:800–806, 1968

33. Swank RL, Putnam TJ: Amyotrophic lateral sclerosis and related conditions. Arch Neurol Psychiatry 49:151–177, 1943

34. Tsukagoshi H, Nakanishi T, Kondo K, et al: Hereditary proximal neurogenic muscular atrophy in the adult. Arch Neurol 12:597–603, 1965

35. Trojaborg W, Buchthal F: Malignant and benign fasciculations. Acta Neurol Scand 41:251–254, 1965

36. Wilkinson M (ed.): *Cervical Spondylosis,* 2nd ed. London, Heineman Medical Books, 1971

37. Zamir R, Kott E, Kuritzky A: HL-A in amyotrophic lateral sclerosis (abstract). In *Proceedings of the 11th World Congress of Neurology.* Amsterdam, Excerpta Medica, ICS #427, 1977, p 43

Commentary

Donald W. Mulder

The diagnosis of ALS depends on recognition of clinical signs and symptoms. There is no laboratory marker that will identify or even confirm the diagnosis. The diagnosis is established when a characteristic pattern of weakness and spasticity that has evolved over months or years is identified. It is not surprising that mistakes in diagnosis are made, and even the most competent clinician may overlook the diagnosis or, more seriously, make an incorrect diagnosis.

In order to establish the diagnosis, it is necessary to demonstrate progressive muscular atrophy and weakness, which should be asymmetric and present with associated hyperreflexia at widely separated segmented levels. There should be no other symptoms or findings. Thus, sensory complaints or findings, dementia, or ocular or bladder symptoms negate the diagnosis.

Laboratory tests may be necessary for confirmation of an alternative diagnosis or to alert the examiner to the possibility of an alternative. There are laboratory tests that will confirm the muscular denervation characteristic of ALS. These tests include the EMG, which has the advantage of being used easily in several muscles and which may be repeated easily, and muscle biopsy, which is a very specific tool for establishing the presence of denervation. All patients for whom the diagnosis of ALS is considered should undergo at least one of these two tests. The exact test that is chosen may depend on the laboratory support available in the area in which the patient is studied. Other laboratory tests, such as spinal fluid examination, routine blood studies, myelography, respiratory function studies, or heavy-metal determinations, must be used as indicated by evaluation of the individual patient. Every effort must be made both to be certain that a benign or treatable condition is not overlooked and to avoid expensive and unnecessary tests.

Because the diagnosis of ALS is a clinical one, a neurologic examination repeated at intervals is often the most satisfactory confirmatory test. The clinical course of the disease over several months to years usually indicates the diagnosis.

In his excellent discussion of the differential diagnosis of ALS, Dr. Norris has focused appropriately on patients who are improperly diagnosed as having ALS. In addition, there is a group of patients with ALS in whom the diagnosis is overlooked and sometimes never made. This group of patients is of interest epidemiologically, even though the missed diagnosis may not be clinically important. The recognition of these patients is of value

2. Sobue I, Saito N, Iida M, et al: Juvenile type of distal and segmental muscular atrophy of upper extremities. Ann Neurol 3:429–432, 1978

Arthur J. Hudson

There are several benign, nonprogressive disorders of the motor neuron that are characterized by fasciculation. It is important that a physician be aware of these conditions before he or she concludes that a patient has a devastating illness like ALS. For instance, traumatic, infective, and metabolic neuropathies and myelopathies may produce fasciculation that can usually be identified by investigation. Benign asymptomatic fasciculation, which we all have experienced, has been described by Dr. Kurland as an occasional symptom that tends to occur in the upper part of the body, especially in the upper limbs and face, but that may be experienced mainly in the lower part of the body, notably in the calves. Benign fasciculation with cramps is a similar condition except that it is more intense; the individual is troubled by cramps and obvious fasciculation. This is seen predominantly in the lower extremities, especially the calves.

The muscular pain–fasciculation syndrome is a condition that was drawn to our attention because the patient complained of pain; examination then revealed fasciculation (2). Pain in this condition is a steady aching or burning and occurs in the legs particularly but also in other parts of the body, especially after activity; cramps also occur. Although fasciculation is found predominantly in the lower limbs, notably the calves, patients complain of fasciculation elsewhere in the body. They may also complain of weakness, but no weakness or atrophy has been demonstrable on examination. I have given serious thought to the possibility that these patients have a forme fruste of ALS, but because complaints of pain suggest sensory involvement, and no spinal cord changes were observed in one autopsied case, they probably have some kind of neuropathy rather than an aborted form of ALS.

Myokymia occurs both as an isolated condition with no associated symptoms and in combination with other features. Myokymia is characterized by undulating movements of muscle due to discharges of the motor neuron that are more rapid than those that occur in fasciculation. Patients with myokymia also have fasciculation, but the two phenomena—with questionable justification in some cases—are generally distinguished in the literature as separate entities. Myokymia as a benign clinical syndrome may be accompanied by muscular pain, cramps, myotonialike muscle spasms, hyperhidrosis, and atrophy (1). Atrophy, when it occurs in these cases, is slowly progressive and generally peripheral, suggesting a neuropathic condition. Spillane et al. have described another disorder that they have called "painful legs and moving toes," which appears to be related to this syndrome (4).

Finally, a benign condition of continuous muscle fiber activity reported by Isaacs, consisting of muscular stiffness and fasciculation, seems to be different from other motor neuron disorders, as suggested by its response to hydantoin therapy (3).

REFERENCES

1. Greenhouse AH, Bicknell JM, Pesch RN, et al: Myotonia, myokymia, hyperhidrosis, and wasting of muscle. Neurology (Minneap) 17:263–268, 1967

2. Hudson AJ, Brown WF, Gilbert JJ: The muscular pain–fasciculation syndrome. Neurology (Minneap) 28:1105–1109, 1978

3. Isaacs H: A syndrome of continuous muscle-fiber activity. J Neurol Neurosurg Psychiatry 24:319–325, 1961

4. Spillane JD, Nathan PW, Kelly RE, et al: Painful legs and moving toes. Brain 94:541–556, 1971

Eric H. Denys

I would like to add two comments. One concerns the differential diagnosis of primary lateral sclerosis as opposed to classic ALS. I have reviewed some 200 EMGs of patients diagnosed as having ALS, including patients who presented with signs of primary lateral sclerosis only, with no evidence of involvement of the lower motor neurons on clinical examination. I have been able to find only four patients in whom there were no signs of lower motor neuron involvement as manifested by positive waves or fibrillations on EMG. Although it is not practical to study every muscle in the body, I should add that a special effort was made to study an adequate sample of muscles. The paraspinal muscles should be examined in such cases.

My second point pertains to the nature of fasciculations, which are so frequently encountered in ALS. I would like to share some preliminary data. One question that has been raised several times is, How long does a fasciculation persist? In order to study this point, we recorded fasciculations in a particular muscle by means of surface electrodes. For several weeks the recordings were repeated from the same site, which had been marked with a skin marker or a tattoo. Figure 1 shows recordings done over approximately four weeks. It can be seen that one fasciculating unit can be observed for up to 17 days, while another unit occurs for the first time on 1/21.

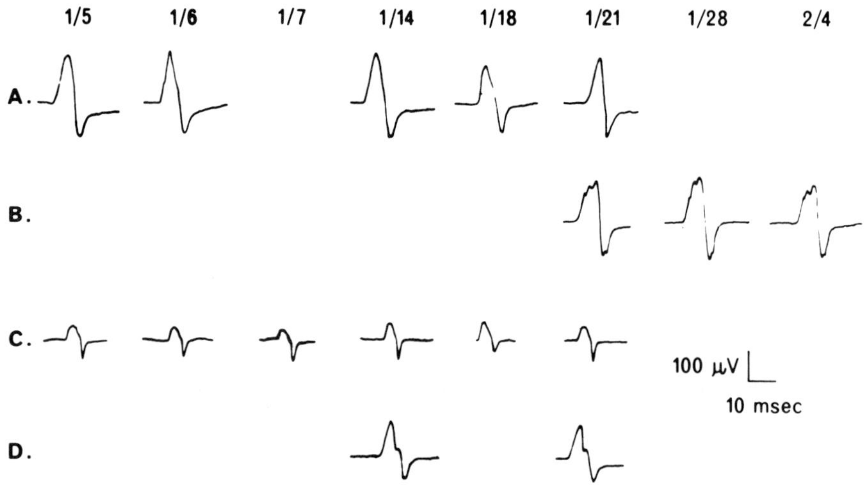

Figure 1 Series of fasciculating motor units recorded in a single site over a period of approximately four weeks. Fasciculations were recorded with surface electrodes over the hypothenar eminence on successive days as indicated. Each recording session lasted two minutes; temperature was controlled. Only fasciculation potentials that recurred during the study period were identified. Four different recurring wave forms (A, B, C, D) were noted. Form B appeared for the first time on 1/21, and A and C disappeared after 1/21.

Fasciculating units, in my opinion, are representative of the underlying motor unit and, as such, give some information on that particular motor neuron. Long-term follow-up studies would be necessary for determination of the differences between various motor units and their ability to manifest fasciculations.

Fasciculations are only a symptom, and their shape, whether normal or polyphasic, depends on the underlying motor unit. Thus, attempts to differentiate benign fasciculations from the malignant ones seen in ALS will not be fruitful because the presence of large polyphasic fasciculations will also be reflected in the changes in motor unit potential on examination with needle electrodes. In Figure 1 (line A), two motor unit potentials look slightly different from the others. This difference can be explained by a slight change in temperature during the recording session. Muscles affected by ALS and the potentials evoked seem to be extremely sensitive to slight changes in temperature, as I have shown in a different study (1). I would emphasize that these findings are preliminary.

REFERENCE

1. Denys EH: The effect of temperature on evoked responses. Electroencephalogr Clin Neurophysiol 4:598, 1977

Theodore L. Munsat

Dr. Norris and others have discussed the wide variability of different diseases that may initially appear to be ALS. I would like to take a more narrow and restricted view toward the diagnosis of ALS. A narrow definition is important in terms of prognosis, particularly for construction of drug trials. Unless we focus sharply on the nature of the disease and its definition, we may create false impressions. In my opinion, a loose definition has resulted in the presumed 20% incidence of benign ALS (see Dr. Juergens's commentary, chapter 3). I do not believe 20% of ALS patients have a benign course, perhaps because I define the disease differently. I suggest that ALS be defined as a disease with clinical upper and lower neuron involvement. Even though a patient may present with lower motor neuron involvement, we should not diagnose ALS until he develops clear evidence of upper motor neuron involvement. This definition would exclude patients with focal amyotrophy and late-onset Kugelberg-Welander disease. The disease should also be disseminated at two or more levels of the nervous system, thus excluding patients with cervical spondylosis and tumors of the foramen magnum. The diagnosis should include the fact that the disease is progressive and that results of the usual laboratory screening tests have ruled out other definable causes. Certain excluding criteria are important: there should be no sensory deficit, and intellect, extraocular muscles, and bladder and bowel function should be spared.

If this strict view is adopted, we can focus on patients for whom we can provide a very accurate prognosis. These patients will deteriorate over a period of a few or several years, although an occasional patient may have an atypical course. These new diagnostic criteria will enable us to construct drug trials and talk about epidemiologic data with more certainty. I do not want to exclude the atypical patients; they are important. In fact, from the point of view of uncovering etiopathogenesis, patients with atypical ALS may be even more important than patients with typical disease.

William R. Kennedy

I must disagree with Dr. Norris about diabetic amyotrophy, at least as far as I understood his chapter. I do not think this condition is rare. Rather, I think it is quite common, and I am certain that I see at least one such patient each month. However, my definition of diabetic amyotrophy may be different than Dr. Norris's. These patients are usually known diabetics with a mild symmetric polyneuropathy. However, a significant number are not overtly diabetic and, as Dr. Sullivan points out, one might have to observe them for as long as two years to prove them diabetic by glucose tolerance tests (3).

The onset of the diabetic amyotrophy is sudden and is dominated by pain; the patient can often recall the exact day or hour. Pain is usually followed by weakness, which on clinical examination is found primarily in the quadriceps and iliopsoas muscles; however, the adductor group innervated by the obturator nerve may also be involved. The degree of sensory change is variable but is most often mild; these changes affect the anterolateral thigh. Bilateral involvement is not rare, but occurrences may be separated by months or years. There is evidence on EMG of partial denervation in the weak muscles; in more than half of these patients, the paraspinal muscles also show denervation. This denervation is unilateral or occasionally bilateral and may extend to many spinal segments, even to the lower thoracic levels. This description refers to the lumbosacral syndrome investigated by Raff et al. (2), Calverly and Mulder (1), and others. In the presence of electrophysiologic and clinical findings along with a history of sudden onset, I have always suspected that this syndrome has a vascular etiology that affects anterior roots more than posterior roots at several levels, occasionally bilaterally.

Patients with this syndrome usually recover over a long period of time, perhaps as long as a year, because reinnervation must occur; however, intramuscular collateralization by surviving motor fibers provides some more immediate increase of function.

I would also like to comment on the question of lead being involved in the etiology of ALS. Since I recently have dealt with this area in relation to a medicolegal case involving a man who had worked in an industry that exposed him to lead for many years and who developed ALS, I have read a great deal of literature on the subject. I have no argument with Dr. Rowland or others who described the 12 or so patients who had had heavy exposure to lead, developed symptoms that suggested ALS, and excreted high quantities of lead after a provocative dose of a chelating agent. We are obligated to treat these patients, although we do not have good evidence that their symptoms will lessen or that the symptoms are related to lead. With all workers who have been exposed to lead, the question is whether lead can cause ALS and, if the worker develops ALS, whether the illness is due to the lead. There is no scientific evidence to show that lead causes ALS, and I do not agree that inducing a significant increase in the amount of lead in blood or urine with a chelating agent demonstrates that the patient's symptoms of ALS are caused by lead. In the absence of more objective data, I do not agree that tests for levels of lead and mercury in the blood must be done on every patient or that failure to treat ALS patients with chelating agents is poor clinical practice.

Finally, I agree with Dr. Munsat that perhaps we make the diagnosis of ALS too quickly or without enough evidence of generalized involvement. I am very uncomfortable about some of the cases I have read in the literature.

I know that the authors are good neurologists and I am confident that the patients have ALS, but the diagnosis is not always clear from the evidence that is presented; involvement in some patients is not widespread enough to suggest a definitive diagnosis. For example, I do not know if these neurologists take into account a peroneal nerve involvement in a cachectic patient or whether they accept it as evidence of generalized disease. Could not a cachectic patient with bilateral ulnar lesions and chronic lumbar-root lesion be mistaken for a patient with ALS? These questions are difficult and require further investigation and discussion.

REFERENCES

1. Calverly JR, Mulder DW: Femoral neuropathy. Neurology (Minneap) 10: 963–967, 1960

2. Raff MC, Sangalang V, Asbury AK: Ischemic mononeuropathy multiplex associated with diabetes mellitus. Arch Neurol 18:487–499, 1968

3. Sullivan JF: The neuropathies of diabetes. Neurology (Minneap) 8:243–249, 1958

W. King Engel

It should be pointed out that a careful clinical examination must be the basis for suspecting abnormalities, which can then be verified by laboratory evaluation. As several authors have emphasized, the physician must be both a good listener and a good questioner. Dr. Norris is a good example of that kind of clinician.

Dr. Rowland and I agree about the heterogeneity of the term *motor neuron disease.* However, I find the term unsatisfactory because some actually include in it the infantile and juvenile spinal muscular atrophies. I prefer the term *ALS* but emphasize that ALS may also be heterogeneous, even among patients with disease of short duration—that is, with a total duration of less than three to four years.

5 Laboratory Evaluation

William R. Kennedy

Several diagnostic examinations are available to the physician to supplement the clinical history and neurologic examination. Because the prognosis for patients with amyotrophic lateral sclerosis is so serious, the physician has a special responsibility to explore all reasonable alternatives before making the diagnosis and discussing its implications with the patient and family. The more helpful of these examinations are described in this chapter. (See also chapters 7 and 18.)

ELECTROMYOGRAPHY

The electromyogram (EMG) is the most useful clinical aid for the diagnosis of ALS. It provides a quick, nontraumatic means of acquiring information from a wide distribution of muscles at repeated intervals.

Electromyography is the recording of the electric potentials arising from muscle. A needle electrode is placed into the muscle, and the amplified electric activity is monitored visually on an oscilloscope and acoustically through a loudspeaker. In relaxed muscle, brief movements of the needle through the muscle are accompanied by short bursts of insertion activity followed by electrical silence. Voluntary or reflex contraction of the muscle results in the appearance of motor unit action potentials that are characterized by their amplitude, duration, configuration, and by their number and rate of discharge in relation to the strength of contraction.

Fasciculations

Fasciculation potentials, the electric component of the spontaneous contraction of muscle fibers making up a motor unit, can frequently be recorded in muscles not undergoing voluntary contraction in patients with ALS. Together with muscle cramps, these potentials are often the first indication of the disease and may appear in the absence of abnormal electric activity. Many patients are first made aware of fasciculations through the observations of family, associates, or sometimes the physician-electromyographer. Fasciculation potentials are observed less often in other diseases affecting the anterior horn cell of peripheral nerve, in some metabolic diseases, and in normal persons. The recording of fasciculation potentials, especially those of increased amplitude and duration or those polyphasic in contour, should increase the suspicion that the patient is afflicted with ALS, but it does not establish the diagnosis.

Fibrillations

Degeneration of anterior horn cells results in denervation of muscle fibers in the affected motor units. The insertion activity accompanying needle movement in such muscle is followed by a train of positive waves and short-duration, diphasic potentials called *fibrillation potentials* (38). These potentials, like the clinical weakness in some ALS patients, may be localized to a few muscles in one extremity or may appear in a generalized distribution. They are most abundant in rapidly progressive disease, in which the number of denervated muscle fibers is greatest. If muscle reinnervation through the growth of collateral sprouts from axons of intact motor axons is adequate to compensate for the progressive loss of anterior horn cells, then fibrillation potentials and positive waves may not be a prominent feature of the EMG.

Motor Unit Action Potentials

Recordings of the motor unit action potentials during a voluntary contraction reveal a loss in the number of potentials elicited in comparison to the strength of the muscle contraction (38). In muscles that are less severely involved, collateral reinnervation of denervated muscle by surviving axons may be sufficient to maintain normal strength, yet the EMG is decidedly abnormal (12, 35, 60). Severely affected muscles have only a few recordable motor units.

The amplitude and duration of the motor unit potentials in ALS are among the largest to be seen in neurologic disorders (38). This reflects the progressive increase in the number and density of muscle fibers in the motor unit. A greater contraction effort by the patient results, not in the appearance of more units as in normal muscle, but in an increased firing rate of the motor units that are already active. This is a compensatory mechanism for the loss of recruitable units and an indication that the patient is indeed attempting to make a strong contraction. Some motor unit action potentials in patients with ALS vary in amplitude from moment to moment (38), suggesting that a proportion of the muscle fibers in the motor unit are not excited by each nerve impulse. This interesting neuromuscular defect helps to explain why some ALS patients receive temporary benefit from physostigmine therapy (46).

The EMG is usually abnormal weeks to months before the onset of clinical weakness in patients whose disease is progressing slowly. This allows the electromyographer to uncover evidence of a generalized neuromuscular disorder in individuals who present clinically with localized weakness. Caution must be exercised to avoid drawing incorrect conclusions regarding the existence of a generalized process based on recordings made from muscles innervated by nerves commonly subjected to trauma or involved in entrapment neuropathies. Thus, reliance on information obtained from the small muscles of the hands or feet as the sole criterion for the existence of anterior horn cell disease in an extremity is hazardous.

Nerve Conduction Velocity

Motor nerve conduction velocities are usually within the normal range, even for patients in whom the disease has reached a stage where the diagnosis is easily established by clinical means. With time, as atrophy increases, the motor conduction velocity may decline to slightly below the normal values. Sensory nerve conduction usually remains normal in the median and sural nerves, providing limb temperature is normal (37).

Electromyographic findings of fasciculations and high-amplitude, long-duration motor unit action potentials in the appropriate distribution, plus normal nerve conduction values, are good corroborating evidence for the diagnosis of ALS. However, none of the electrophysiologic abnormalities is specific for this disease. Other anterior horn cell disorders such as Kugelberg-Welander disease (36), hereditary spinal and bulbar muscular atrophy (34), primary muscular atrophy, and chronic residual poliomyelitis often produce similar findings. The EMG findings in some chronic polyneuropathies, such as Charcot-Marie-Tooth disease, are also similar to those of ALS; here the low conduction velocities of the nerves aid in the distinction. Differentiation of ALS from the axonal neuropathies found in patients with severe renal disease, various chronic intoxications, carcinomas, neuronal forms of peroneal muscular atrophy, or those undergoing chemotherapy for carcinoma can be especially difficult (19, 20). However, the distribution of the findings may be helpful in these cases, because patients with ALS have proportionally more ab-

4. Bjornskov EK, Dekker NP, Norris FH Jr, et al: End-plate morphology in amyotrophic lateral sclerosis. Arch Neurol 32:711–712, 1975

5. Boothby JA, DeJesus PV, Rowland LP: Reversible forms of motor neuron disease. 'Lead Neuritis.' Arch Neurol 31:18–23, 1974

6. Bosma JF, Brodie DR: Disabilities of the pharynx in amyotrophic lateral sclerosis as demonstrated by cineradiography. Radiology 92:97–103, 1969

7. British Medical Journal: Diagnosis of inorganic lead poisoning: A statement. Vol 4, 1968, p 501

8. Brody JA, Hadlow WJ, Hotchin J, et al: Soviet search for viruses that cause chronic neurologic diseases in the USSR. Science 147:1114–1116, 1965

9. Campbell AMG: Calcium versonate in motor-neuron disease. Lancet 1:376–377, 1955

10. Campbell AMG, Williams ER: Chronic lead intoxication mimicking motor neuron disease (letter). Br Med J 4:582, 1968

11. Campbell AMG, Williams ER, Barltrop D: Motor neuron disease and exposure to lead. J Neurol Neurosurg Psychiatry 33:877–885, 1970

12. Cöers C: Les variations structurelles normales et pathologiques de la jonction neuromusculaire. Acta Neurol Belg 55:741–866, 1955

13. Cöers C, Woolf AL: *The Innervation of Muscle.* Oxford, Blackwell, 1959

14. Collis WJ, Engel WK: Glucose metabolism in five neuromuscular disorders. Neurology 18:915–925, 1968

15. Conradi S, Ronnevi L-O, Vesterburg O: Abnormal tissue distribution of lead in amyotrophic lateral sclerosis. J Neurol Sci 29:259–265, 1976

16. Conradi S, Ronnevi L-O, Vesterburg O: Increased plasma levels of lead in patients with amyotrophic lateral sclerosis compared with control subjects as determined by flameless atomic absorption spectrophotometry. J Neurol Neurosurg Psychiatry 41:389–393, 1978

17. Cremer NE, Oshiro FJ, Norris FH Jr, et al: Culture of tissues from patients with amyotrophic lateral sclerosis. Arch Neurol 29:331–333, 1973

18. Currier RD, Haerer AF: Amyotrophic lateral sclerosis and metallic toxins. Arch Environ Health 17:712–719, 1968

19. Dyck PJ, Lambert EH: Lower motor and primary sensory neuron diseases with peroneal muscular atrophy. Arch Neurol 18:619–625, 1968

20. Dyck PJ, Lambert EH, Mulder DW: Charcot-Marie-Tooth disease: Nerve conduction and clinical studies of a large kinship. Neurology 13: 1–11, 1963

21. Feldman RG: Urban lead mining: Lead intoxication among deleaders. N Engl J Med 298:1143–1145, 1978

22. Feldman RG, Hayes MK, Younes R, et al: Lead neuropathy in adults and children. Arch Neurol 34:481–488, 1977

23. Felmus MT, Patten BM, Swanke L: Antecedent events in amyotrophic lateral sclerosis. Neurology 26:167–172, 1976

24. Friedman AP, Freedman D: Amyotrophic lateral sclerosis. J Nerv Ment Dis 111:1–18, 1950

25. Gardner MB, Henderson BE: Lower motor neuron disease in mice and amyotrophic lateral sclerosis in man (letter). Lancet 2:952, 1974

26. Gibbs CJ Jr, Gajdusek DC: Amyotrophic lateral sclerosis. Parkinson's disease, and the amyotrophic lateral sclerosis–Parkinsonism dementia complex on Guam: A review and summary of attempts to demonstrate infection as the etiology. J Clin Pathol 25 (Suppl):132–140, 1972

27. Goldblatt D: Treatment of amyotrophic lateral sclerosis. Adv Neurol 17:265–283, 1977

28. Green VA, Wise GW, Callenbach J: Lead poisoning. Clin Toxicol 9:33–51, 1976

29. Hirano A: Pathology of amyotrophic lateral sclerosis. In *Slow Latent and Temperate Virus Infections.* Edited by DC Gajdusek, CJ Gibbs Jr, M Alpers. NINDB Monographs No. 2, Washington DC, NINDB, 1965, pp 23–27

30. Hudson AJ: Amyotrophic lateral sclerosis and toxic hydrocarbons (letter). Arch Neurol 34:721, 1977

31. Ionasescu V, Luca N: Studies on carbohydrate metabolism in amyotrophic lateral sclerosis and hereditary proximal spinal muscular atrophy. Acta Neurol Scand 40:47–57, 1964

32. Kehoe RA: Occupational lead poisoning. 2-Chemical signs of the absorption of lead. J Occupational Med 14:390–396, 1972

33. Kennedy WR: Innervation of muscle spindles in amyotrophic lateral sclerosis. Mayo Clin Proc 46:245–257, 1971

34. Kennedy WR, Alter M, Sung JH: Progressive proximal spinal and bulbar muscular atrophy of late onset. Neurology 18:671–680, 1968

35. Kugelberg E, Edstrom L, Abbruzzese M: Mapping of motor units

in experimentally re-innervated rat muscle. J Neurol Neurosurg Psychiatry 33:319–329, 1970

36. Kugelberg E, Welander L: Heredity of familial juvenile muscular atrophy simulating muscular dystrophy. Arch Neurol Psychiatry 75: 500–509, 1956

37. Lambert EH: Diagnostic value of electric stimulation of motor nerves. EEG Clin Neurophysiol 22 (Suppl):9–16, 1962

38. Lambert EH, Mulder DW: Electromyographic studies in amyotrophic lateral sclerosis. Mayo Clin Proc 32:441–446, 1957

39. Lebo CP, Ü KS, Norris FH Jr: Cricopharyngeal myotomy in amyotrophic lateral sclerosis. Laryngoscope 86:862–868, 1976

40. Lehrich JR, Oger J, Arnason BGW: Neutralizing antibodies to poliovirus and mumps virus in amyotrophic lateral sclerosis. J Neurol Sci 23: 537–540, 1974

41. Livesley B, Sissons CE: Chronic lead intoxication mimicking motor neuron disease (letter). Br Med J 4:387–388, 1968

42. Mallette LE, Patten BM, Engel WK: Neuromuscular disease in secondary hyperparathyroidism. Ann Intern Med 82:474–483, 1975

43. Miller RD: Pulmonary disability as a symptom of amyotrophic lateral sclerosis. Mayo Clin Proc 32:436–437, 1957

44. Mills CP: Dysphagia in pharyngeal paralysis treated by cricopharyngeal sphincterotomy. Lancet 1:455–457, 1973

45. Mueller PS, Quick DT: Studies of glucose, insulin, and lipid metabolism in amyotrophic lateral sclerosis and other neuromuscular disorders. J Lab Clin Med 76:190–201, 1970

46. Mulder DW, Lambert EH, Eaton LM: Myasthenic syndrome in patients with amyotrophic lateral sclerosis. Neurology 9:627–631, 1959

47. Namba T, Aberfield DC, Grob D: Chronic proximal spinal muscular atrophy. J Neurol Sci 11:401–423, 1970

48. Oshiro FJ, Cremer, NE, Norris FH Jr, et al: Virus-like particles in muscle from a patient with amyotrophic lateral sclerosis. Neurology 26:57–60, 1976

49. Palo J, Jokelainen M: Geographic and social distribution of patients with amyotrophic lateral sclerosis (letter). Arch Neurol 34:724, 1977

50. Patten BN, Bilezikian JP, Mallette LE, et al: Neuromuscular disease in primary hyperparathyroidism. Ann Intern Med 80:182–193, 1974

51. Pederson L, PerPlatz C, Jersild C, et al: HLA (SD and LD) in patients with amyotrophic lateral sclerosis (ALS). J Neurol Sci 31:313–318, 1977

52. Petkau A, Sawatzky A, Hillier CR, et al: Lead content of neuromuscular tissue in amyotrophic lateral sclerosis: Case report and other considerations. Br J Indust Med 31:275–287, 1974

53. Quick DT: Pancreatic dysfunction in amyotrophic lateral sclerosis. In *Motor Neuron Diseases.* Edited by FH Norris, LT Kurland. New York, Grune & Stratton, 1969, pp 189–198

54. Simpson JA, Seaton DA, Adams JF: Response to treatment with chelating agents of anemia, chronic encephalopathy, and myelopathy due to lead poisoning. J Neurol Neurosurg Psychiatry 27:536–541, 1964

55. Smith AWM, Mulder DW, Code CF: Esophageal motility in amyotrophic lateral sclerosis. Mayo Clin Proc 32:438–441, 1957

56. Steinke J, Tyler HR: The association of amyotrophic lateral sclerosis (motor neuron disease) and carbohydrate intolerance. A clinical study. Metabolism 13:1376–1381, 1964

57. Vicale CT: The diagnostic features of a muscular syndrome resulting from hyperparathyroidism, osteomalacia owing to renal tubular acidosis, and perhaps to related disorders of calcium metabolism. Am Neurol Assoc 74:143–147, 1949

58. Williams ER, Buford A: Creatine phosphokinase in motor neuron disease. Clin Chem Acta 27:53–56, 1970

59. Wilson SAK: The amyotrophy of chronic lead poisoning—amyotrophic lateral sclerosis of toxic origin. Rev Neurol Psychiatry 5:441–455, 1907

60. Wohlfart G: Collateral regeneration from residual motor nerve fibers in amyotrophic lateral sclerosis. Neurology 7:124–134, 1957

61. Woolf AL, Alberca-Serrano R, Johnson AG: The intramuscular nerve endings and muscle fibers in amyotrophic lateral sclerosis. In *Motor Neuron Diseases.* Edited by FH Norris Jr, LT Kurland. New York, Grune & Stratton, 1969, pp 166–174

62. Zil'ber LA, Bajdakova ZL, Gardaš'Jan AN, et al: Study of the etiology of amyotrophic lateral sclerosis. Bull WHO 29:449–456, 1963

Commentary

W. King Engel

The EMG does not provide the diagnosis in terms of specific findings, rather it tells us the extent of disease. If one is worried about cervical syringomyelia or foramen magnum meningioma, then one searches for electrical evidence of denervation in the lower extremities. Likewise, the upper extremities are examined more carefully if there is an obvious clinical denervation in the lower extremities. The same is true of muscle biopsy. We even biopsy a clinically normal muscle looking for subtle evidence of denervation, as Dr. Mokri mentions in chapter 7, if we are trying to rule out disease extending beyond the cervical region or beyond the lumbar region (8). There is, however, the interpretive problem that if one finds denervation it might be due to concomitant spondylosis disk disease and may not be related to a generalized ALS. One must exercise interpretive judgment. Electromyography allows sampling of many more sites of the muscles being evaluated than biopsy, but biopsy histochemistry can detect more subtle changes.

In regard to the syndrome of benign focal amyotrophy (1, 8), we have found by EMG a few enlarged or fasciculating motor units outside the area of clinical involvement, indicating that this finding in itself does not mean that the disease is going to be rapidly progressive. In spite of the slight dissemination evident by EMG, we have given the diagnosis of benign disease based on clinical data and, fortunately, have been proven correct by time. Thus, subclinical involvement does not necessarily presage immediate clinical involvement.

In spite of all the discussion about the differential diagnosis of ALS, we, like Dr. Mulder and others, are still seeing patients who have been diagnosed as having ALS but who have either a treatable disease or a benign untreatable one. Recently, we have seen two patients with syringomyelia and one with a foramen magnum meningioma who was considered to have postpolio progressive amyotrophy. (Even if a patient has postpolio residua, the development of progressive motor disease means that the neurologist has to use all the neuroanatomic analyses that we teach our students in the first year of neurology.)

In ALS there is no selective muscle fiber type of involvement, and therefore by inference there is probably no selective involvement of one subset of alpha motor neurons (8). [Neither we nor others have yet demonstrated histochemically different types of alpha motor neurons (3–5, 7) although different alpha motor neurons may well exist to control distinct histochemical types and subtypes of muscle fiber.] Whatever is the cause of ALS, it must be related to a factor common to all alpha motor neuron types, rather than to any subtle differences among them. It must also relate to a commonality between lower motor neurons and upper motor neurons (and some other neurons) (13).

In the histochemical studies we did with Dr. Campa, distinct differences were observed between the motor neurons of the cat ventral horn that measured about 30 μ in diameter and the ones measuring less than 30 μ. We implied that the group below 30 μ consisted of the gamma efferents, internuncials, and Renshaw cells. They were, for example, low in phosphorylase and glycogen content and high in oxidative enzyme activity. The ones above 30 μ in diameter, which were considered to be alpha motor neurons, had opposite profiles with those reactions. If the gamma efferents are indeed involved in ALS, then one has to extend the commonality of neuron involvement to that group, too.

In terms of laboratory diagnosis, even if it is postmortem, the spinal cord involvement should be mentioned. It is curious that the hereditary form of ALS, although clinically indistinguishable from the sporadic form, always, I believe, has the pattern of middle root zone involvement in the posterior columns (10). I have never seen a case without it. One has to look for it, though, in tissue sections that have not been dehydrated. In other words, one should have frozen sections of the cord stained with a myelin stain and not simply a paraffin section stained with a so-called myelin stain (paraffin sections stained with Luxol fast blue are not satisfactory). Also, one should have a neutral lipid counterstain such as oil-red-0. Enzyme histochemistry of fresh-frozen sections of spinal cord is also helpful to show gliosis of the middle root zone (9).

The question of sensory findings in ALS always arises. We can turn that question around. In view of the demyelination of the entire anterolateral column, which is not so complete as in the corticospinal tracts but nevertheless causes pallor throughout the anterolateral column, the relative absence of sensory findings is remarkable.

With HL-A typing, we, too, have not found any groups preferentially represented in ALS patients (unpublished observations). The Zil'ber study of transmission of ALS to primates (14) was not entirely convincing. I believe it was Dr. Kurland who many years ago organized the showing of the film of the Zil'ber monkeys that had received ALS neural tissue. The paraparetic monkeys appeared to me to have probable transverse myelitis because, as I recall, there was lack of evidence of discomfort in response to painful stimulation of the lower extremities. I do not think those monkeys had ALS as we recognize it.

Abnormalities have been noted in the spinal fluid of ALS patients. The level of homovanillic acid is low basally and can be raised to normal or above with L-dopa, but the elevation does not benefit the patients (11). Levels of cAMP and cGMP are low in the spinal fluid; cAMP, but not cGMP, can be raised to normal with phthalazinol (which inhibits cAMP phosphodiesterase more than cGMP phosphodiesterase), but that does not help the patient in the vast majority of cases (2). In one case, bulbar ALS was arrested while the patient was taking phthalazinol, but whether this was an effect of the drug or spontaneous is not yet known (unpublished observation). These biochemical abnormalities are not specific enough to be of diagnostic value.

I think a creatine phosphokinase value more than 5–10 times the patient's top normal value should provoke one to suspect a disease other than ALS. Certainly the patient should be placed in an atypical group. Likewise, a major elevation of cerebrospinal fluid protein is suspicious. I would not consider 150 mg/100 ml part of "ordinary" ALS but would allow an upper limit of 100, and even that is high; in fact, above 90 is high and should be somewhat suspect. Usually, it is not more than about 80 mg/ml in ALS. If the CSF protein is more than 100 mg/ml, one certainly has to seek other explanations such as another basic disease, collateral major spondylosis, or a previous myelogram. One of our recent ALS-referred patients with a CSF protein level of 150 mg/ml had a foramen magnum meningioma.

We studied three patients with Dr. Patten who had both hyperparathyroidism and "ordinary" ALS. In them, treatment of the hyperparathyroidism per se was successful but did not ameliorate the ALS (unpublished observations). These patients contrast with others we have studied, also with Dr. Patten, who had hyperparathyroidism accompanied by some muscle weakness, fatigability, and brisk reflexes, but not clear-cut ALS; these abnormalities did respond to treatment of the hyperparathyroidism (12).

It is true that we are no longer seeing acute poliomyelitis. However, one has to wonder what live polio vaccine might be doing. Is there or is there not an increased incidence of ALS? If so, is there any relationship to the widespread use of polio vaccine? A major point against such an association is that ALS virtually always involves upper motor neurons and tracts while poliovirus essentially never does.

Another question is whether patients will be able to recover if the ALS disease is stopped by some medication. I believe different laboratory studies have indicated that they should improve. First, it is known from work with poliomyelitis patients that there can be remarkable recovery of lower motor neuron functions over the first few weeks; this is probably a metabolic recovery of the neurons themselves. Second, there can be collateral sprouting from intact neurons to "rescue" denervated muscle fibers, which accounts for the muscle fiber–type grouping (6) that Dr. Mokri discusses in chapter 7; there should be functional improvement of strength from that. Third, a person can probably make more muscle fibers by hypertrophy and splitting of existing fibers and having those fibers then become innervated by collateral sprouting. Thus, as in poliomyelitis, even if lost motor neurons cannot be brought back there should be distinct functional improvement if the progression of ALS is stopped.

Finally, I would like to mention the question of diabetic amyotrophy. What is it, and how can one be certain of the diagnosis? Is the diagnosis only made in retrospect by whether or not the patient benefits significantly from antidiabetic treatment? I share Dr. Norris's uncertainty as to whether a diabetic amyotrophy really exists in addition to diabetic sensorimotor neuropathy and variants of it and diabetic mononeuritis multiplex. If so, how can we be certain of the diagnosis?

REFERENCES

1. Adornato BT, Engel WK, Kucera J, et al: Benign focal amyotrophy. Neurology 28:399, 1978

2. Brooks BR, Engel WK, Sode J, et al: Cyclic nucleotide phosphodiesterase (PDE) inhibitor therapy with phthalazinol in amyotrophic lateral sclerosis (ALS). Neurology 28:402, 1978

3. Campa JF, Engel WK: Histochemical and functional correlations in anterior horn neurons of the cat spinal cord. Science 171:198–199, 1971

4. Campa JF, Engel WK: Histochemistry of motor neurons and interneurons in the cat lumbar spinal cord. Neurology 20:559–568, 1970

5. Campa JF, Engel WK: Histochemistry of motor neurons innervating slow and fast motor units. In *New Developments in EMG and Clinical Neurophysiology.* Edited by JE Desmedt. Basel, S Karger, 1973, pp 178–185

6. Engel WK: Histochemistry of neuromuscular disease—significance of muscle fiber types. Neuromuscular Diseases. In *Proceedings of the VIII International Congress of Neurology,* Vienna, Austria, 1965, Vol II. Amsterdam, Excerpta Medica, pp 67–101

7. Engel WK: Introduction to disorders of the motor neuron nerves and related abnormalities. In *Scientific Approaches to Clinical Neurology*. Edited by GM Shy, ES Goldensohn, SH Appel. Philadelphia, Lea & Febiger, 1977, pp 1250–1321

8. Engel WK: Motor Neuron Disorders. In *Scientific Approaches to Clinical Neurology.* Edited by GM Shy, ES Goldensohn, SH Appel. Philadelphia, Lea & Febiger, 1977, pp 1322–1346

9. Engel WK: Motor neuron histochemistry in ALS and infantile spinal muscular atrophy. In *Motor Neuron Diseases.* Edited by FH Norris Jr, LT Kurland. New York, Grune and Stratton, 1969, pp 218–234

10. Engel WK, Kurland LT, Klatzo I: An inherited disease similar to amyotrophic lateral sclerosis: An intermediate form? Brain 82:203–220, 1959

11. Mendell JR, Chase TN, Engel WK: Modification by L-dopa of a case of progressive supranuclear palsy. Lancet 1:593–594, 1970

12. Patten BM, Bilezikiar JP, Mallette LE, et al: Neuromuscular disease in primary hyperparathyroidism. Ann Intern Med 80:182–193, 1973

13. Smith MC: Nerve fibre degeneration in the brain in amyotrophic lateral sclerosis. J. Neurol Neurosurg Psychiatry 23:269, 1960

14. Zil'ber LA: Study of the etiology of amyotrophic lateral sclerosis. Bull WHO 29:449, 1963

Richard T. Johnson

Caution must be taken in interpreting serologic studies. For example, poliovirus antibody levels are not higher in patients who have had paralytic poliomyelitis than in patients who have had asymptomatic gastrointestinal infection. Antibody levels are not dependent on site of replication but may be elevated abnormally if there is continuous antigenic stimulation, as in subacute sclerosing panencephalitis.

Absence of measurable antibody is not conclusive evidence against infection. Atypical agents such as in Creutzfeldt-Jakob disease fail to evoke any discernible immune response. Even the murine leukemia virus strain causing chronic polioencephalomyelopathy, although a fully antigenic virus, evokes little antibody in the mouse, and this antibody is hard to detect. The absence of antibody in humans in no way argues against an analogous type of virus in ALS.

6 Motor Nerve Conduction Velocities

Eric H. Denys

Classic amyotrophic lateral sclerosis is a system disease involving the motor pathways. It can affect both the upper and the lower motor neurons, and the diagnosis usually can be made or suspected during a careful clinical neurologic examination. The finding of muscle atrophy and hyperactive reflexes in the same extremity is a main indication, although ALS can also present with focal weakness and atrophy in the absence of hyperreflexia or can involve only the lower motor neurons. In the latter case, the term *progressive muscular atrophy* has been used.

Electromyography (EMG) is one of the most useful diagnostic tests employed to complement the clinical neurologic examination. It provides determinations of motor and sensory nerve conduction velocities as well as a needle electrode examination of the muscles. The majority of the motor nerve conduction velocities obtained in patients with ALS are within normal limits. The sensory nerve conduction velocities are always normal, and the finding of a normal sensory nerve potential in an extremity with marked atrophy is very useful in establishing that the disease is limited to the motor system. The findings on needle electrode examination include spontaneous activities such as fibrillations; positive waves; fasciculations; bizarre high-frequency discharges; changes in the motor unit potentials as the number of motor unit potentials under voluntary control decreases secondary to either lower or upper motor neuron involvement; and abnormalities in the size, duration, configuration,

Supported by a grant from the Muscular Dystrophy Association of America.

and amplitude of the motor unit potentials. The sprouting of healthy nerve terminals to reinnervate previously denervated muscle fibers creates so-called giant motor unit potentials. None of the described abnormalities is specific for ALS. They can also be seen in other diseases involving the anterior horn cell (e.g., poliomyelitis, Werdnig-Hoffmann disease, or Kugelberg-Welander disease), in peripheral neuropathies, and in cases where osteoarthritic changes of the vertebral column cause pressure on the nerve roots. Electromyographic examination therefore should not be limited to the clinically involved extremity but should be used to detect pathologic changes in clinically unaffected extremities. Abnormalities in at least three extremities in the appropriate clinical setting make the diagnosis certain.

Although normal motor and sensory nerve conduction velocities are the rule, slow motor nerve conduction does occur in ALS and, if taken in context, does not preclude a diagnosis of ALS. Several previous studies have dealt with this problem. One of the earliest was reported by Lambert and Mulder in 1957 (9); this study was expanded by Lambert in 1962 (10) and again, with a state-of-the-art review of 322 patients, in 1969 (11). The slowing of motor nerve conduction generally correlated with the degree of atrophy in the muscle from which the recording was done. Conduction in the distal segment of the nerve behaved in a similar manner. Similar findings were reported by Isch et al. (8). Ertekin found motor and sensory nerve conduction velocities and distal latencies to be within normal limits in a sample of 15 patients with ALS (7).

Lambert added that unusual precautions had not been taken to maintain the nerve at a standard temperature, but, since slow conduction velocities were seen only in motor nerves and not in sensory nerves, it was most likely a valid observation (11). A low temperature may indeed cause a decrease in the nerve conduction velocity. De Jong et al. found a reduction of 1.84 m/sec per degree centigrade between 36° C and 23° C for the peroneal nerve (4). DeJesus et al. studied the effect of temperature on the median nerve conduction velocity in 15 normal volunteers and found a linear relationship (3). A low temperature (as low as 29° C) is not unusual in an atrophic extremity even when the room temperature is normal [personal observation, see also (3)]. Despite these reports, slow motor nerve conduction velocities in patients with ALS continue to raise doubt about the correct diagnosis.

CLINICAL STUDY

A review of the motor and sensory nerve conduction velocities in 186 patients with ALS at the Institutes of Medical Sciences in San Francisco confirms the previous observation that although slow motor nerve conduction can occur in ALS, it is usually seen in the context of muscle atrophy. Analyses of the distal latencies and computations of the residual latencies show a similar correlation but also point to the possibility of selective involvement in the distal part of the motor nerves.

Only patients with a firm diagnosis of classic ALS or progressive muscular atrophy with steady progression of clinical symptoms were included in this study. There were 107 men and 79 women. Their average age was 56 years. Ulnar, median, and peroneal nerves were studied using the Mayo Clinic technique and surface electrodes. Recordings were done from the hypothenar, thenar, and extensor digitorum brevis muscles. Patients in whom proximal nerve stimulation revealed a marked drop in amplitude of the evoked muscle response (>2.0 mV), which was not present with stimulation 10 cm more distally, were not included, as this was indicative of a localized conduction block. One or more of the three nerves was tested.

Responses were recorded on photographic paper for the determination of latencies. The distal motor latency was corrected for a standard distance of 6.5 cm for both the ulnar and the median nerves and 9.0 cm for the peroneal nerve according to the formula:

$$\text{corrected latency} = t_m - \frac{d - ds}{v}$$

(t_m = measured latency, d = distance between stimulation and recording electrode, ds = standard conduction distance, v = conduction velocity in the proximal segment of the nerve). The upper limits of normal for the distal latencies of the median, ulnar, and peroneal nerves were 4.6, 4.2, and 6.5 msec, respectively; these values represent the maximum values observed in a large control population (12). The amplitude of the M-wave was measured from the baseline to the peak of the negative potential. Temperature was controlled at 35°–37° C for the arm and 33°–36° C for the leg. Control subjects were normal volunteers free of neurologic disease.

Sensory nerve conduction velocity was determined by orthodromic stimulation of the second digit and surface recording at the wrist with a standard interelectrode distance of 13.0 cm. The latency was measured to the peak of the potential.

CONDUCTION VELOCITIES AND M-WAVES

The motor nerve conduction velocities and M-wave amplitudes are summarized in Tables 1–3. The maximum motor nerve conduction velocity is slower in patients with ALS than in controls (Table 1) by an average of 11% (11% for the ulnar, 14% for the median, 8% for the peroneal nerves). These values are quite similar to the ones reported previously (8, 11). The M-wave, which gives an approximation of the number and

Table 1 Motor Nerve Conduction Velocity (NCV) versus M-Wave Amplitude in Patients with ALS and in Controls

Nerve	Group	No. of Patients	Age (years)		Motor NCV (m/sec)		M-Wave Amplitude (mV)	
			Mean	Range	Mean ± SD	Range	Mean ± SD	Range
Ulnar	ALS	167	55	26–82	52.9 ± 6.5	34–68	5.7 ± 3.7	0.1–14.5
	Control	16	35	15–72	59.5 ± 2.6	55–63	12.0 ± 2.5	8.4–17.0
	Mayo Clinic data	174			59.8 ± 5.5	47–75	11.1 ± 2.6	5.6–20.0
Median	ALS	107	56	28–82	51.6 ± 7.8	25–65	4.5 ± 3.6	0.1–13.5
	Control	13	42	15–72	59.8 ± 3.0	57–66	10.8 ± 2.7	6.8–14.5
	Mayo Clinic data	113			59.1 ± 5.2	49–79	10.7 ± 3.7	4.2–21.4
Peroneal	ALS	66	56	26–82	45.4 ± 5.1	30–59	3.6 ± 2.4	0.1– 9.0
	Control	8	35	15–45	49.4 ± 2.5	46–54	7.7 ± 2.5	5.2–12.0
	Mayo Clinic data	90			50.7 ± 3.7	41–59	7.3 ± 2.6	2.2–14.6

Table 2 Motor Nerve Conduction Velocity (NCV) versus M-Wave Amplitude in Patients with ALS

Nerve	M-Wave (mV)	No. of Patients	NCV Mean ± SD	NCV Range
Ulnar	>10	21	57.6 ± 5.2	50.0–68.4
	5–10	66	55.3 ± 4.6	45.5–67.5
	<5	80	49.7 ± 6.5	34.2–61.6
Median	>10	11	57.9 ± 2.3	54.4–61.5
	5–10	30	54.9 ± 4.2	43.5–63.9
	<5	66	49.1 ± 8.4	25.3–64.6
Peroneal	>5	21	47.2 ± 4.7	33.7–53.8
	<5	45	44.6 ± 5.1	30.0–59.4

Table 3 Motor Nerve Conduction Velocity (NCV) versus M-Wave Amplitude in ALS Patients with M-Wave Amplitudes below 5 mV

Nerve	M-Wave (mV)	No. of Patients	NCV Mean ± SD	NCV Range
Ulnar	4–5	19	53.0 ± 3.4	46.1–59.1
	3–4	12	53.7 ± 5.1	44.9–61.6
	2–3	13	49.6 ± 7.4	35.6–57.8
	1–2	15	49.5 ± 5.6	38.4–60.5
	<1	21	44.6 ± 6.4	34.2–56.2
Median	4–5	8	55.7 ± 6.7	43.8–64.6
	3–4	10	54.0 ± 2.2	51.1–57.6
	2–3	16	51.6 ± 4.7	43.6–59.5
	1–2	7	51.1 ± 5.0	44.4–56.9
	<1	25	42.7 ± 9.3	25.3–60.2
Peroneal	4–5	6	46.1 ± 3.0	40.3–48.6
	3–4	11	45.5 ± 4.1	38.0–50.8
	2–3	9	43.5 ± 3.2	39.8–48.0
	1–2	4	46.7 ± 6.7	38.6–55.0
	<1	15	43.3 ± 6.7	30.0–59.4

size of the muscle fibers under the recording electrode, is also smaller in patients with ALS, and the difference from controls is 53%, 58%, and 53% for the hypothenar, thenar, and extensor digitorum brevis, respectively. The influence of such an important variable as atrophy is shown in Tables 2 and 3. This analysis shows that successively slower nerve conduction velocities are recorded when the M-wave becomes smaller. Of interest also is the increasing standard deviation with decreasing nerve conduction velocity and M-wave amplitude.

Although the nerve conduction velocity diminishes with increasing atrophy, it usually remains within the normal range (85% for the ulnar, 72% for the median, 79% for the peroneal nerves) until marked atrophy is present, as manifested by M-waves below 5.0 mV for the ulnar and the median nerves (Table 3). The scattergrams in Figure 1 show the relationship between conduction velocity and M-wave amplitudes for all the data points. These findings again are in agreement with previous reports (10).

The values for the ulnar and median nerves show the most striking trends. The analysis of variance (ANOVA) between the subgroups of the ulnar and the median nerves was highly significant ($P < 0.001$). The findings in the peroneal nerve, although similar, were less significant; the ANOVA between the two groups with M-waves above or below 5 mV was significant ($P < 0.05$), but no statistical correlation was found for the subgroups. Slight to moderate slowing of conduction velocity in the peroneal nerve can be present in the absence of severe atrophy as determined by M-wave amplitude.

Nerve conduction velocities are directly proportional to the diameter of the myelinated nerve fibers (13). The standard test to determine conduction velocity records the speed of conduction in the fastest-conducting fibers. The maximum motor nerve conduction velocity in patients with ALS will therefore depend on the size of the largest remaining nerve fibers.

In most patients with ALS, nerve conduction velocities stay within the normal range even when atrophy is present, so it is unlikely that preferential early involvement of large neurons occurs, as has been suggested (16). A random loss best explains the widening range of nerve conduction velocities seen with advancing disease. The finding of slow conduction velocities simply indicates that the fastest fibers have been lost. The same type of loss might also occur at the slow end of the spectrum, but this is not detected by standard nerve conduction studies. The tendency, therefore, is for the lowest conduction velocities to be seen in the most severely atrophied muscles, where the M-wave is of very low amplitude.

Atrophy is reflected in a decrease in the amplitude of the M-wave, which depends mainly on the number and size of innervated muscle fibers under the recording electrode. The M-wave is only an approximate indicator of neuronal loss, however. The sprouting of nerve

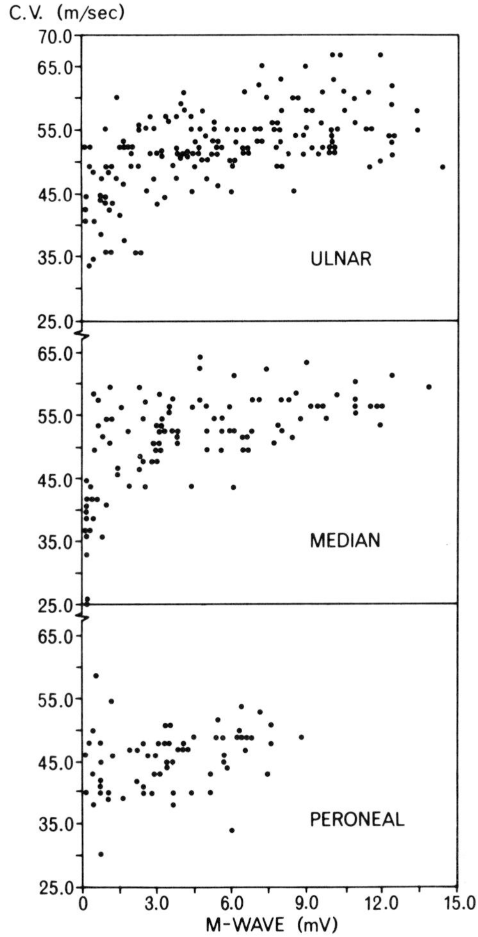

Figure 1 Motor nerve conduction velocity in the ulnar, median, and peroneal nerves in 186 patients with ALS are represented as a function of the amplitude of the M-wave in the thenar, hypothenar, and extensor digitorum brevis muscles, respectively. Each dot represents one set of data. Temperature was controlled (see text). Slow nerve conduction velocities were seen only in the presence of a low-amplitude M-wave.

terminals may temporarily prevent muscle atrophy; marked disease of the upper motor neurons may result in disuse atrophy and account for a decrease in M-wave amplitude without concomitant loss of lower motor neurons.

The clear correlation between M-wave and conduction velocity in the median and ulnar nerves contrasts with findings in the peroneal nerve, where the trend is less obvious. A possible explanation could be the frequent finding of chronic neurogenic changes in the extensor digitorum brevis (which are sometimes associated with denervation changes such as fibrillation and positive waves) during needle electrode examinations of even asymptomatic control populations. This finding is presumed to be secondary to local trauma caused by pressure from footwear around the ankle and the dorsum of the foot. Such preexisting changes can be associated with atrophy and render the M-wave a less reliable correlate of conduction velocity.

Conduction velocities tend to become slower with increasing age (6). However, when the data were analyzed with age as a covariant, no significant influence of age was detected for the ulnar or peroneal nerve. This means that any effect of age is overshadowed by the disease process itself. However, an age factor was found for the median nerve ($P < 0.001$), and the overall correlation between M-wave and conduction velocity remained significant when age was included as a covariant.

DISTAL AND RESIDUAL MOTOR LATENCIES

Lambert found conduction in the distal section of the motor nerve to become slower as the degree of atrophy increased (11). With amplitudes of less than 1 mV, the distal latency was, on the average, 40% greater than normal for the ulnar nerve with similar values for the median and peroneal nerves. However, most individual values were still within the normal range, although some were slightly prolonged.

In the current series, the distal latencies also showed a significant inverse relationship to the amplitude of the M-wave ($P < 0.001$ for the ulnar and the median nerves, $P < 0.05$ for the peroneal nerve). The distal latencies (corrected for a standard distance) in the median, ulnar, and peroneal nerves, however, were within normal limits in most patients. The patients whose corrected distal latencies were outside the normal range are represented in Tables 4 and 5. The corresponding M-wave

Table 4 Increased Distal and Residual Latencies in Patients with ALS

Patient No.	*Corrected Distal Latency (msec)*	*M-Wave (mV)*	*Conduction Velocity (m/sec)*	*Residual Latency (msec)*
Median Nerve[a]				
1	6.6	0.1	38.8	4.9
2	5.7	0.1	42.3	4.1
3	10.9	0.1	37.3	9.2
4	5.9	0.2	42.2	4.4
5	4.8	0.2	40.3	3.1[b]
6	5.3	0.2	36.6	3.5
7	4.9	0.2	40.6	3.3

Table 4 Increased Distal and Residual Latencies in Patients with ALS (*continued*)

Patient No.	*Corrected Distal Latency (msec)*	*M-Wave (mV)*	*Conduction Velocity (m/sec)*	*Residual Latency (msec)*
8	4.8	0.2	25.5	2.2[b]
9	4.8	0.3	40.0	3.3
10	5.6	0.3	43.8	4.1
11	5.4	0.4	39.2	3.7
12	5.2	0.6	54.0	4.0
13	6.5	0.7	52.2	5.3
14	6.6	0.7	35.7	4.8
15	4.9	1.0	51.0	3.6
16	5.8	1.4	47.3	4.4
17	4.9	1.8	44.4	3.4
18	5.0	2.2	59.5	3.9
19	5.0	2.4	48.1	3.7
20	5.1	2.5	43.6	3.6
21	5.0	3.0	51.0	3.7
22	5.5	3.3	52.6	4.3
23	5.0	4.3	43.8	3.5
24	5.0	5.2	54.9	3.8
25	5.5	5.6	52.8	4.3
26	6.4	6.4	58.4	5.2
Ulnar Nerve[c]				
1	4.3	0.1	40.5	2.7
2	7.1	0.1	44.6	5.7
3	4.7	0.1	53.4	3.6
4	6.7	0.3	52.8	5.5
5	4.4	0.4	35.0	2.5
6	4.4	0.5	40.7	2.8
7	9.5	0.9	45.0	8.1
8	6.5	1.0	50.0	5.2
9	5.6	1.0	35.9	3.8
10	4.5	3.8	47.6	3.1
11	4.6	9.6	62.2	3.5
Peroneal Nerve[d]				
1	9.0	0.5	50.0	7.2
2	7.6	0.8	30.0	4.6
3	7.3	1.0	40.0	5.0

[a] Distal latency values are corrected for 6.5 cm (maximum, 4.6 msec). Normal values for the residual latency are 1.4–3.1 msec. Sensory nerve potential was normal in this group of patients.
[b] These values are within the normal range.
[c] Distal latency values are corrected for 6.5 (maximum, 4.2 msec). Normal values for the residual latency are 0.9–1.8 msec.
[d] Distal latency values are corrected for 9.0 cm (maximum, 6.5 msec). Normal values for the residual latency are 2.4–4.3 msec.

Table 5 Proportion of ALS Patients with Latencies Outside the Normal Range

Nerve	Percentage of Patients with Abnormal Conduction Velocity	Patients with Increased Corrected Distal Latency		Patients with Increased Residual Latency	
		Fraction	Percentage	Fraction	Percentage
Ulnar	15	11/167	6.6	58/167	34.7
Median	28	26/107	24.3	33/107	30.8
Peroneal	21	3/66	4.5	3/66	4.5

amplitudes and motor nerve conduction velocities in the proximal segment are included. The residual latency was obtained by subtracting from the distal latency the time it takes for the nerve impulse to travel over the distal segment, assuming the velocity is the same as in the proximal nerve segment. In healthy individuals, that residual time is taken up by slowing caused by tapering of nerve fibers, slowing at branching points, and delays at the neuromuscular junction. Additional slowing can occur if there is a pathologic conduction block; blocks are caused by an area of myelin damage, as commonly seen in the carpal tunnel syndrome. Normal upper values for the residual latency in the median, ulnar, and peroneal nerves are 3.1, 1.8, and 4.3 msec, respectively (E.H. Lambert, personal communication). Median sensory latencies were always within the normal range according to age-adjusted values.

Two observations can be made. First, prolongation of corrected distal latencies was found more often (24.3%) in the median *motor* nerve than in the ulnar nerve (6.6%) or the peroneal nerve (4.5%), whereas median *sensory* nerve latencies were normal in all the patients. Second, the mean amplitude of the M-wave in the group with prolonged distal latencies was very low (1.7 ± 1.9 mV) and, as expected from our findings, associated with conduction velocities below the lower limit of normal in a large number of them (18 of 25 patients for the median nerve, 6 of 11 for the ulnar nerve, and 2 of 3 for the peroneal nerve). Some patients had increased distal motor latencies in the median nerve but normal motor nerve conduction velocities in the proximal segment and a normal sensory latency, which raises the question of whether other factors contribute to the slowing observed in the distal segment.

Assuming that the characteristics of the distal part of the nerve are the same as those in the proximal segment for all nerves regardless of size, the increased distal latency should be proportional to the degree of slowing in the proximal segment of the nerve. However, to explain an increase in the distal latency over a given distance solely on the basis of a reduced conduction velocity in the nerve, the conduction velocity would have to decrease markedly. For example, a 1.0-msec increase in the distal latency (from 3.5 to 4.5 msec) over a distance of 6.5 cm would require the conduction velocity to decrease from 55 m/sec to 29.8 m/sec or from 65 m/sec to 32.5 m/sec. These low values were rarely seen in this group of patients with ALS. Moreover, if the longer distal latencies were due solely to the slow conduction velocities of the remaining nerve fibers, one would not expect to find an increased residual latency. When the residual latency was used as a criterion, even more patients had abnormal values (Table 5). The median and the ulnar nerves showed a similar pattern, which argues against a local entrapment. The peroneal nerve findings were, with a few exceptions, normal.

Without histologic and morphometric data, one can only speculate about the factors operating in ALS. Nerve sprouting in an effort to compensate for the loss of motor neurons is a prominent feature (17). The slower conduction times found in immature sprouts (15) cannot explain the increased latencies recorded, but additional branching points could cause an increased number of impulse blockings (14). There is neurophysiologic evidence that neuromuscular transmission fails increasingly as the disease progresses (5); the marked morphologic change in the neuromuscular endplates of patients with ALS (1) could increase synaptic delay.

An attractive hypothesis, based on the fact that ALS can be considered a dying-back neuronopathy, would be that some abnormalities occur preferentially in the most distal part of the nerve. It does not explain why a long nerve such as the peroneal should be less involved.

Whatever the mechanism, the changes detected are rather modest. Nevertheless, a relatively short lifespan of a diseased motor neuron would prevent abnormalities from accumulating.

SUMMARY

Motor nerve conduction velocities in the ulnar, median, and peroneal nerves were reviewed in 186 patients with amyotrophic lateral sclerosis. The average nerve conduction velocity in patients with ALS was lower than that in a control population and became progressively slower with advancing disease, as represented by the amplitude of the M-wave. Most individual motor nerve conduction velocities were within the normal range, but abnormally low values tended to occur in the presence of marked atrophy. The distal latencies were usually within normal limits, although the median nerve exhibited a higher frequency of prolonged distal latencies than the ulnar or peroneal nerve. Increased residual latencies, however, were found to the same degree in median and ulnar nerves. This finding could not be explained solely on the basis of slow conduction because of neuronal loss. The findings were less obvious in the peroneal nerve. In general, slow motor nerve conduction velocities do not rule out ALS if the amplitude of the M-wave is low. The abnormal residual latencies in the median and ulnar nerves could represent selective distal neuronal disease.

It is therefore important, when determining motor conduction velocities in patients suspected of having ALS, to pay special attention to the temperature of the extremity. If, despite this, a slow conduction velocity is found, its significance will depend on the amplitude of the response evoked. A slow conduction velocity in the presence of a very low amplitude response does not necessarily indicate disease of the anterior horn cells, however; it can also be seen in peripheral neuropathies. The ultimate diagnosis will depend on the total clinical presentation.

REFERENCES

1. Bjornskov EK, Dekker NP, Norris FH, et al: End plate morphology in amyotrophic lateral sclerosis. Arch Neurol 32:711–712, 1975

2. Blom S, Hagbarth KE, Lundberg PO: Motor conduction velocities in amyotrophic lateral sclerosis, polyradiculoneuritis and Charcot-Marie-Tooth's disease. Acta Neurol Scand 40:6–12, 1964

3. DeJesus PV Jr, Hausmanowa-Petrusewicz I, Barchi RL: The effect of cold on nerve conduction of human slow and fast nerve fibers. Neurology 23:1181–1189, 1973

4. De Jong RH, Hershey WN, Wagman IH: Nerve conduction velocity during hypothermia in man. Anesthesiology 27:805–810, 1966

5. Denys EH, Norris FH: Amyotrophic lateral sclerosis: Impairment of neuromuscular transmission. Arch Neurol 36:202–205, 1979

6. Electromyography–sensory and motor conduction findings in normal subjects. Compiled by P Rosenfalck. Copenhagen, Rigshospitalet, Laboratory of Clinical Neurophysiology, 1975

7. Ertekin C: Sensory and motor conduction in motor neuron disease. Acta Neurol Scand 43:499–512, 1967

8. Isch F, Isch-Treussard C, Jesel M: La mesure de la vitesse de conduction des fibres nerveuses motrices dans les atrophies neurogènes chroniques progressives. Rev Neurol 115:122–129, 1966

9. Lambert EH, Mulder DW: Electromyographic studies in amyotrophic lateral sclerosis. Mayo Clin Proc 32:441–446, 1957

10. Lambert EH: Diagnostic value of electrical stimulation of motor nerves. Electroencephalogr Clin Neurophysiol 22 (Suppl):9–16, 1962

11. Lambert EH: Electromyography in amyotrophic lateral sclerosis. In *Motor Neuron Diseases.* Edited by FH Norris, LT Kurland. New York, Grune & Stratton, 1969, pp 135–153

12. Ohta M, Ellefson RD, Lambert EH, et al: Hereditary sensory neuropathy, type II. Arch Neurol 29:23–37, 1973

13. Patton HD: Special properties of nerve trunks and tracts. In *Neurophysiology.* Edited by TC Ruch, HD Patton, JW Woodbury, et al. New York, WB Saunders Co, 1961, pp 71–74

14. Stalberg E, Thiele B: Transmission block in terminal nerve endings: A single fiber electromyographic finding in man. J Neurol Neurosurg Psychiatry 35:22–29, 1972

15. Stalberg E, Ekstedt J: Single fiber EMG and microphysiology of the motor units in normal and diseased human muscles. In *New Developments in Electromyography and Clinical Neurophysiology,* Vol 1. Edited by JE Desmedt. Basel, S Karger, 1:113–129, 1973

16. Wohlfart G, Swank RL: Pathology of amyotrophic lateral sclerosis. Arch Neurol Psychiatry 46:783–799, 1941

17. Wohlfart G: Collateral regeneration from residual motor nerve fibers in amyotrophic lateral sclerosis. Neurology 7:124–134, 1957

7 Muscle Biopsy

Bahram Mokri

The diagnosis of amyotrophic lateral sclerosis is usually made by careful clinical evaluation and electromyographic (EMG) examination. Thus, the need for muscle biopsy in order to establish a diagnosis of ALS arises only infrequently.

Muscle biopsy in ALS will point to the involvement of the lower motor neurons by demonstrating evidence of denervation, reinnervation, or both in the muscle tissue. These changes are not specific for ALS and are also seen in many other neurogenic disorders. However, certain patterns of change are more likely to be seen in some of the neurogenic diseases. From examination of the muscle biopsy, it is virtually impossible to determine reliably the level of the lower motor neuron involvement in order to localize it to the spinal, radicular, or peripheral nerve levels. Such attempts at localization should be based on clinical and EMG findings. In ALS, as in many other progressive neuromuscular diseases, the degree of histopathologic change varies with the severity of the weakness and the rate of progression and duration of the illness. Thus, the severity of the changes may vary not only from patient to patient but also from muscle to muscle in a given patient. Sometimes a clinically uninvolved muscle shows early changes of denervation, reinnervation, or both, or histologic examination (14). This is similar to the detection by EMG of signs of denervation in clinically unaffected muscles. Ideally, moderately weak muscles should be biopsied. Stronger muscles may not show sufficient changes to confirm the diagnosis, and the advanced disease may obscure the basic pathologic process in very weak muscles.

Muscle histochemistry can identify neurogenic changes in muscle that are not readily detectable by routine pathologic methods (6).

CHARACTERISTIC CHANGES IN MUSCLE

One or more characteristic changes are seen in muscle with disease of the lower motor neurons (neurogenic atrophy). The severity of each change varies with the degree of weakness, duration of the disease, and rate of progression of the disease. Thus, various patterns may be observed. On cryostat sections of fresh-frozen muscle, the following characteristic changes are found.

Muscle Fiber Atrophy

Denervated muscle fibers shrink and on cross-section usually appear angulated, often with concave borders (Fig. 1). The fiber atrophy is not associated with any significant change in fiber architecture. The cross-striations of these atrophic fibers are generally preserved until the atrophic process is far advanced. As muscle atrophy increases and the fiber diameter decreases, the subsarcolemmal nuclei lie closer together. In advanced stages, clumps of pyknotic nuclei may be seen with

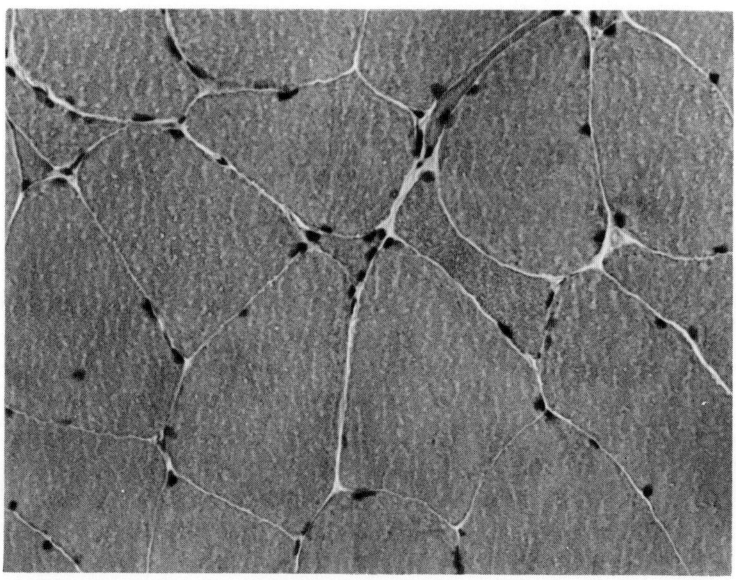

Figure 1 Atrophic angulated fibers. Fresh-frozen section, triceps muscle. (Hematoxylin and eosin stain, original magnification ×400.)

very little associated cytoplasm (Fig. 2). The atrophic fibers often, although not always, show high oxidative enzyme activity and react strongly for NADH dehydrogenase (Fig. 3) or menadione-linked α-glycerophosphate dehydrogenase. When sparsely scattered, the denervated atrophic fibers can be more readily identified by these histochemical reactions. As judged by myofibrillar ATPase reactions, both type 1 and type 2 fibers show atrophy, although at times one fiber type may be involved more often than the other. Demonstration of atrophic fibers of both major histochemical types distinguishes between atrophy due to denervation and selective fiber-type atrophy (6, 11, 13). In ALS, as in most neurogenic diseases of muscle, not all motor neurons are involved simultaneously. Fibers innervated by intact motor neurons will not atrophy, and some may even show compensatory hypertrophy. As a result, three populations of fibers occur: atrophic, normal, and hypertrophic. Thus, the muscle histogram curve may show a bimodal or trimodal configuration (1).

Grouping of Atrophic Fibers

The grouping of the atrophic and usually angular fibers is a prominent feature of neurogenic atrophy. In some neurogenic diseases,

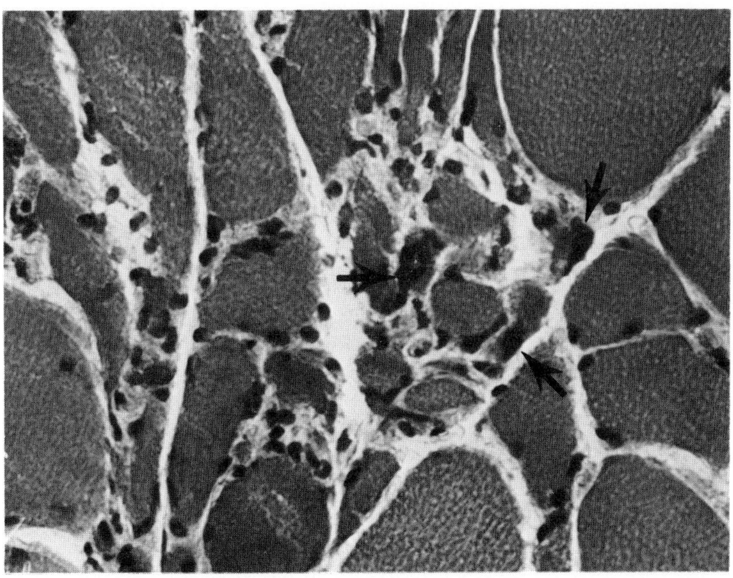

Figure 2 Group of atrophic fibers, some with clumps of pyknotic nuclei and with little associated cytoplasm (*arrows*). Fresh-frozen section, triceps muscle. (Hematoxylin and eosin stain, original magnification ×400.)

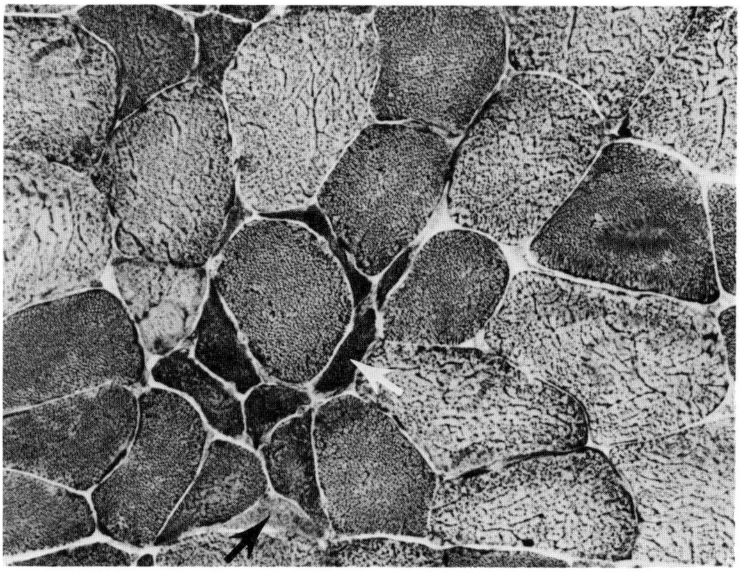

Figure 3 Group of atrophic angulated fibers. Most of the atrophic fibers (*white arrow*) but not all of them (*black arrow*) show high oxidative enzyme activity. Fresh-frozen section, triceps muscle. (NADH dehydrogenase reaction, original magnification ×250.)

such as certain spinal muscular atrophies or certain chronic peripheral neuropathies, large groups of atrophic fibers are commonly seen. In ALS, however, the groups of atrophic fibers are usually small (Fig. 4). Nevertheless, in advanced stages of the disease, larger groups of atrophic fibers are common.

Histochemical Fiber-Type Grouping

Reinnervation of denervated muscle fibers by collateral sproutings from nearby motor axons leads to the formation of large motor units (7). The histochemical profile of the muscle fiber is determined by its innervation, and all the fibers in a single motor unit are of the same histochemical type (2, 4, 8, 9, 19, 20). Thus, the histochemical characteristics of fibers reinnervated by one motor neuron become identical. The histochemical correlate of large motor-unit formation is histochemical type grouping and loss of the normal checkerboard pattern of fiber types (Fig. 5). Type grouping is thus a sign of reinnervation of previously denervated fibers and points to a neurogenic process (12, 16, 18). The extent of fiber-type grouping may have prognostic significance. Considerable type grouping, especially when there is little fiber atrophy,

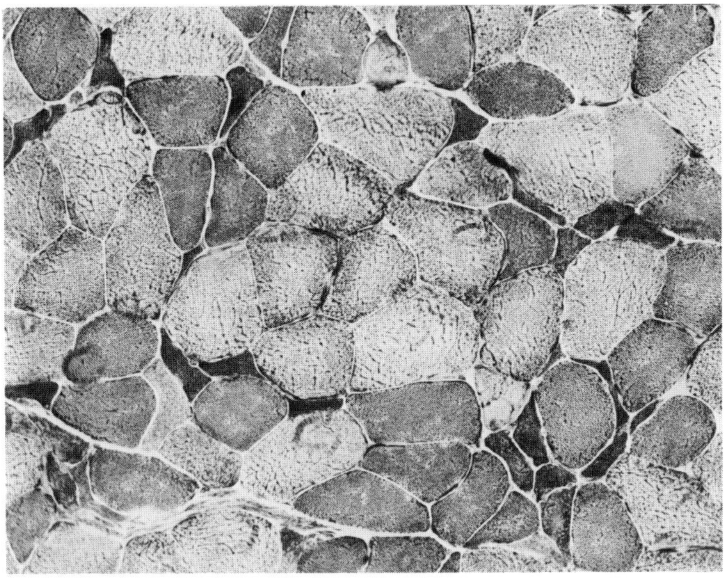

Figure 4 Small groups of atrophic angulated fibers. Fresh-frozen section, triceps muscle. (NADH dehydrogenase reaction, original magnification ×160.)

suggests effective compensation for denervation and points to a milder, more chronic, and less aggressive course.

Target Fibers

Target fibers, first described by W. K. Engel (10), have three concentric zones and are usually associated with neurogenic disease, although they are also seen in association with tenotomy under experimental conditions (15). The target fibers may or may not be atrophic, and they probably signal reinnervation rather than denervation (5). They are difficult to identify in sections stained with hematoxylin and eosin. In paraffin sections, target fibers are best shown by Mallory's phosphotungstic acid–hematoxylin stain or Gomori's stain. In histochemical preparations, they are best demonstrated by reactions for oxidative enzyme (Fig. 6).

The targets are found almost exclusively in type 1 fibers, and usually the target can be traced over a short distance in longitudinal sections. Usually there is only one target per fiber at a given level of sectioning. Although there are similarities between targets and cores, the cores (at least those with the NADH dehydrogenase reaction) can be followed along the entire length of the fiber on longitudinal sections, and more than one core per fiber may be seen.

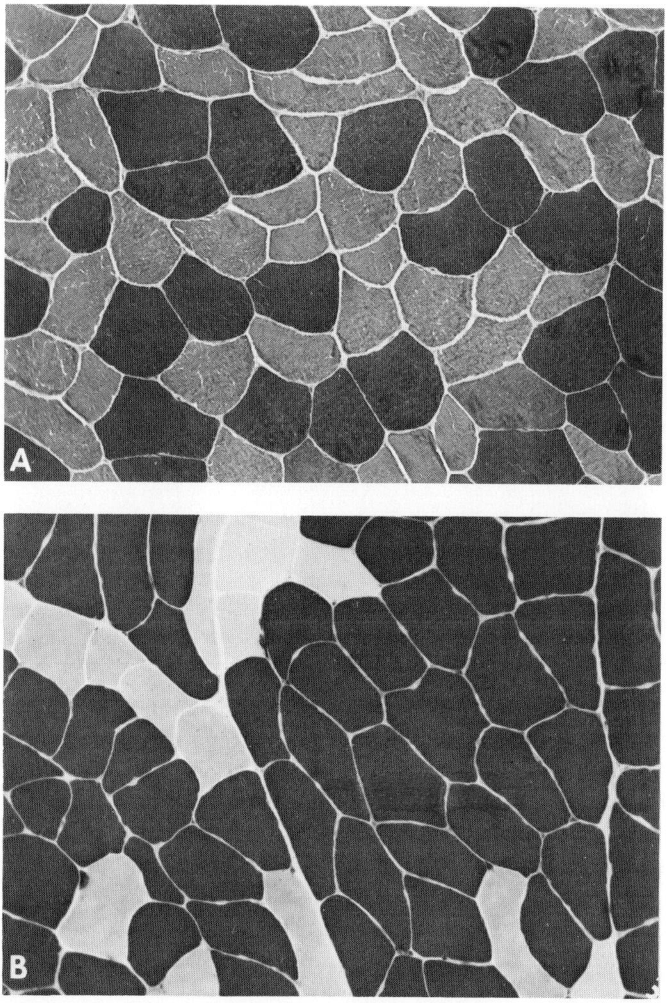

Figure 5 **(A)** Usual checkerboard pattern of fiber types. Fresh-frozen section, vastus lateralis muscle. (ATPase reaction, pH 9.3, counterstained with eosin; original magnification ×160.) **(B)** Loss of the usual checkerboard pattern and grouping of histochemical fiber types. Fresh-frozen section, peroneous longus muscle. (ATPase reaction, pH 9.3; original magnification ×160.)

In ALS, the target fibers are usually sparse, although occasionally they are abundant. They are typically quite frequent during the recovery from acute neuropathy or neuronitis and in chronic peripheral neuropathies.

The structure of the target fibers, as determined by light and electron microscopy (6, 10, 14, 17), can be divided into the central, intermediate, and outer zones.

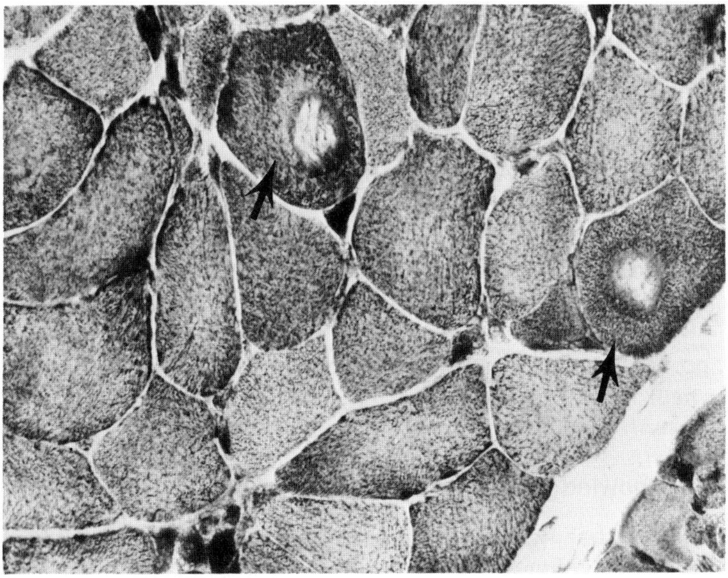

Figure 6 Target fibers (*arrows*). Fresh-frozen section, gastrocnemius muscle. (NADH dehydrogenase reaction, original magnification ×250.)

The *central zone* stains bright red with Gomori's trichrome stain and consists of condensed, disorganized myofilaments. Myofibrils are indistinct or absent. The banding pattern is lost because of myofilamentous disorganization and extension of the Z-disk material into I and A bands. This zone may show collections of triads, tubules, and vacuoles. However, it is devoid of or contains only sparse mitochondria and glycogen. The central zone has no demonstrable enzyme activity, and in histochemical preparations it appears to be unstained.

The myofilament arrangement is mildly disturbed in the *intermediate zone.* Myofibrils are sparse. Usually there is an increase in mitochondria and sarcoplasmic reticulum–like membranous structures. In paraffin sections, the intermediate zone appears to be virtually unstained, whereas on histochemical preparations it appears as a darkly stained rim surrounding the unstained central zone.

The *outer zone* has an essentially normal structure.

Fiber Hypertrophy

Hypertrophic fibers are common in many neurogenic diseases of muscle. They occur frequently in ALS but less often than in chronic neuropathies. Presumably they represent an attempt to compensate for the atrophy. Fiber hypertrophy is more common in milder than in more severe forms

8 The Initial Patient Interview

Rita A. Roelofs

Donald W. Mulder

Treatment of the patient with amyotrophic lateral sclerosis begins with the initial diagnosis and discussion of the disorder with the patient. The discussion greatly influences the patient's understanding of the disorder, and the patient will ask many questions that he or she may not ask again during the course of the illness. Therefore, the discussion must be planned before the patient is seen. Despite the importance of this initial session, the interview frequently is brief, and the patient may be left with a feeling of rejection by the health care system. The medical literature is of little help in solving the problem of what to tell the patient with ALS. There is extensive literature dealing with whether or not the patient with terminal illness should be told the truth about the disease (1–4, 6). However, this literature is concerned with cancer almost exclusively, and little has been written specifically about ALS.

In the initial interview, we attempt to include not only the specifics of the disease (e.g., effects on the body, possible outcomes), but also the limitations of our knowledge (lack of information about cause or cure). We have found it most satisfactory to allow the patient to set the limits of the discussion. It is not totally under our control what information about ALS is given or withheld, particularly the knowledge of the fatal character of the disorder. As others have stated, and we agree, most patients in whom a diagnosis of a serious disease has been made can sense the situation, whether or not they consciously recognize this awareness or discuss it (8). Thus, we assume that when we have arrived at a diagnosis the patient is at least partially aware of the seriousness of the problem. Often the patient has made an unconscious decision as to how much information he or she wishes to hear at that time. In our discussion with the patient, we attempt to be cognizant of this inner awareness or readiness and to respect the unspoken limits that we sense the patient has placed around the discussion.

Patients may signal their wishes in many ways, for example, by declining the opportunity to ask further questions, by changing the subject of discussion, by physically preparing to leave the room, and, in some cases, by simply stating that they do not want more information at this time. In the few instances in which the patient clearly does not wish to know about the severity of the illness, we inform the relatives separately about the implications of the diagnosis, usually after requesting the patient's permission and often at the patient's suggestion.

We begin to discuss the illness with the patient after the diagnosis has been established. All testing should be complete, and we must be sure that the diagnosis is certain before we undertake full discussion with the patient. When the diagnosis is questionable, we inform the patient that we do not, as yet, know the answer to his or her condition. If no further testing is indicated at that time, we often suggest reevaluation in three to six months. We are very careful not to discuss a tentative diagnosis with the patient, because we have observed that patients often assume that the tentative diagnosis is the established diagnosis.

Once the diagnosis has been established, we use a team approach in the discussion. The team usually includes a physician, nurse, and physiatrist. In some cases a dietitian, speech pathologist, medical student, or resident who has been involved in the diagnostic studies will be present. We always include significant members of the patient's family, if they are available, or significant friends. Our initial statement to the patient refers to the illness as one that involves the anterior horn cells, much as in poliomyelitis. We then describe it as possibly affecting all the musculature except the heart, the eye muscles, the bladder, the bowel muscles, and sexual function. We then give the patient and his or her family an opportunity to ask questions. The questions that are asked vary greatly with the patient's understanding, but usually, given sufficient time, most of the important questions are asked by the patient with the family present. Once the discussion has been terminated by the patient (perhaps by declining the opportunity to ask further questions or by silence) we have found it useful for the physician to leave the room and allow the discussion to proceed with the nurse alone. This usually occurs when the patient does not wish to accept more information from the physician about the illness. The patient usually regards the nurse as a sufficiently different person, probably less authoritarian, and further discussion almost invariably begins just as the physician leaves the office. Topics that arise at this time include: What caused the disease? What should I do about activity? Can my children get this?

Is there anything else I should be doing? Would you contact me if a new treatment were discovered? The nurse frequently can answer many of the questions that the patient had but apparently felt insecure about asking the physician.

Another important role for the nurse is that of sharing emotions with the patient and the family. The interview ideally allows expression of feelings that may need to be shared if the patient is to completely understand the illness; the nurse can help by answering simple questions or by sharing tears. Thus, the nurse frequently can maximize this human aspect of the disease problem. The patient as a person is stressed, and he or she often gains insight into what the diagnosis really means. The nurse can also provide the patient with written information about ALS and suggest other sources of information (adequate information about ALS is often difficult to obtain).

This initial discussion may take only 10 minutes or may last an hour or more. We always give the patient the opportunity to return to ask additional questions or to call us at a later date. Whenever possible, the patient's family is present during the initial discussion; this prevents the patient or the family from hiding knowledge of the severity of the illness from one another, in an attempt to spare the other from distressing information. Rarely, significant family conflicts make it improper to include some family members in the discussion. However, in spite of previous disagreements, most families unite after this serious illness has been diagnosed, and they are most supportive to the patient and to each other.

The information requested by the patient varies depending on his or her age, intellectual capacity, education, severity of disease, occupation, and other factors. Questions—such as, What is wrong with me? What can I do about this? What does all this mean? What do we do now?—may have different meanings to the patient and to ourselves as medical personnel. We try to respond to the patient's emotional needs in addition to providing the information that he or she is prepared to assimilate. The questions must be answered in terms that each patient can understand; this may necessitate drawing simple illustrations of a neuron and its branches on a note pad, writing down key words for the patient, etc.

It is important to ascertain what information the patient can comprehend, because it is difficult to correct misconceptions that the patient and the family may develop during the initial discussion. For example, an illiterate patient who was unable to grasp the meaning of written information was too proud to tell us of his difficulty in reading, and we learned about the problem only later. Another patient and his wife, whom we thought had an adequate understanding of the illness, interpreted our comments about the patient's weakness to mean that he should have his legs amputated.

We allow the patient to focus on questions of interest to him or her and to set the limits of the discussion. If, as happens only rarely, another member of the family insists on taking over the interview and asks questions the patient does not wish to have answered, we ignore these questions. In many instances, the patient will excuse himself/herself at this point. For example, one elderly man told his wife when she began asking pointed questions about the cause of death that all that was happening to him was what happened to all older people, and that he did not see much point in discussing it further but that he would leave the room and let her speak with the nurse alone if she wished. In a small percentage of patients (about 5%–10% in our practice), we find that it becomes necessary to give the patient's family more information than is obtained in the initial interview with the patient.

Most patients have never heard of ALS before the diagnosis. They usually begin the discussion with a set of similar questions: What is it? What caused it? What can be done? After they have obtained the answers to these, they ask another set of questions, such as: How do I live with this disease? Will there be other areas involved? Will it get worse and how will it get worse? What can I do to help? and Is there any treatment? Finally, they may ask more specific questions such as: Is this a hereditary disease? Will it affect my breathing? How common is this disorder? Is it similar to multiple sclerosis?

In answering these questions, we usually begin by referring to the illness as a motor neuron disease, if for no other reason than that the term amyotrophic lateral sclerosis seems a clumsy grouping of words to the average patient. If the patient asks us about Lou Gehrig's disease, we verify that this is the same illness. The patient and the family often are most insistent on understanding the cause. They usually ask whether diet, physical activity, trauma, emotions, or toxins may be related to the illness. In our experience, it is important to tell the family and the patient how little we know about the cause of ALS. It may be helpful to explain that there are a number of theories about the cause, but that we do not know the cause. Frequently, we find that it is particularly important to help families recognize that certain things they did or that the patient did are not, as far as we know, the cause of the illness.

In answering the questions about progression of the disease, it is essential to ascertain what the patient means by progression. He or she may want to know about the symptoms, about disability, or about the actual prognosis, but sometimes he or she means something quite different. Once the question has been clarified, the information that the patient wishes to know can be provided. We usually point out that, although the illness is a progressive one, there are instances in which the disease seems to reach a standstill. We explain that all muscles are involved but that sexual function, bladder and bowel function, the eyes, the mind, and the heart are spared. We report that the symptoms may become worse but that pain is not a symptom of this disease and that loss of sensation or loss of intellect is not a part of the problem. Although this latter information may not be specifically requested by the patient, we have invariably seen an expression of relief by both the patient and the family after hearing that there is no pain and no disturbance of the intellect.

We also attempt to stress other positive aspects of the illness, for example, that many patients continue to work and that it is necessary for them to do what is important to them. Sometimes the patient or the family may ask how long the patient has to live. We respond by pointing out how difficult it is to know how long any of us will live and speak in terms of averages. We tell the patients that, in our experience, one-half of the patients who come to see us with this illness are alive three years after the onset of the disorder and that many live for a much longer time (5).

The patient often describes fatigue and asks what he or she should do. We stress that each patient needs to set his or her own limits, avoiding only excessive fatigue. During the visit to the clinic, the patient is given a physical therapy program to maintain the musculature and avoid disuse phenomena (7). If the patient is in a work situation that is obviously inappropriate, we explain that he or she is disabled from a medical point of view and allow the patient the opportunity, with the help of his or her employer, to make the decision whether to stop working or to continue.

In response to questions about therapy, we state that, although there is no cure, symptomatic treatments—such as physical therapy, speech therapy, dietary advice regarding types of and preparation of foods—can be helpful. We emphasize that there is ongoing research, and often give the patient the names of persons who are carrying out therapeutic trials or offer the patient a chance to enter into a research program with which we are currently involved. We also provide the patient with information about available symptomatic treatment.

In spite of our original anxiety about this direct approach to the patient's illness, we know of only one patient who committed suicide after the diagnosis of ALS was established. He was one of several thousand patients on whom we have used this approach. This patient had previously had disk surgery for weakness of his legs. Unfortunately, his weakness progressed after surgery, and it became apparent that he had ALS. He was angry with the physicians who had not recognized his problem originally. Another physician who was a friend of his asked us to see him, and, in the interim, the patient received some psychiatric help. On arriving for his consultation, he informed us that he wanted us to tell him the truth about his illness, and he also stated that if it were ALS he would commit suicide. Unfortunately, the diagnosis of ALS was apparent, and after a complete evaluation we discussed the problem with him and with his physician friend in some detail. We offered him psychiatric help because it was obvious that he was seriously depressed. However, he and his friend decided to return home and, as he had threatened, he did commit suicide. It was our impression, however, that his depression antedated his ALS and that the ALS served only as a trigger.

The written information that we give patients covers much the same topics as the discussion but in greater depth and provides additional sources of information (for example, the *Brochure for Patients* from the Amyotrophic Lateral Sclerosis Society of America). We have observed that the patients always take this information with them. It is our observation that some of them do not use the information themselves, but we know that their families do.

In summary, our approach has been to tell the patient the truth and to allow the patient to set the limits on the discussion. We have chosen to do this by giving him or her an opportunity to talk with a physician and a nurse and by providing additional information in pamphlet form. We believe that by offering these patients an opportunity to learn about their disorder in a supportive situation in which they are able to voice their anxieties and their questions, first to the physician and then to a nurse, we have been able to help them learn to live with their disease in a more satisfactory fashion.

In this chapter, we have assumed the answers to a number of questions based on clinical impressions. We believe our approach has been helpful, and a limited preliminary effort to evaluate this approach has received positive responses from patients. We believe that the initial counseling of patients with ALS may have significant positive or negative therapeutic implications. Thus, we urge that additional attempts to evaluate the best approach to this important initial interview be undertaken.

REFERENCES

1. Aitken-Swan J, Easson EC: Reactions of cancer patients on being told their diagnosis. Br Med J 1:779–783, 1959

2. Hackett TP, Weisman AD: The treatment of the dying. Curr Psychiatr Ther 2:121–126, 1962

3. Kelly WD, Friesen SR: Do cancer patients want to be told? Surgery 27:822–826, 1950

4. Kübler-Ross E: *On Death and Dying.* New York, Macmillan Co, 1969

5. Mulder DW, Howard FM Jr: Patient resistance and prognosis in amyotrophic lateral sclerosis. Mayo Clin Proc 51:537–541, 1976

6. Novack DH, Plumer R, Smith RL, et al: Changes in physicians' attitudes toward telling the cancer patient. JAMA 241:897–900, 1979

7. Sinaki M, Mulder DW: Rehabilitation techniques for patients with amyotrophic lateral sclerosis. Mayo Clin Proc 53:173–178, 1978

8. Wilson JM: Should the patient be told the truth? Patient Counseling and Health Education 1:70–74, 1978

Commentary

Katharine M. Donohoe

Ms. Roelofs has identified an area of great concern to patients with the diagnosis of ALS. I would like to emphasize several points.

First, the *manner* in which the diagnosis is initially communicated may be as important as the *content.* The facts about ALS may be presented in a variety of ways, both verbal and written, as Ms. Roelofs has described. Assessment of the patient's readiness to learn is often difficult but, by the approach she outlines, most misconceptions can be clarified and most questions answered. Although there may still be questions that the patient does not ask, and answers that he or she does not fully comprehend, the supportive tone of the initial discussion will allow the patient to return for further clarification. The manner in which information is presented will affect the way in which the diagnosis is received by the patient. A good "manner" would entail a clear, honest presentation by a care provider who is perceived as a competent clinician, who allows for hope, and who confirms his or her caring attitude. The caring and the attitude of open awareness on the part of the care provider will enable the patient to return for additional information as he or she is ready for it. Providing literature may also help the patient and family review the information discussed during the first and subsequent interviews.

Second, patients ask many questions of, and confide in, health care providers other than the specialty physician or neurologist who makes the diagnosis. This confidant can be a family physician, lay person, nurse, or other professional. Ms. Roelofs, a nurse, cites her experience in dealing with the many questions that ALS patients ask. Nurses are viewed as being different from physicians, yet knowledgeable about health and illness. Approaching them may be less threatening to the patient, and they are often described as empathic listeners. These characteristics allow the patient the freedom to ask serious questions while maintaining the option of denying the information received. The confidant needs as much accurate information about ALS as the specialist can provide. Such persons can also benefit from the literature that the patient receives, for example, the pamphlet provided by the ALS Society of America.

Health care providers will need to answer questions as they arise throughout the course of the patient's illness. By providing nurses and others with adequate knowledge and support, we will decrease the nurse's anxiety (which might lead her to avoid the patient) and, thus, increase the quality of support for the patient. Therefore, I would advocate ongoing education for the patient, the family, *and* for any health care providers who might interact with the ALS patient (e.g., public health nurses, physical therapists, social workers, family physicians, and lay counselors).

I am certain that we do not know the best way to respond to all the questions that these patients might ask. Additional research may be needed to help us learn how to present the factual information to patients and their families in the best possible manner.

Christine Cassel

Whether or not to tell the truth to a patient with a fatal disease is one of the most important ethical issues in the health professional–patient relationship. I agree strongly with the approach that has just been described. Clearly, further studies need to be done because almost all of our discussions on the subject are theoretic or anecdotal. Most of the literature on telling patients the truth has concerned cancer and cancer patients. It has been pointed out that doctors have strong assumptions about what will happen to patients if they are told the truth about their disease, especially if the disease has a poor prognosis. However, there have been no studies to substantiate these assumptions, which are often based on the doctor's own conscious and unconscious feelings.

Dr. Donald Oken polled a series of internists in 1961 regarding the question of disclosure of prognosis (2). He found that 65%–90% of them would not tell the patient of the diagnosis of a fatal disease and, yet, when he asked them if they would want to be told, 80% of them said "yes." A recent study shows that this attitude has changed significantly since that time (1).

It is important, I think, to explore further the reasons for this discrepancy. The training in medical schools is only one place to begin trying to change these attitudes. There is a prevalent opinion, as mentioned previously, that if the patient is told of a fatal disease, he or she will become depressed and is more likely to commit suicide. Yet there are no studies showing that this actually occurs. In fact, Cicely Saunders, who is Medical Director of St. Joseph's Hospice in London, reports that *uncertainty* about diagnosis more often than knowledge leads to despair. Knowledge seems to give the patient some sense of power over what is happening and some sense of working together with the medical team in his or her care.

The issue of truth telling is very closely related to the issue of patients' rights, a phrase we are hearing more of these days. I think that almost all philosophers in the field would agree that the right of the patient to know as much as possible about his or her disease is so strong that the burden of proof lies with the physician who decides not to tell. A paternalistic attitude often begins with the projection of the physician's or the family's own fears of what might happen to the patient if the patient is told the truth. We cannot listen only to the families either in this regard. Except in extreme, mitigating circumstances, it is the patient's right to know as much, and as little, as we ourselves do, because it is his or her body and his or her own fate. The patient should be given every chance to let us know if, when, and how he or she wants to know the truth. Wherever there are rights there are usually duties that correspond to those rights. If the patient has a right to know, the physician and the health care team have a duty to tell him or her. Along with the duty of disclosure goes the duty to continue support, both emotional support and symptomatic support. This is the one chance we have to sustain the patient's hope without telling lies.

I think that the outcome of the interview has a great deal to do with *how* that information is transmitted. The main thing that causes despair in patients is the feeling of abandonment. This is something that sociologists have written about. If we project the despair we feel because of our powerlessness to cure this disease, the patients are going to pick up on that and likewise feel it. Despair and hopelessness are extremely contagious. If we have some positive feeling about what we *can* do for them, and, of course, never absolutely deny hope, we can create a better emotional atmosphere for both ourselves as health professionals and for the patients. At the same time, we are obliged not to give them a false hope or to deceive ourselves with Polyanna-ish optimism. It is a very delicate job, and it needs to be done with careful coordination of everyone involved.

The truth in modern medicine is that we can never say "never." I think everyone would agree with that. But, it is very important not to use that fact as a way of skirting the issue and saying: "Well, maybe tomorrow we will find a cure and everything will be all right." I think that it is important to admit our own ignorance and in that way to make the patients our partners in the endeavor so that their hope, although it may not be for themselves, may be for some larger sense of progress.

REFERENCES

1. Novack DH, Plumer R, Smith RL, et al: Changes in physicians' attitudes toward telling the cancer patient. JAMA 241:897–900, 1979

2. Oken D: What to tell cancer patients: A study of medical attitudes. JAMA 175:1120–1128, 1961

H. Richard Tyler

As physicians, we attempt to care for patients and hope to cure their diseases. Some of us have the conviction that we are here to cure all diseases. If the physician assumes that he or she will cure the patient with ALS, the patient and the physician both become distraught as the disease worsens.

At the present stage of our knowledge of this disorder, the true role of the physician is to serve as a counselor. He or she explores with the patient the options that will allow the patient to live with the disease with as much dignity and hope as possible. If, in addition, the physician is carrying out clinical trials for the treatment of ALS, management becomes much easier for patient and physician. A valid clinical trial is a real expression of hope.

H. Eames Bishop

It was almost six years ago that my wife was diagnosed as having ALS. I was told at that time (and have since learned that most other ALS patients' spouses are told the same by the diagnosing neurologist):

1. Your spouse will be gone within three years.
2. There is currently no known cure.
3. There is no organized research to find the cure.
4. We are not sure how many persons have the disease.
5. No heroic endeavors are justified.
6. Take your spouse home and make her as comfortable as possible until her time is up.

Six years have now gone by, and the disease has run its full course: she is totally paralyzed, on life-support equipment, and cannot swallow or speak. She communicates by eye movement; she is in no pain; she is mobile with a wheelchair equipped for air and can be transported by van to her children's homes and elsewhere; she still runs her home; she is a mentally alert, functioning individual; and she has hope that medical science somehow, some day, will help her to increase her functioning capacity.

Mary Frances has a chance because she has not given up, nor has her family or doctor given up. We have been blessed with dedicated nursing, and, at long last, a vigorous research effort to find the cause and cure has been mounted. Moreover, clinicians now know that the symptoms of the disease can be treated successfully and that a prognosis of early demise is not warranted.

The mail received by the Amyotrophic Lateral Sclerosis Society of America and my personal contact with patients reveal hundreds of ALS patients living 5, 10, and even 25 years after diagnosis. Robert Dicus, the Board Chairman of ALSSOA, has lived with the disease for 17 years and is a vital, productive individual.

I am convinced that the original prognosis of ALS by the neurologist should be softened significantly. The prognosis should allow for a measure of hope. That little bit of hope, a slim sliver, can make a marked difference in the life span of an ALS victim as well as in the quality of the remaining life.

9 Home Care

David Goldblatt

Katharine M. Donohoe

Kathleen Landon

The clinical course, physical and functional abilities, and coping mechanisms vary a great deal among patients with amyotrophic lateral sclerosis. In spite of this variability, several features of care remain constant:

1. Most patients will live at home and can be cared for there.
2. They will have to adapt to many changes and crises.
3. They will come in contact with many agencies and care providers.
4. There will be a continuous educational process throughout the course of illness.

The existing literature on chronic debilitating illness focuses primarily on the care of the cancer patient, who rarely has the physical and functional impairments that ALS patients have, or not for such a long time (3, 5). The duration of ALS, with its resultant changes and constant stress, can severely tax the resources of the patient and his or her family. There are other changes in addition to the physical and functional disabilities. One study identified the major fears of a group of chronically ill and dying cancer patients as abandonment by others, pain, and shortness of breath (1). Other concerns were losing autonomy, being

---

The essay on home care was written entirely by K.M. Donohoe; case report 1 is by D. Goldblatt, case report 2 by K.M. Donohoe, and case report 3 by K. Landon.

disfigured and physically repulsive, being a burden, and not knowing the future of their families. Many of these fears are undoubtedly shared by patients with ALS.

In view of all these factors, how do we meet the patient's need for comprehensive home care? We must begin with family assessment. Most providers of health care concentrate on the diagnostic process: historic, clinical, and laboratory findings that culminate in the diagnosis of a health problem. But family, social, and psychosocial problems also need careful review if the correct type of intervention is to be prescribed (6, 9).

Smilkstein describes a system of family assessment during a period of crisis that can be applied to patients with ALS and their families (6). It includes: assessment of communication patterns; present illness and adaptations; past history of illness and adaptation; review of social, cultural, educational, financial, and health status; and the family's functional status in the areas of commitment, maturity, differentiation, and intimacy. Previous experience with caring for patients at home and the family's reaction to it also provide valuable information.

Before deciding that home care really is best for a given family, one should evaluate the members of the family *at home*. In our practice, the nurse clinician and patient-service coordinator usually make these visits. Public health nurses with extensive experience or educational preparation in the care of neurologic patients are of invaluable assistance. The evaluation of family functioning cannot be made on a single visit, but attention to specific areas of functioning can provide valuable clues. In the home visit, we try to define:

1. Current health status of patient and family.

2. Need for equipment, community services (public health nurse, organized home care), and home renovation.

3. Learning needs regarding all aspects of the illness and patient care.

4. Effectiveness of previous teaching, particularly with regard to physical therapy, pulmonary care, and the use of equipment.

5. Dietary adequacy and compliance with instructions for medications.

6. Family functioning, communication, and home supports.

The visit also increases bonding and trust, showing that someone cares and has not given up in spite of the patient's progressive illness. If our assessment leads us to believe that home care is feasible even if it will be difficult, we approach the patient and the family to help or to reassure them that it will succeed.

The four themes of feasibility of home care, crisis management, continuity and coordination of care, and educational needs are intermingled, and each will receive more or less attention at different stages of illness.

FEASIBILITY OF HOME CARE

Home care *feasibility* means that the problems or major obstacles to home care identified by the patient, family, or health-care provider can be solved. It means that even when the solution to a problem is denied or deferred, the obstacle does not create enough change in the patient/family system to necessitate taking the patient out of the system. The home visit and family and physical assessments are tools to discover which problems are treatable. The intervention should be based on these assessments and can range from obtaining a piece of equipment to adding a night nurse or placing the patient in extended or "respite" care. The patient and his or her family make the choice. Our job is to give them as much support and information as they need to allow them to continue as they have planned.

Other major considerations determining the feasibility of home care are derived from the family assessment. A spouse who has a chronic illness or is the sole support of the family may not be able to provide the physical care that the patient may need. A lack of nearby extended-family members may also be a problem. The availability or lack of a family member with nursing education or previous experience in caring for patients in the home can be a major variable. Identifying all the positive and negative factors requires teamwork, as does arriving at the decision that, *at this time, home care can work.*

CRISIS MANAGEMENT

A crisis can occur whenever there is change. It can be precipitated by physical or emotional and social factors. Some crises can be anticipated, but it is important to remember that a crisis is dependent on the family's own definition of an event (7). For example, crises can develop over anything from changes in daily activities to poor nutrition or respiratory impairment. Often, home visits can detect impending problems, such as exhaustion in the care provider or the need for equipment and services. By making clear plans as to *whom* the patient can call with questions and problems, needless worry can be alleviated. Many patients have more than one illness and should understand the responsibilities of each care provider—neurologist, family physician, and nurse (8). A contingency plan, particularly in regard to problems that must be resolved rapidly, should be developed in advance. Listing the telephone numbers of ambulance services, care providers, and information services is a basic aspect of such a plan. Our patients can call a special 24-hour answering service to obtain the assistance of persons who are familiar with them.

CONTINUITY AND COORDINATION OF CARE

The previously independent ALS patient will have to face a series of losses throughout the course of his or her illness. Abandonment by care providers only heightens feelings of loss and hopelessness. The results of a survey in a neuromuscular specialty clinic indicate the need for maintaining continuity of care. Over half of the patients sampled did not have a consistent source of care other than the specialty clinic (2). Many patients said that, although they have a family doctor or have had one in the past, they do not have the architectural access, financial means, or interest to continue the relationship. Abandonment can also occur when the patient or care provider feels that there is nothing to offer the patient in terms of care or palliation. Supportive care, emphasized in this volume and elsewhere (4), needs to be communicated to the patient and to other care providers. Several sources point out that the *quality* of the time spent with the patient is far more important than the *quantity*, particularly in view of the emotional and social isolation of patients with a chronic debilitating illness (1). This may mean listening to a series of frustrating problems that may often seem to defy solution. The consistency and perseverance of all care providers, be they family members or professionals, are important aspects of dealing with frustration and hopelessness.

Coordination of patient care requires knowledge of community services, including financial assistance, transportation, home care, respite and day care, social and emotional support groups. There are many problems with today's complex health-care system. One of the most often cited is that available community services are poorly utilized—often because the health care providers do not know enough about them. Red tape can also slow delivery of needed services.

Another problem is fragmentation and lack of coordination among existing care providers who may be aware of community supports and patient needs. Someone must communicate with the multitude of professionals (public health nurses, doctors, therapists, etc.) as they need to be educated, supported, and advised. These people may be giving conflicting messages to the patient and to each other.

EDUCATIONAL NEEDS

Many families will never have experienced the problems that can accompany ALS, a disease that requires a tremendous amount of physical care and utilization of techniques such as suctioning, pulmonary care, tube feeding, physiotherapy, and the use of equipment such as Hoyer lifters and suction machines. Use of these techniques and devices requires continuous reinforcement and support. In view of the technical care required, we often overlook the importance of teaching the family how to provide basic comfort.

Technical care requires additional knowledge and expertise, and in the setting of acute illness can be more rewarding. Comfort care takes energy, ingenuity, patience, and creativity. It takes experience and skill to be able to teach a family how to position the patient comfortably, how to achieve basic hygiene, how to exercise a sore limb to avoid pain. There are books written on such aspects of care and diagrams to give the patient after the office demonstration. Home visits continue to be the best way of teaching both comfort and technical aspects of care. Videotapes may also be a method of demonstrating new techniques and are unique because they are standardized and can be repeated as necessary. The patient and his or her family need extensive education about the disease process, but the pace of the educational effort is usually set by the patient. The provision of literature opens up many questions and informs the patient about societies such as the Amyotrophic Lateral Sclerosis Society of America (ALSSOA) and their services.

To summarize, we believe that by using the described assessment and educational techniques, by planning for crisis and change, and by directing attention to continuity and coordination, home care can be made feasible.

CASE REPORTS

To examine the ways in which the principles of home care can be successfully or unsuccessfully applied, we will present three cases. The first is an example of failure for home care. The second is an example of an intermediate or somewhat ambiguous situation in which the patient moved in and out of an institutional setting and was at the center of conflicting opinion as to where she would be cared for best. The third patient remained at home with his family until his death. We will try to identify the principal factors that determine how a given patient can be cared for best.

Patient 1

Daniel is a 30-year-old man who expects to spend the rest of his life in a Veterans Hospital about 100 miles from his home. He sleeps in a large ward. In the bed opposite his, an old man with a stocking cap pulled down over his eyes talks to himself incessantly. Daniel is largely confined to a wheelchair and his speech is impaired, but he is mentally alert and fully cognizant of his situation. At home, he has a wife and three little girls, aged 2, 4, and 6. He sees them about once a month, although their visits may be prevented by bad weather in the winter. Daniel and his wife were high school sweethearts from the age of 16, and they married at 20. After a separation imposed by his service overseas in the Army, he returned home and got a job in the factory where his mother worked. He was steadily employed, and they were able to buy their own house. His wife was pregnant with their youngest child when he first began to notice that a bowling ball would slip from his hand.

When Dan became disabled, it seemed, at first, as if the family were doing everything right: his mother-in-law used money from an unexpected inheritance to build a ramp from the patio, remodel the sunporch into a downstairs bedroom, and add a larger bathroom with a safety rail for the tub. He had a hospital bed with side rails, an overbed table, a raised toilet seat, and a wheelchair with a tray and gel cushion.

It was only after he entered the hospital that we realized fully what had caused Dan to leave his home. He had been unaccepting of his illness and increasingly frustrated as he shifted from one job to another in the factory, trying to find something he could still do. He thought of himself as a provider and as a disciplinarian to his children. When he could no longer punish them physically, he felt that he had failed as a father, and his wife agreed. He kept trying to walk, refused to use his wheelchair, and fell frequently. He said he would like to go to live with his mother and let his children think he was dead.

While Dan was in the service, his wife, alone and insecure, had attempted suicide. Now she again felt insecure, and they quarreled. Dan had never had an interest in sex, and felt more comfortable with men. His wife and her mother wondered if he were bisexual.

In the Veterans Hospital, Dan seemed happy; he had his CB radio, bowled by using a ramp for the ball, and went on outings where he enjoyed the food and the companionship of other patients. On visits home, he quickly ran out of things to talk about. It was not long before his wife was "dating," and trying to gather the courage to tell him that her new boyfriend had moved in with her and the children.

Clearly, the interpersonal relationships in this marriage were poor before the illness began, and ALS served only to intensify the strain. We helped to provide the mechanics of home care, the physical equipment and techniques, but nobody took any direct measures to prevent the breakup of the marriage. The failure of our initial family assessment was apparent. With proper counseling and support, perhaps this couple might have been able to stay together. As it was, the thousands of dollars spent on remodeling the home were wasted. The failure of home care was a secondary result of a failed marriage.

Patient 2

Theresa had symptoms of ALS for three years before her death. The diagnosis was established about a year before she died at the age of 38. This relatively short period of her life was one of great personal, physical, and emotional change for both the patient and her family.

Theresa was a single woman, the oldest of three children. Her medical history began when she was 13, when she developed insulin-dependent diabetes mellitus. She remained relatively healthy and, after completing her education, was employed as a secretary-bookkeeper. When she was 20, her father died suddenly of a myocardial infarction. Her mother developed a brain tumor when Theresa was 34 and died a year later. The mother lived at home throughout her illness and required an increasing amount of care, which Theresa provided. Theresa's younger sister, who is married, helped. When their mother died, Theresa lived on in the family home.

In its early stages, Theresa's illness was considered to be diabetic neuropathy. It progressed until her hands became useless and she was largely wheelchair-bound and dependent in all activities of daily living. She was admitted to the rehabilitation unit of the county hospital, a chronic care facility, where, after two months of intensive efforts, she gained some independence, although she did not gain strength. A repeat neurologic examination suggested that ALS was the proper diagnosis.

Eleven months before she died, Theresa returned home with the support of organized home care, which provided a home health aide, physiotherapy, and a community health nurse who coordinated these services. Theresa felt that the home health aide did not have enough to do and, in general, she was happy only with the physical therapy. She said that she would rather have her boyfriend care for her, as he had the year before, with her sister as backup. Although she was alone during the day, she was able to manage with the assistance he provided when he returned from work. Traveling in a van, she and her boyfriend were able to take a three-month vacation in Florida. They returned seven months before she died.

When she returned, she continued to live with her boyfriend, who was an alcoholic. Theresa said, "He's wonderful when he's sober but I'm afraid of him when he's drunk." During her visits to the clinic, she discussed her problems, which included difficulty in sleeping because she could not roll over in bed without help. An alternating pressure mattress somewhat alleviated that problem. She also had pain during intercourse because of spasm in the adductor muscles of her legs. This problem was managed by a frank discussion of positioning and by use of diazepam (Valium).

Theresa became increasingly apprehensive about living with her drunken, unreliable boyfriend and began to plan for the possibility that she would live with her married sister. They obtained a Hoyer lifter and a hospital bed with these plans in mind and, during visits to the clinic, both were able to air their feelings of insecurity and doubt. Joan, the sister, was fearful of being unable to provide care and about the effect of Theresa's progression on her children. Joan and her husband attended a marriage encounter, and she felt that this improved her relationship with her husband and her ability to communicate in general. Finally, in spite of her ambivalence, Theresa put her house up for sale in June 1978, four months before she died, and went on vacation with her sister and family for the summer. The fears that they had both expressed subsided in this setting. The children helped to feed and transfer Theresa, and the oldest gave Theresa her daily insulin injection. They installed an intercom system to let Theresa make her needs known immediately.

They returned home about a month before Theresa died and planned to buy a larger home to accommodate Theresa. Shortly thereafter, she was admitted to the hospital because of her breathing problems. She spent the last month of her life in the neurology unit. There was a legitimate difference of opinion among the staff as to whether she should stay in the hospital. On admission, and intermittently throughout her hospitalization, she was short of breath, uncomfortable, and anxious. After she had stabilized somewhat, each time her discharge was discussed, the idea was met with considerable resistance from the house staff and nurses. She expressed the desire to die and refused respiratory aids, but was afraid of suffocation. Her vital capacity fell to 340 ml. A methadone-amphetamine mixture helped to ease her anxieties during the final days of her life.

When one of us (K.D.) visited Joan, Theresa's sister, several months after Theresa's death, the conversation helped to put Theresa's illness into perspective: Joan felt that having taken care of their terminally ill mother together enabled her and Theresa to speak freely about Theresa's increasing needs. Joan accepted the fact that Theresa had to make the decisions, and they were discussed openly. Another positive factor was Joan's ability to share her feelings and to receive support from her husband—an ability she attributed to the marriage encounter they had attended.

Joan also named the Muscular Dystrophy Association and the ALS Clinic as major supportive factors. Theresa and Joan's previous interaction with other community agencies was hampered by architectural barriers, large volumes of paperwork, equipment arriving too late to be of use, and lack of communication and coordination regarding financial planning. They appreciated the ability of the Muscular Dystrophy Association and the ALS Clinic to meet their needs for services and provide information immediately.

Finally, Joan felt the major problem Theresa faced was her fear of abandonment. She had a caring family in the strictest sense. She was single and had no formal bond or commitment from her boyfriend, whose care of her was erratic and did not inspire confidence. Theresa repeatedly stated that she felt she was a burden. Her previous experience, caring for her dying mother, emphasized the responsibility of caring for someone around the clock. This colored her perception of her sister's taking on the task of caring for her and caused feelings that this was a burdensome responsibility. Her sister felt just the opposite way: she felt that her ability to participate made the whole experience a positive thing.

An additional aspect bears discussion. As is usually appropriate, discharge plans were started soon after Theresa's admission to the hospital. Joan was prepared for the change in the amount of care Theresa would need at home, and all support services, from equipment to organized home care, were mobilized. Nursing home placement was not an option they wanted to consider, but the topic was discussed. A hospice center in Rochester is in the planning stages, but, at present, 24-hour skilled nursing coverage for terminally ill patients is provided for only short periods of time (and is dependent on insurance coverage). No one was certain what course Theresa's illness would take. Therefore, taking this option was not advocated by the staff. Instead, the staff tried to make her hospital room more homey by encouraging frequent visitors, home movies, voice tapes from relatives and the minister, special foods from home, and maintenance of her routines for personal care. Our hospital believes in the primary nursing system, in which the same nurse provides, directs, and evaluates a patient's care from admission to discharge. In this way, the nurses provide continuity as well.

The more Theresa's weakness progressed, the more reluctant she became to go home. This reluctance was increased by some of the house staff, who felt death was imminent. (She lived 33 more days.) The choice between home and hospital was a difficult one. Theresa felt confident with the care she received and enjoyed our frequent visits and those of the house staff, nursing staff, friends, and family. If, at the end, she had been given the same confidence in the care she would receive at home, home care would have been feasible.

Theresa was shifted about during her illness from her living arrangement with her boyfriend, to the community hospital for chronic care, to her sister's home, and then to the university hospital, where she remained for prolonged terminal care, although that was not the most appropriate place to live out her last month of life. In retrospect, we could see that Theresa had been given conflicting messages from the many people who took care of her concerning the appropriateness of each of these various situations while she was in it. On the other hand,

Theresa's own ability to express her thoughts and exchange feelings with others helped her to overcome the drawbacks of what might otherwise have been inappropriate home situations—depending on a boyfriend or on a sister already busy with her own family. She made the most of the time she had left, making her physical situation less important, and we remember her admiringly for that.

Patient 3

Harry, a barber, was diagnosed as having ALS in May 1977. He died 15 months later at the age of 63. Harry had two married daughters and one son. His wife was a nurse at the state school for retarded children in the small community in which they lived. Harry also worked at the state school to supplement his income. The fact that both worked for the state and had Blue Cross–Blue Shield health insurance with major medical benefits proved very helpful when help was needed for home care.

After his diagnosis had been established, one of Harry's daughters wrote to the national office of the Muscular Dystrophy Association in New York City asking for information on where they could go for help and what treatment, if any, was available. Subsequently, he became a patient in the ALS Clinic at Strong Memorial Hospital. The clinic is sponsored by the Muscular Dystrophy Association.

As Patient Service Coordinator for the Muscular Dystrophy Association, one of us (K.L.) was able to obtain for the family various pieces of equipment, including a suction machine, a wheelchair with headrest, a hospital bed, a Hoyer lifter, a commode, and an alternating-pressure pad. These items and the patient's orthopedic collars were provided at no cost to the family.

The first home visit took place about four months before Harry died. He was a constant care. He could no longer talk, drooled constantly, and had fits of crying. He frequently requested that his neck brace be removed or changed. He could stand with help but it was almost too much for his wife to pull him up. It was obvious that they needed a Hoyer lifter. They were eager to have it but fearful of using it. The Patient Service Coordinator promised to return to demonstrate the equipment and also provided measurements and suggestions for a ramp which was needed for the wheelchair.

The living room became Harry's bedroom. He stayed in the family room most of the time so that he was not cut off from family activities. He went for rides and shopping until the last few months of his life. One of his daughters, a teacher for special education, made a speaking board for him. He used a pointer held in his teeth to spell out words. For the last few weeks of his life, one of his daughters moved back home to share the burden of his care.

Harry knew from the beginning that he would die of his disease. His speech was affected first, and this caused much frustration. He and his friends were embarrassed by this, as they thought he had taken to drinking. He accepted his disease and, in the first stages, helped to solve many of his own problems. However, at a later stage, his personality changed, and he became very demanding and irritable.

Progression of illness was very rapid. Through the skillful care of his wife and the help she was able to obtain from the family and from home health care aids, he remained at home. His medical insurance policy paid 80% of the cost of having a registered nurse at night. Registered nurses were hard to find in their small community, and, finally, a note from their doctor allowed them to obtain the services of a licensed practical nurse. A physical therapist visited the home once, but there was not much she could offer in the final stages.

His constant demands to have his limbs moved or to have his collar taken off and then put back on would probably have been too much for a woman weaker than his wife. Her training as a nurse, the support of her children, and her being able to obtain nurses for the night so that she could rest all helped Harry's wife to keep her husband at home.

It was hard for many of his family and friends to see the progression of the disease. They stopped going to see him, and, in fact, for the last few weeks the family asked people not to come, and it was easier for everyone.

Harry died with his wife and daughter by his side, neither of them aware that the time had come. His death was easy. There was no last struggle to breathe. The family expressed a sense of relief not to see him suffer further.

After his death, Harry's wife said that the support she had received from the clinic and its personnel helped her to survive. The equipment, suggestions, and moral support were offered before she needed them, so that she always knew what was available.

Three months after Harry's death, the patient service coordinator and the nurse clinician met with Harry's wife and his daughter, Susan. They were very enthusiastic about the visit, which occupied most of the morning. It was their feeling that they had been able to handle the problems that the disease imposed because they were a close family. Specific mention was made of having members of the family living at home to assist with Harry's physical care and social activities, as well as maintaining the home and yard. The biggest barrier was "figuring out the system" of health care and services in their area, particularly after his diagnosis but before he came to the ALS Clinic, and when they needed home health services.

Because they lived 15 miles from Rochester, finding an available nighttime nurse to relieve them was a constant struggle. They felt strongly that if they had not had family and home health aides and nurses, they would not have been able to manage. Being able to have the necessary equipment (e.g., suction machine, hospital bed) *when* they needed it was cited as a big plus, as was the constant support we gave them. They independently volunteered to assist other patients and families in any way possible, including participation in our research. They suggested one additional support, an encounter group, to help both patients and families deal with the emotional strain. We will try to get one started in our area in the near future.

It was also interesting to note that during our last visit, Harry's wife ended our conversation by saying, "I don't think I could have gone on any longer." Our personal opinion is that, yes, she could have gone on. This family had all the ingredients needed to help her cope with a severely disabled patient, and she could not have let him go to be cared for in a place other than his own home.

The idea that a sick person should be taken care of by his family at home is certainly nothing new (5, 9). But, with all the technologic advances of modern medicine, is the home *still* the best place to keep someone with ALS, a chronic, progressive illness? We believe that it is, and our view appears to coincide with the view of most health care providers and families. For the victims of ALS in this country, there is no widely developed, satisfactory alternative to home care.

REFERENCES

1. Cassem NH, Stewart RS: Management and care of the dying patient. Int J Psychiatry Med 6:293–304, 1975

2. Donohoe KM: Primary health care delivery in the specialty clinic. Presented at the American Nurses Association Council of Nurse Researchers Meeting, Health Promotion: Illness Prevention. San Antonio, Texas, December 7, 1979

3. Garfield CA (Editor): *Psychosocial Care of the Dying Patient.* New York, McGraw-Hill, 1978

4. Goldblatt D: Treatment of amyotrophic lateral sclerosis. In *Advances in Neurology,* Vol 17. Edited by RC Griggs, RT Moxley. New York, Raven Press, 1977, pp 265–283

5. Kassakian MG, Bailey LR, Rinkar M, et al: The cost and quality of dying: A comparison of home and hospital. Nurse Pract 4:18–23, 1979

6. Kolb LC, Crawford M, Damrosch D: *Psychosocial Aspects of Terminal Care.* New York, Columbia University Press, 1972

7. Smilkstein G: The family in trouble: How to tell. *J Fam Pract* 2:19–24, 1975

8. Strauss A: *Chronic Illness and the Quality of Life*. St Louis, CV Mosby, 1975

9. Weller C: Home health care. NY State J Med 78:1957–1961, 1978

Commentary

William R. Kennedy

What are the roles of the physician and the neurologist in the care of patients with amyotrophic lateral sclerosis? What are the roles of other health care professionals? The answers depend on our individual professional situations, talents, and personalities. Some of us are probably taking very different approaches to the care of our patients, but probably the approach of each of us is consistent from patient to patient. Notice that I have not mentioned the patient or the family in determining what our roles will be. I think that they accept whatever we think our role should be, and they modify it only slightly. With them, it is a one-time experience, so they are not exactly sure what we should be doing.

I am only going to answer the question for myself. I am a university-based physician with an unusually heavy commitment to diagnosis and laboratory research in neuromuscular disease. I am not in frequent contact with patients in their home environment. In this situation, I cannot in good conscience undertake the primary care of the ALS patient. I have taken the position of friend and advocate for the patient and the family, equally. If the patient does not have a physician that will be available when needed for medical care, I find one. If the patient is still working and has problems with his or her job, or if the spouse has problems with his or her job, I will make phone calls or attend a meeting to help. When the problem of finding nursing assistance arises, or the necessity of finding devices or funding for such, I take on that task. I do not assist with the use of the devices. I do not prescribe for the patient or for the family; I do not act as their physician. I do talk to the physician they have found, or I have found for them; I apprise him or her of my self-assigned role, and I offer my assistance and advice. I answer, as fully as I can, the questions raised by patients and their families concerning the disease and the many problems that arise, always attempting to leave hope, but never false hope. If you raise false hope, you are usually found out. I think what I consider to be my most important or useful function is serving as intermediary at family meetings in the home. For some reason, it seems that the patient, spouse, or children (usually teenagers) will ask me questions that apparently are not brought out in family conversations. For example, a teenager will ask, "What am I supposed to do when Dad is so irritable and wants his hands moved every three or four minutes?" This role does not require me to give many answers. The answers are better supplied by the family members. I relay, sharpen, direct, or try to interpret the question. I just facilitate the emergence of attitudes and questions. Frustrations are vented, solutions to frustrating problems are planned, and, eventually, I find out whether the solution is worked out on my next visit—when different questions or the same questions are raised.

I consider it important not to form an alliance with either the patient or the family, except on a very temporary basis on a specific issue. For example, an issue that always arises is: how much should a high school student help in the care of the patient or in household work? I don't know; each situation is different. I suppose the teenager should do enough to be of help to the family and, more importantly, enough to avoid developing a sense of guilt for not having helped—a guilt that could carry through for the rest of his or her life. However, I do not feel that so much should be required of teenagers that life is no longer fun, or that they would be isolated from their peer group. This is a heavy assignment for a teenager. It is usually his or her first major trial in life. It is one that is important to pass, because it will continue to affect his or her mental health.

Admittedly, my role as I outlined it is not the traditional role of a neurologist or of most physicians. Yours may be the more commonly visualized role, or you may play other parts. I hope we will find out what other people do. That would be helpful to me.

For the families that do decide to take care of the patient at home, I believe that my particular role has been helpful, but minor when compared with that of another person. That person, usually a woman, is a registered nurse, or licensed practical nurse, whom the family almost inevitably needs for at least eight hours a day. Next to the spouse, she is the essential figure. The family doctor and I provide only back-up for her decisions and a source of advice and added depth of knowledge about the disease. Finding a compatible nurse is essential and may require trying out 2, 5, 10, or more before the "right" one is found. I think Eames Bishop told me they were on number 30 and had found 2 of the 30 who were compatible with the family and the patient.

Some final points can be made. To me, it seems almost a necessity for the spouse to have a legitimate and pressing need to be out of the house for several hours a day. There are probably exceptions; we heard one in the case presentation of Harry. An eight-hour day seems ideal. Spiritual advisors are a tremendous help to give some meaning to this desperate struggle. They are as much a help for the family as for the patient. Any mental challenge that the patient can engage in with a realistic, almost certain chance of meaningful success is a tremendous help—again, as much to the family as to the patient. The family should continue its social life by having friends come into the home; the children's friends should continue to come to play, etc. Anyone who habitually comes in should be cultivated to continue to come, so that the disease is discussed openly. After a short, and admittedly traumatic, interval most people begin to relate directly to the patient as a person who is in trouble but, most importantly, as a person.

It would be very helpful for me to know what part others take in the care of the patient with amyotrophic lateral sclerosis.

Rita A. Roelofs

I believe we have been impressed that, for the patients we have been seeing, the families have seemed to be a definite support system. I do not believe we have noted that the families have fallen apart. While there may be an initial adaptation period, our overall impression is that the family gathers around in a supportive fashion, both emotionally and in coping with the physical needs of the patient with amyotrophic lateral sclerosis.

We have not felt that ALS itself posed any psychiatric problem, but we have observed that existing problems or situations were often intensified by the diagnosis and prognosis of the disease. Perhaps the patient and family could have continued to cope with the preexisting problem, but the development of ALS was a factor that moved the situation over the brink. This is when emotional help may be necessary.

I would like to comment on several other points. One is the fact that the availability of home care may be a real problem. Family members do need time off; they need to know where to go to obtain help in the care of the family member who has ALS. However, is such home care available? We have been speaking of large medical centers where there may be a sizable public health service or home health agency, but what about rural areas? Perhaps there may be a visiting nurse available for a brief weekly visit, but the family may need much more than that. What is available to them?

Another point has to do with the politics of health care. Even if home care is available, will the care providers that these families need be able to receive third-party reimbursement? If not, how will the families be able to pay for these services? This is an issue currently affecting nursing and other allied health professions.

Forbes H. Norris, Jr

Home care, with rare exceptions, impresses me as better than institutional care for patients with advanced paralysis due to amyotrophic lateral sclerosis. A major problem is finding a nearby physician who is willing to make house calls, who knows how to adjust and maintain a respirator (if one is necessary), and who can cope with the major psychologic problems. There are many difficult problems in home care, and each case has to be approached individually. I find that at least one house call, if the patient lives within a reasonable distance, helps a great deal in crisis management, because one can evaluate the patient's and the family's coping mechanisms better in the home than in the hospital. Is the home slovenly and the patient fending for himself, or is the home a well maintained place with good esprit de corps? One cannot always learn this from the family in the hospital, because people figuratively put on a mask when they come to the hospital in order to be seen at their best.

10 Psychiatric Aspects

Brian S. Gould

Despite considerable clinical interest in the personality of patients with amyotrophic lateral sclerosis, there has been little formal investigation in this area by psychiatrists. Many physicians working with ALS patients have the impression that these patients exhibit a certain personality type, the prominent characteristics of which are high life success, extreme self-control, and denial of psychic distress, even under the stress of advanced illness. Unfortunately, in most clinical centers, even those with a research orientation, this illness presents a small population for study; care is transient, and hence patients with ALS have been relatively ignored. New cases of ALS do not confront the practicing neurologist frequently, and typically do not stay in active treatment for long. Combined with the fact of a variable level of interest in the psychologic aspects of ALS on the part of the local neurologist, the opportunity for psychiatric involvement and study is often missed. Consequently, as of 1970, the psychiatric literature concerning the psychologic functioning of individuals with ALS consisted of only one paper, which reported a series of only 10 patients (4 of whom were inpatients at a psychiatric service) (2).

Using the national referral network of ALS patients to Pacific Medical Center, San Francisco, we attempted to replicate and expand this psychologic study in 1975. Our initial findings on 40 consecutive patients were published in 1977 (4). The data collected from this larger, more representative group, however, failed to support Brown and Mueller's earlier conclusions or to suggest any particular personality style typical of patients with ALS. Other findings related to the psychologic impact of severe neurologic disease did emerge, and these are being pursued further. Our series now consists of approximately 60 to 65 patients who have had psychiatric assessments.

Four major areas of psychiatric relevance have emerged: the psychologic experience of ALS, the "death and dying problem" in clinical care, psychiatric intervention within the family unit, and the physician's reactions to ALS.

THE PSYCHOLOGIC EXPERIENCE OF ALS

When ALS patients were examined for general psychopathology, internal versus external locus of control (utilizing Rotter's scale measuring belief in the personal control of events), depression as a feeling state, depression as a clinical syndrome, self-concept, and use of denial as a major defense mechanism, we could not establish any characteristics distinguishing them from other medically ill populations. Similarly, data collected on age, sex, social class, and (surprisingly) severity of illness also failed to show any correlative relationships. Nevertheless, clinical impressions related to the impact of terminal illness in general and data concerning length of illness as a major independent variable do warrant discussion.

One usually finds patients with ALS to be positively motivated, unexpectedly cheerful people who adhere to treatment reliably and who demonstrate compensatory maneuvers that are truly resourceful. It was not unusual in our series, for example, to encounter patients afflicted in the prime of life, unable to either speak or write, who still managed (despite the great effort required) to communicate with the outside world. Typically, they would still be expressing optimistic attitudes despite the burden of their deficits. Within a short time it became easy to understand the reputation these patients have for heroic stoicism.

On nondirected clinical interviews and psychologic testing, however, we witnessed a rather different type of response. These patients easily changed from their posture of positivism and spontaneously expressed considerable discouragement and dysphoria. This change was not so much an abandonment of a nongenuine "front" as it was the sharing of a deeper and more private level of concern; this level is revealed to those who take the time and express an interest in learning about it.

Weisman commented on this phenomenon in his elegant discussion of both the primitive and adaptive aspects of denial (9). What we commonly witness in ALS patients is the dropping of a *second-order denial* defense, which allows the individual to again draw inferences about the extensions and implications of the illness. (*First-order denial* is based on how a patient perceives—or fails to perceive—the primary facts of illness, while *third-order denial* is concerned with the image of death itself: denial of extinction.) The use of denial in such a way blocks awareness of the full impact of the illness and increases the individual's capacity to cope with the threat of annihilation and the inescapable fear of abandonment. It is therefore much more of a healthy, adaptive, dynamic *coping* mechanism than the rigid and primitive defense of denial is usually considered to be. This latter view of denial—as a short-lived period of shocked nonacceptance from which the patient should recover as soon as more mature defenses are mobilized—has been widely popularized among the clinicians of many disciplines by the work of Elisabeth Kubler-Ross (7). We found the common understanding of denial to be inadequate for explaining our clinical findings.

The ALS patients in our series frequently maintained a strategy of partial denial throughout their illness, but in a most healthy fashion. Reality was not denied as much as redefined; the most distressing, immutable aspects of the disease were not part of ordinary conscious functioning, and hope was maintained. Under safe conditions that allowed reflection and ventilation, however, the second-order denial was easily overridden; distressing awareness was allowed to enter the consciousness in a controlled fashion, and considerable dysphoric tension was discharged. At the conclusion of such a catharsis, we witnessed denial reassert itself, composure be regained, and the previous jaunty "I will persevere" attitude reestablish itself.

Clinicians who fail to appreciate the adaptive function of even flagrant denial run the risk of interfering with it by ill-considered or poorly timed confrontation and actually (albeit unintentionally) work against their patient's success.

Weisman further points out that while "a potential danger is apt to evoke denial, a common threatened danger is a *jeopardized relationship with a significant key person* (author's emphasis). Hence, the purpose of denial is not simply to avoid a danger, but to prevent loss of a significant relationship. This explains why patients tend to deny more to certain people than to others" (9). Paradoxically, they will often speak most candidly about their diagnosis and prognosis with the more peripheral members of the staff, i.e., those with less authority and involvement such as ward aides, medical students, and consultants.

Since an expression of doubt or discouragement could be considered to imply criticism or lack of confidence in the treatment or hospital, we found that it was seldom shared with family members, nurses, or house staff and almost never revealed to the neurologist in charge, but was easily mobilized by ourselves. The psychiatric consultant was perceived as a relatively superfluous and powerless figure (i.e., he or she made no treatment decisions), and therefore was in effect an insignificant person to whom the patient could risk revealing deeper concerns. It is a role with considerable potential for enhancing treatment effectiveness and worth considering even when the patient does not seem to require psychiatric consultation based on manifest psychopathology.

Although we found underlying despair to be more or less ubiquitous, only 22% of the initial study population warranted a diagnosis of clinical depression based on cognitive distortion with negative expectations, motivational disturbance, somatic dysfunction, or sustained change in emotional state. As a group, they responded well to a brief psychotherapeutic approach that combined both supportive and interpretative elements in the inpatient setting (5). Slightly fewer than half of these (10% of the studied population) also demonstrated "endogenomorphic features" (6) (anhedonia, early morning awakening, diurnal variation, or psychomotor retardation) predictive of "probable tricyclic antidepressant (TCA) responsiveness." We believe these ratios (20%–25% of patients with significant depression, 10% with TCA responsiveness) are typical of the ALS population overall. Other varieties of psychopathology were rare and irregular.

An unanticipated and highly provocative finding was the relationship among duration of illness, anniversary events, and locus of control. *Locus of control* can be defined as the quality of seeing oneself as either the mover of events or the victim/beneficiary of events controlled by external forces. It is commonly considered to be a psychologic trait that is relatively constant for an individual personality. Clinical findings such as ours, however, suggest that one's perception of control-dominance is more fluid, being influenced by life events such as serious illness, and is therefore more of a transient state than a fixed characteristic.

The ALS population yielded data suggestive of a three-phase, bimodal distribution of scores for locus of control. Those patients who were within a year of initial diagnosis scored as *externalizers.* We interpreted this as indicating that their confidence was invested in medicines, doctors, and hospitals. "I will follow medical instructions and get well."

As the first anniversary passes without cure, however, there is a shift into *internality:* "If I am going to beat this thing, I will have to do it myself." Although treatment compliance is maintained, year 2 of illness is frequently characterized by intense personal effort to maintain activities, exercises, nutrition, etc., and patients often scout out new experts and treatment programs on their own.

With the passing of the second anniversary date without cure, however, there seems to be a shift back toward a perception of external control. This time though, it is in a direction of existential fatalism or religious faith—"I've done all I can, my fate is in God's hands now." Survival to successive anniversaries serves to bolster hope but does not significantly influence locus of control scores.

Although we would like to follow a number of individuals longitudinally to confirm the existence of these shifts (hypothesized from studying subpopulations homogeneous for length of illness), we believe this three-phase pattern to be of great potential importance. If confirmed in patients with ALS and other chronic progressive diseases, it suggests that length of illness must be a controlled variable in future studies of psychologic adaptation to medical illness (it seldom is at present) and that a patient's perception of locus of control—a critical personality characteristic with high impingement on attitude, mood, and treatment motivation—will vary in a regular, predictable way.

THE DEATH AND DYING PROBLEM

Amyotrophic lateral sclerosis is a fatal illness. Patients with this disease are therefore subjected to all the activities engendered by the new interest in the dying patient (1, 3, 7–9). Although this reappraisal of our attitudes and treatment of patients with terminal disease has had undeniably positive benefits, it has also suffered from elements of faddism, reductionism, and glamorization. The glorification of death as a "special" life event may itself represent a cultural reaction formation against our own overwhelming fear of it, which is not much different from our previous avoidance of the subject. Weisman again cautions us that the disruption of personal relationships by severe illness causes more psychologic distress than does the "spectre of death itself" (9).

Approaching all fatally ill patients as if their eventual death were the central concern is a fashionable conceit that robs the patient of individuality, and even identity. We have found that most of the current recommendations for "death counseling" are at best imprecise and at worst frankly inappropriate for patients with ALS.

Since the publication of Dr. Kubler-Ross's watershed book in 1969, cancer death has served as the medical model for all major studies of terminality (7). We feel that much of what is now "understood" about death and dying, while true for cancer, is simply not applicable to other terminal diseases; ALS is an excellent case in point.

While cancer is so well known as a terminal illness as to be almost a synonym for it (leading many practitioners to find a euphemistic diagnosis to avoid patient panic), ALS remains almost totally obscure to the general public. The newly diagnosed ALS patient usually has no personal knowledge of the disease's major symptoms or prognosis. In contrast to the newly diagnosed cancer patient, who immediately confronts a "death sentence," the ALS patient has an uncontaminated psychologic field in which fantasies of treatment and cure can develop, take root, and grow before the truth is learned. Contemplation of death comes later, as a second-stage phenomenon.

The cancer patient is often asymptomatic or at least untroubled at the time of diagnosis; a spot on a chest film, a small lump, or a spot of blood may be the only sign of malfunction—abstract, seemingly trivial, but fatal. The ALS patient, on the other hand, has sought evaluation because of disturbing symptoms, usually limb weakness or dysarthria/dysphagia. The illness is "real" from the start and, again, less likely to produce terror.

The course of the cancer patient is typically complicated by considerable ambivalence toward the treatment: chemotherapy and radiation produce massive iatrogenic secondary illness, surgery is mutilating, and there is often considerable preconscious rage at the physician(s) who failed to make the diagnosis early and give the patient a "better chance." Much of Dr. Kubler-Ross's renowned five-stage defensive behavior (denial, anger, bargaining, depression, and acceptance) seems engendered, or at least potentiated, by the conflicts imposed by this intensely ambivalent relationship with the treatment itself. In ALS, treatment is either flatly unavailable or discouraged as ineffectual. Rather than feeling ambivalent, patients feel fortunate if they can make their way to a research center to receive experimental treatment. In almost all cases, the drugs and procedures are relatively benign with few side effects and limited invasiveness. Even where treatment is completely ineffective, we still observe dramatic positive placebo effects from the clinical interest, general hospital care, and aggressive physical therapy. This beneficial psychologic impact is in marked contrast to the impact of therapy on the cancer patient, in whom the rigors of treatment can cause severe psychologic distress which, in turn, can become the major factor limiting treatment tolerance.

Finally, the longitudinal course of the cancer patient is usually one of preserved function (except for the side effects of therapy) until the terminal stages, which are characterized by generalized weakness, malaise, obtundation, and great pain. In fact, fear of pain is perhaps the most frequently voiced anxiety in the cancer patient (probably more common than fear of death per se). Narcotic analgesics can diminish the level of pain, but at a cost of increasing obtundation and therefore further accelerating loss of function.

The course of the patient with ALS is one of progressive weakness with totally preserved cognitive clarity and psychic energy. This preservation of intellectual stamina allows the creation of *symbolic action systems* which can compensate for the loss of strength and kinetic control with increased (or at least maintained) social control. For example, a mother with ALS may be too weak to walk or prepare meals but might continue to occupy her role by planning the family menus, preparing the shopping list, directing the cooking, eating with the family, etc., from her bed or chair. By the time the mother with cancer becomes bedridden, she is generally too sick and cognitively impaired to maintain any of her family responsibilities or ties.

Our basic observation is that a patient dying of ALS undergoes a significantly different process on the psychologic level than a patient dying of cancer and that these differences should lead to a reappraisal of much of the current thought and conventional wisdom pertaining to death and dying.

PSYCHIATRIC INTERVENTION WITH THE FAMILY

It is an often neglected truth that illness affects families, not just individuals. We have yet to see a family that has not had significant psychiatric symptoms develop in a member other than the ALS patient.

Amyotrophic lateral sclerosis usually strikes one of the productive adult partners of the nuclear family. The emotional, financial, and social consequences to the spouse and children of this attack on the family foundation cannot be overstated. The modifications in family life required by this prolonged, crippling, expensive, eventually fatal neuromuscular disease are far more extensive than if the family member had suffered an equally tragic but sudden death. Families invariably profit from education regarding what to expect and intermittent therapy when signs of crisis or breakdown appear.

This illness robs its victims of various physical abilities while preserving their personality and intellect. They are the "same person," but trapped in a body that allows progressively diminishing levels of physical competence, autonomy, independence of action, and social interaction. There is no specific treatment. This constellation of features universally creates feelings of powerlessness on the part of family members. Because powerlessness is particularly threatening, it is defended against with unrealistic guilt. (We hide from the fact that there is nothing we can do by believing that there is something, but that we are just not good enough—a slightly more optimistic position.) Guilt then leads to overinvolvement and overextension. Eventually, anger and resentment build but cannot be tolerated consciously. If these feelings are untreated and unmodified, we will witness various manifestations of rationalized abandonment, unconscious sadism, or the displacement of this anger onto a scapegoated family member who is healthy and "can take it."

Necessary psychiatric intervention for the family involves instructing and assisting family members in acting to preserve the maximum degree of autonomy for the patient (this usually requires an outside perspective to balance unrealistic expectations against premature invalidism); uncovering and exploring family fantasies of responsibility, guilt, and omniscience; assisting them in establishing and maintaining appropriate limits; facilitating and legitimizing the ventilation of angry feelings concerning the patient; identifying and working through individual conflicts precipitated by the illness (as, for example, when an adolescent boy must deal with the conflicts created by the progressive weakness of his father); and supporting the family through its ordeal with knowledge, experience, and empathy. We have also found that our willingness to schedule periods of hospital-based treatment gives unusually stressed families a period of rest and can be a particularly effective primary prevention technique.

THE PHYSICIAN'S REACTIONS TO ALS

In addition to the other aspects of terminal illness that have been studied in recent years, the physician's own reactions to the dying patient have not escaped attention (8). The need to see oneself as a powerful healer, when present to an exaggerated degree, prohibits calm, responsive, and empathetic treatment of the terminal patient. Such physicians, when confronted with this situation, often adopt the manner of a technician who concentrates on the details of a technical treatment program until the situation is clearly hopeless and then bows out by abandoning the self-expectation of care, and hence the patient. ("There is nothing more that can be done.") Since all physicians are motivated to some degree by the need to help and to heal, the terminal phase of any patient's treatment is a difficult one.

Since ALS is widely understood to be untreatable, the "terminal phase" associated with physician ineffectuality can be seen as spanning the entire duration of illness. In our interviews of ALS patients we were impressed with the large number of reports of physicians who allegedly instructed the patient to "go home and wait to die." While we believe that such quotations involve a specific variety of distortion, the records of these patients speak for themselves. In case after case, even minimal hospital treatment, nutritional enrichment, and physical therapy have been completely withheld. The only possible explanation for such irrationality would have to reside at the level of the physician's own emotional needs.

Physicians tend to be overachievers. They are people who bind anxiety with active obsessional defenses. They also have scholastic records of high achievement, at least partially motivated by a competitive avoidance of "failure." Clinical "failure" elicits strong feelings of personal inadequacy and is therefore strongly defended against. A preconscious awareness of the destructive potential of these competitive defenses can break through and serve as a rationalization for withholding treatment and actually rejecting the ALS patient (who represents a certain failure regardless of treatment). Although couched in reasoned statements such as "Anything we give you will have greater likelihood of hurting you than helping you," the patient (not incorrectly) perceives the message of "We decline to treat you; go home to your own devices; eventually you will die." Physicians often have to be reminded that the equation between the availability of active, efficacious agents and all treatment is recent (and lamentable). Medicine was a healing art long before there were specific effective agents for any illness. However, to administer nonspecific care and tolerate the patient's inexorable course of deterioration, the physician must possess the capacity to redefine his or her concepts of success and failure and make them less dependent on cure or symptom abatement. Psychiatric support to the *physician* often facilitates this process.

Conversely, in our program we have found that our carefully worded promise, "We will treat you with a series of experimental agents of unproven value," is frequently distorted and exaggerated through a strong rescue fantasy to, "We will find something to help you," or even, "We will cure you." Fairly frequent treatment review and reexplanation of reasonable expectations help to retard this process, but misquotes and unfortunate disappointments occur anyway.

We have attempted to demonstrate that psychiatric involvement in each of these four areas is a useful adjunct to the care of patients with ALS. While functioning collaboratively with the neurology service, we have found the ALS patient group to be an unusually rewarding one with which to work. The contributions of a psychiatrist on the clinical team have been both well received and personally satisfying.

REFERENCES

1. Becker E: *The Denial of Death.* New York, Free Press, 1973

2. Brown WA, Mueller PS: Psychological function in individuals with amyotrophic lateral sclerosis (ALS). Psychosom Med 32:141–152, 1970

3. Feifel H (Editor): *The Meaning of Death.* New York, McGraw-Hill, 1959

4. Houpt JL, Gould BS, Norris FH: Psychological characteristics of patients with amyotrophic lateral sclerosis (ALS). Psychosom Med 39:299–303, 1977

5. Karusu TB: Psychotherapy of the medically ill. Am J Psychiatry 136: 1–11, 1979

6. Klein DL: Endogenomorphic depression: A conceptual and terminological revision. Arch Gen Psychiatry 31:447, 1974

7. Kubler-Ross E: *On Death and Dying.* New York, Macmillan, 1969

8. Spikes J, Holland J: The physician's response to the dying patient. In *Psychological Care of the Medically Ill.* New York, Appleton-Century-Crofts, 1975

9. Weisman AD: *On Dying and Denying.* New York, Behavioral Publications, 1972

Commentary

Robert D. Currier

Dr. Gould's chapter shows a perceptive analysis of the patient's attempt to cope with amyotrophic lateral sclerosis and the physician's response to the patient with this disorder. It is a thoughtful and provocative paper that should be studied by everyone attempting to treat patients with ALS.

Dr. Gould tells us, as others have, that patients with ALS are not unique psychiatrically (1). Even though we might expect them to be depressed, few are. Their basic fears center more on loss of loved ones than on the idea of death itself. The patient tends to conceal his or her feelings from the physician, but this can be overcome if we spend enough time in our discussion with the patient. Dr. Gould describes the common difficulty physicians have in discussing the diagnosis and stresses the harmful effect of a poorly timed confrontation.

I wonder what the ideal method of caring for patients with ALS is. It is obvious that this will vary in each situation. In my clinical practice in Mississippi, we have available a very active and able group of general practitioners who are willing to accept responsibility for the treatment of patients with ALS, and we turn to them for the follow-up care.

One other area in which we need help as neurologists is in the proper evaluation of therapeutic trials. There are drugs and treatments that should be tried in ALS and probably are not being tried. At present, in our nonsystem, we try three or four patients on a drug, find they get worse, and we do not report our findings. I may well have tried the same eight or nine things you have tried, and there is no record of these trials anywhere in the literature. I would like to suggest that a central data center for ALS treatment trials be established. Just the recording of trials that failed would be helpful, and, ideally, such a center might help coordinate trials of treatment. Then, in the future, it might be possible for all neurologists to use such a data center to make more meaningful therapeutic trials. This would be of potential benefit to both patient and physician. I refer our readers to chapter 22 for additional comments.

REFERENCE

1. Peters PK, Swenson WM, Mulder DW: Is there a characteristic personality profile in amyotrophic lateral sclerosis? A Minnesota Multiphasic Personality Inventory study. Arch Neurol 35:321–322, 1978

11 Rehabilitation

Mehrsheed Sinaki

Amyotrophic lateral sclerosis is a relentlessly progressive disease that has no known cure. Thus, its diagnosis is often equated with a death sentence by the patient's physician, and frequently no therapy is offered. We have observed, as others have (7, 14), that physical therapy and rehabilitation can help many patients with ALS by improving their ability to live with their disease. These patients should be kept active and independent as long as possible. We will outline the physical therapy and the rehabilitation techniques that we have employed in recent years in the management of our patients with ALS.

GENERAL RECOMMENDATIONS

The success of rehabilitation efforts depends on the active participation of the patient. This requires that the physician discuss the illness and its clinical course directly and frankly with the patient. It is always difficult for the physician to discuss this fatal illness, but we have found, as have others, that the patient can live most effectively with his or her handicap when a direct and open approach is used. All questions should be answered, and the physician should try to give the patient adequate information about the disease and its clinical course. The goal of therapy in ALS is to help the patient cope with his or her disability and be independent as long as possible.

The progressive nature of ALS and the variability in the distribution of weakness from patient to patient require that rehabilitation techniques be individualized after careful neurologic and physiatric evaluations. We have found it useful to classify patients by the rapidity of the clinical course, the site of onset of the disease, the age of the patient, and the stage of the disability. In our experience, approximately one-half of patients with ALS live for more than 3 years from the onset of their illness, and 10% live for 10 years or more (9). The treatment of patients with a long clinical course obviously differs from that of the 50% who die within 3 years of onset. The patients with long clinical courses have a remarkable capacity to compensate for motor unit loss, and this may enable them to continue their daily activities for years (3).

We have also found it helpful to differentiate patients according to whether the symptoms began in the bulbar musculature or in the axioappendicular musculature. In the axioappendicular group, we have found it useful to classify the severity of illness according to stages when outlining a therapeutic program (13).

During the initial stage of the illness, patients are advised to avoid fatigue but to continue with their daily activities. We encourage range-of-motion exercises and exercises to strengthen muscles that are unaffected. When muscle weakness becomes apparent, the patient must be warned to avoid development of contractures in muscles that are antagonistic to the weakened ones. The patient should be encouraged to do stretching exercises that will prevent this problem. In most patients, no exercise other than that inherent in everyday ambulatory activities is indicated. A prolonged program of strengthening exercises is not warranted unless the patient has the slowly progressive form of the disease. We continue to believe that the exercise regimen of each patient must be individualized and do not agree with Norris et al. that vigorous daily exercise is appropriate for all patients with ALS (11). We have observed patients in whom weakness first became apparent after vigorous exercise of an affected limb and the weakness remained. This suggested to us that the severely involved anterior horn cells are adversely affected by excessive fatigue. In any event, the patient must remain as active as possible without overly fatiguing the involved muscles. Appropriate physical therapy will prevent disuse atrophy, keep muscular power at the maximal level during the changing stages of this chronic illness, and, in general, maintain the patient as a functioning human being for long periods.

Rehabilitation techniques for the management of ALS are aimed at maintaining the patient at his optimal functional level for as long as possible and at preventing the complications secondary to disuse of muscles and immobilization (1, 2). Lack of activity and immobilization cause loss of muscle strength. In the absence of any contraction of a muscle, muscle strength decreases 5% per day in normal subjects (10). One contraction each day at half the maximal strength is enough to prevent this decrease. Muscle contractions involved in daily activities act as stimuli regulating the muscle strength. When these stimuli are not sufficient, optimal strength is not maintained.

The patient who has limited walking endurance because of weakness should be encouraged to use a wheelchair or another appropriate supportive device whenever the affected muscles become unduly fatigued, as in attending sporting events, shopping, and other activities.

The patient's family should be included in these therapeutic programs because they also must learn to cope with the illness and they need to be informed about what can be done and what help is available for such patients. The family will have an important role in the patient's therapy. As weakness progresses from one group of muscles to another, requirements for assistive devices change, and new problems arise in the handling of activities of daily living. With an adaptive management process, the physiatrist and the family can be very helpful to the patient. With the proper aids, some patients can realistically expect to maintain a satisfactory lifestyle for a decade or more after the onset of illness. Other patients can be helped to function, in spite of their disease, for briefer but reasonably productive periods.

STAGING OF ALS PATIENTS WITH AXIOAPPENDICULAR INVOLVEMENT

Patients with predominant involvement of the axial and appendicular muscles are candidates for the application of rehabilitative techniques. The illness generally can be divided into the following stages, each of which requires a somewhat different rehabilitative approach.

Stage I

In stage I, patients are ambulatory and can care for themselves and accomplish the activities of daily living. There is mild weakness or clumsiness of the musculature. The patients usually do not need any therapy beyond psychologic support and encouragement, but it may be necessary to instruct them in the development of auxiliary muscles to support the muscles that are already weakened. Normal physical activities and general range of motion exercises are usually advised. Patients should be advised against performing strenuous exercises in a misguided attempt to build up already weakened muscles. Such exercise may result in extreme fatigue of the muscles and increase the patient's disability. For strengthening, we usually recommend isometric exercises. A daily program consisting of six maximal isometric contractions, each lasting 6 seconds with a 20-second interval of relaxation, increases muscle strength (8). With continued exercise, the increase in strength will continue for six weeks before a plateau is reached. In other words, the patient would strengthen the muscle to its maximal strength in six weeks. After this period, the patient may continue with the exercises every other day or twice a week to maintain the strength that has been achieved. The patient also should attempt to strengthen unaffected muscles to compensate for those that have been impaired.

Stage II

In stage II the patient has moderate weakness in selected muscle groups. For example, such a patient may have mild foot-drop on one or both sides. He or she often has difficulty climbing stairs, elevating the arms, or using the hands—especially for fine activities such as buttoning garments. The patient may need proper support, in the form of braces or splints, for joints poorly supported by weakened muscles. Otherwise, sprain of the ill-supported joints secondary to weakness of muscles would cause mechanical pain and irreparable wear and tear of the joints.

The patient may require such measures as ankle-foot orthoses to assist with dorsiflexion of the feet. Such devices help the patient to walk better and also provide good mechanical support for the stability of the ankles. The supports can be made of unobtrusive lightweight materials (Fig. 1). The posterior leaf-spring types of ankle-foot orthoses are, in essence, braces, and because they have to be custom-made, they are expensive. Such braces are used for patients who cannot dorsiflex their ankles or who have very weak dorsiflexor muscles. Alimed is a less

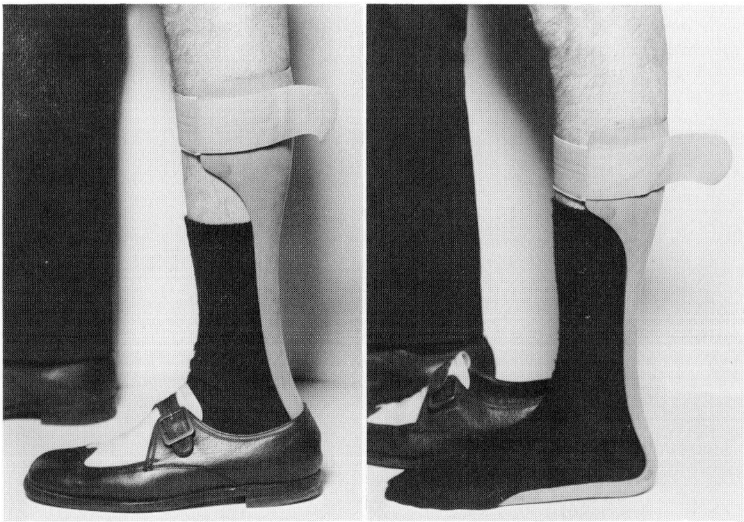

Figure 1 Example of a lightweight ankle-foot orthosis. This is a custom-made posterior leaf-spring brace.

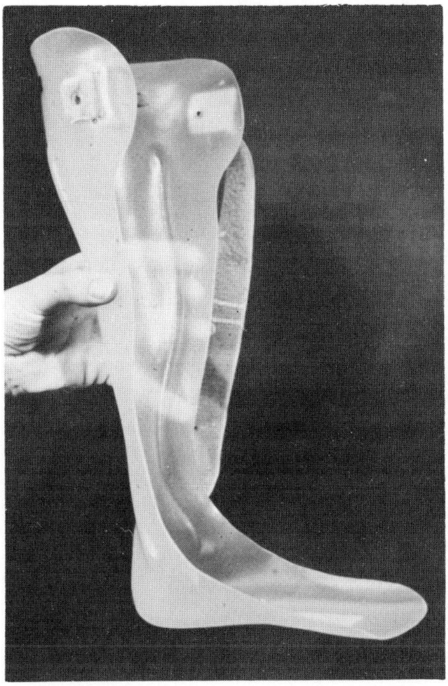

Figure 2 Example of a lightweight ankle-foot orthosis (Alimed) that is commercially available in small, medium, and large sizes. (Reprinted with permission from Sinaki M, Mulder DW: Rehabilitation techniques for patients with amyotrophic lateral sclerosis. Mayo Clin Proc 53:173, 1978.)

expensive type of ankle-foot orthosis that is available commercially in three sizes (Fig. 2). These are used mainly as splints for patients who have weak but not totally paralyzed or severely affected dorsiflexor muscles (Fig. 3).

The double-upright short leg brace with a Klenzak ankle joint is heavy, weighing 1 kg (Fig. 4). This brace can be used by patients who have strong hip flexor muscles and strong quadriceps muscles. Otherwise, its use is not advisable. Because the posterior leaf-spring weighs less than 0.2 kg, it is helpful even in the presence of weak proximal muscles.

If the upper extremities are involved, the patient may benefit from wrist supports, which facilitate extension of the wrist and thus enable the patient to grip better (Fig. 5). Weakness of the abductor pollicis brevis muscle may be aided by the addition of an extra splint that places the thumb in opposition to obtain more effective use of the hand for small movements (Figs. 6 and 7). With this method, the patient has a stronger grip and can use his or her hand more effectively (Fig. 8).

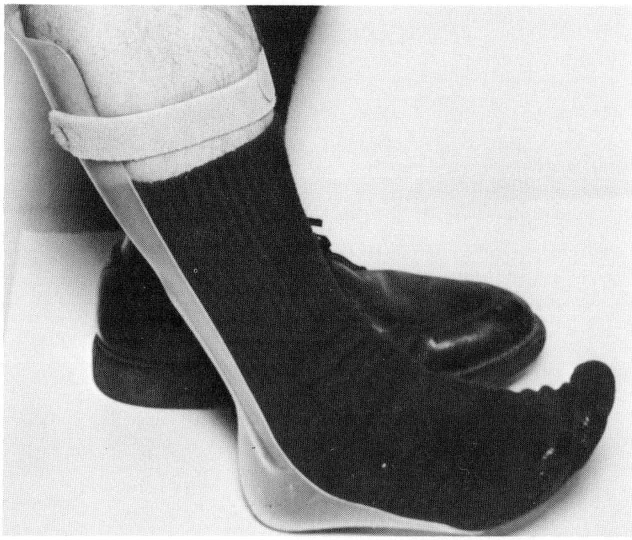

Figure 3 Alimed can be used by patients who have foot-drop but not complete paralysis of foot dorsiflexor muscles. Patient can attempt some dorsiflexion. Alimed splints are not so strong a support as the posterior leaf-spring brace. (Reprinted with permission from Sinaki M, Mulder DW: Rehabilitation techniques for patients with amyotrophic lateral sclerosis. Mayo Clin Proc 53:173, 1978.)

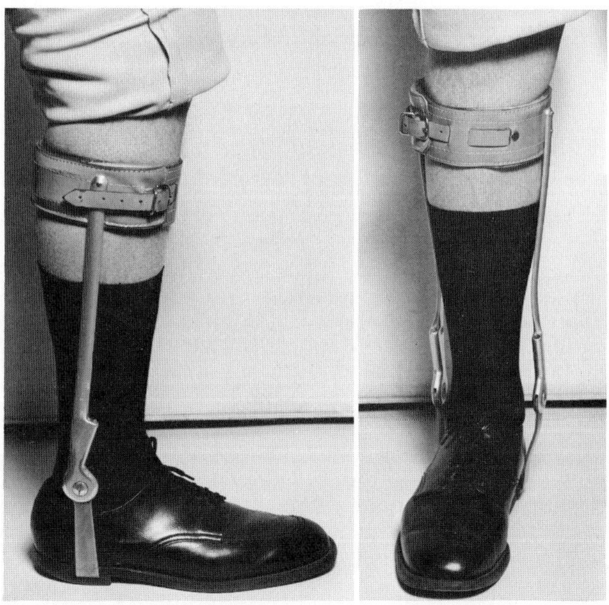

Figure 4 Double-upright short leg brace. These braces are heavy (about 1 kg) and obtrusive.

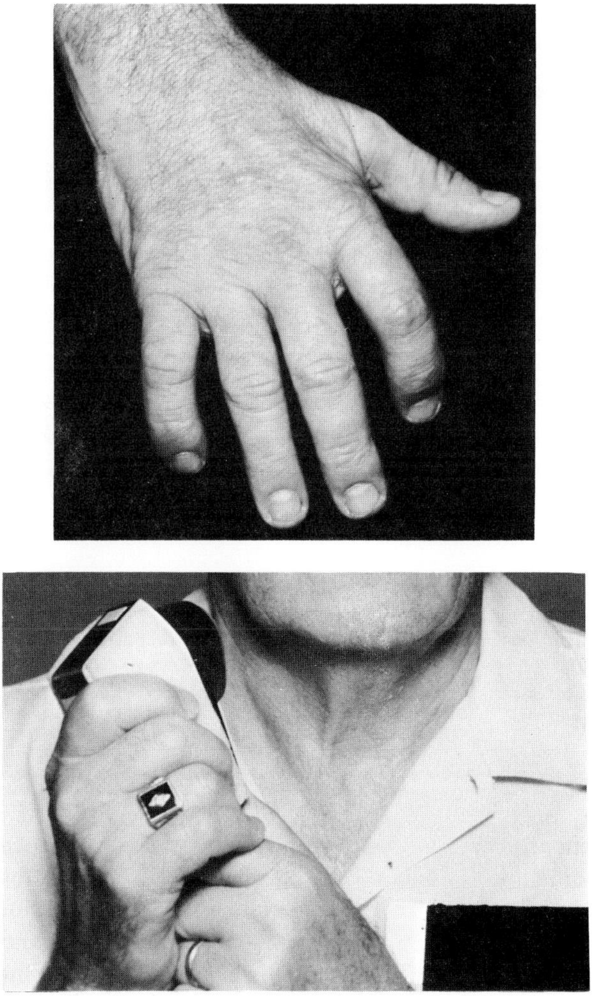

Figure 5 Patient with weakness of wrist extensor and intrinsic hand muscles is unable to hold an electric razor with one hand. (The bottom figure is reprinted with permission from Sinaki M, Mulder DW: Rehabilitation techniques for patients with amyotrophic lateral sclerosis. Mayo Clin Proc 53:173, 1978.)

The dynamic finger-extension splint can be very helpful to patients with weak finger extensors. This splint facilitates the extension of the digits that initiate the grasp (Fig. 9). Patients are often aided by simple instruction in the use of clothing that has been altered so that it can be more conveniently taken off and put on. For example, the use of a Velcro fastening rather than buttons for shirts and other garments may be particularly helpful.

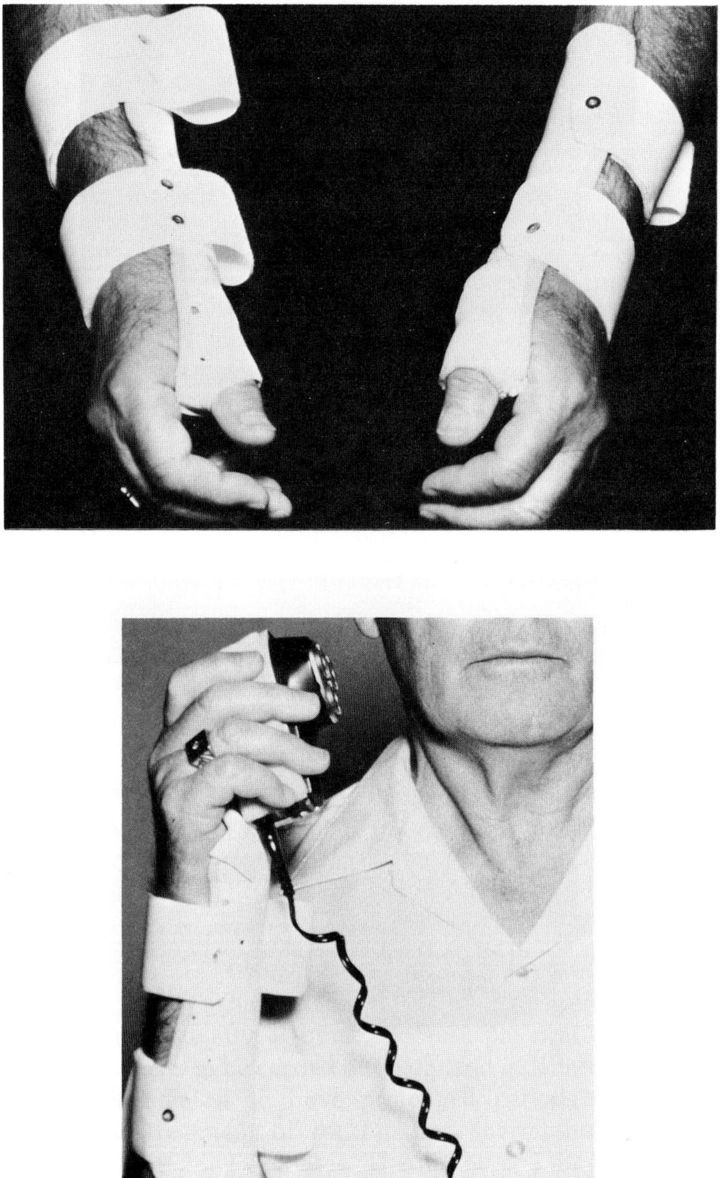

Figure 7 Application of wrist extension splint with thumb shell addition. This splint enabled the patient shown in Figure 5 to hold an electric razor effectively with one hand. (The figure on the right is reprinted with permission from Sinaki M, Mulder DW: Rehabilitation techniques for patients with amyotrophic lateral sclerosis. Mayo Clin Proc 53:173, 1978.)

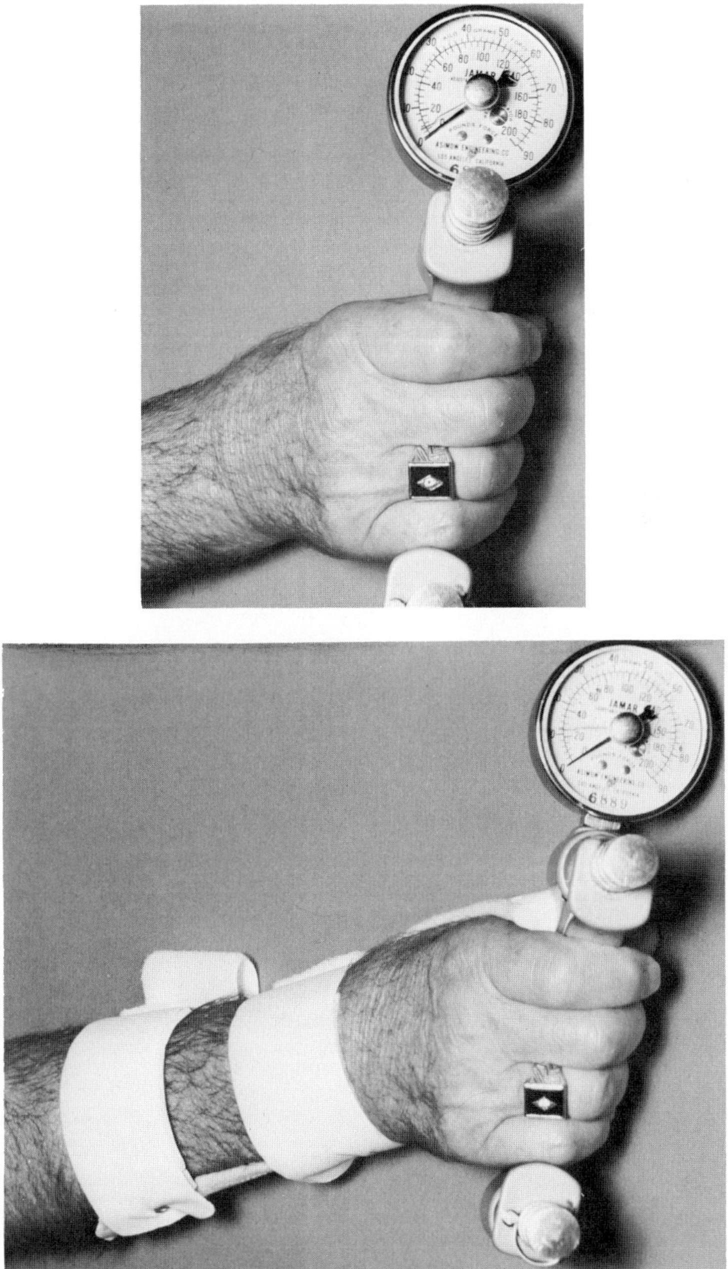

Figure 8 Without a splint, the patient's power grip, measured by a Jamar dynamometer, was 3.5 kg on maximal effort. After application of the static wrist extension splint, the power grip was increased to 12 kg (same patient as in Figs. 5 and 7). (Reprinted with permission from Sinaki M, Mulder DW: Rehabilitation techniques for patients with amyotrophic lateral sclerosis. Mayo Clin Proc 53:173, 1978.)

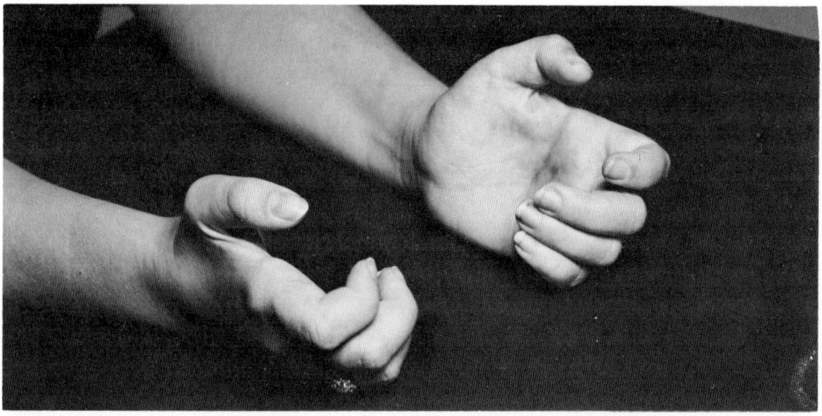

A

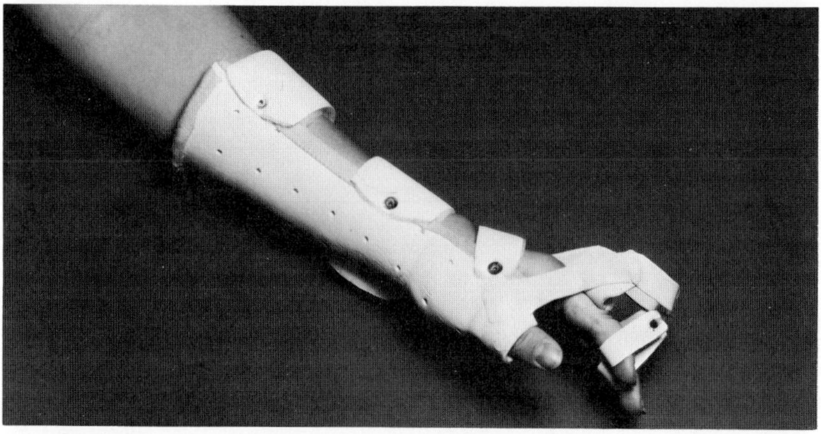

B

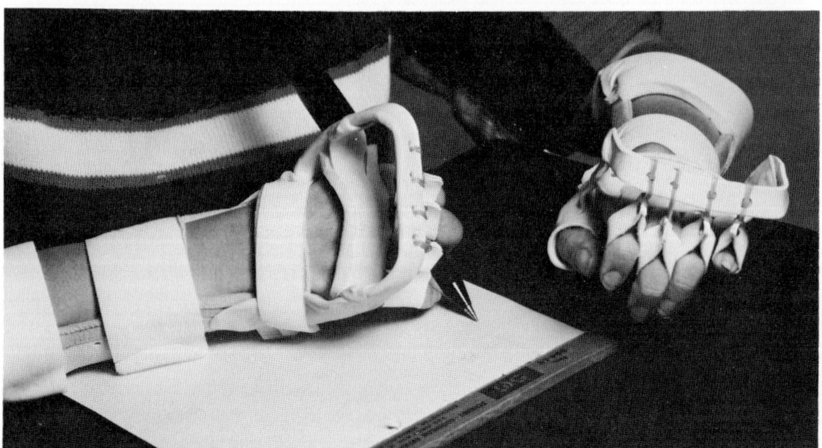

C

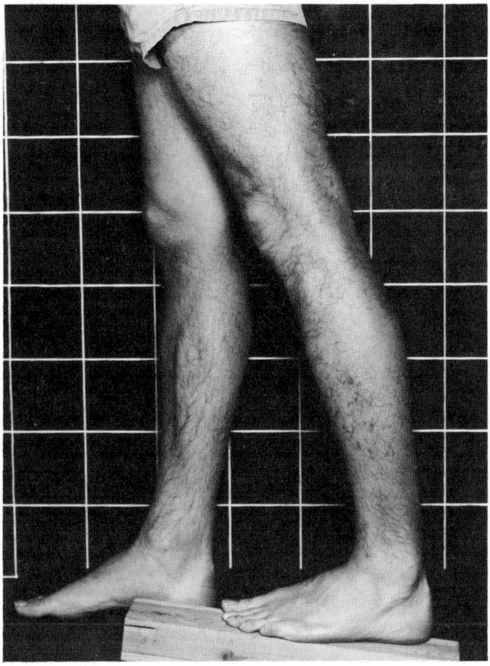

Figure 10 A practical maneuver for stretching the Achilles tendon.

Stage III

In stage III, the patient is ambulatory but has severe weakness in selected muscle groups. Such a patient often has severe foot-drop and pronounced weakness and atrophy of the intrinsic muscles of the hand. Often, he or she cannot rise from a chair without help. The patient at this stage requires, in addition to the previously described techniques, such devices as lightweight ankle-foot orthoses, wrist splints, and high-seated or electrically powered height-adjustable chairs to assist in sitting and rising from the sitting position. Every attempt must be made to keep the patient physically independent. As the weakness advances, deep-breathing exercises should be encouraged to enhance the use of auxiliary muscles of respiration. Assistive respiratory exercises with the aid of a

---

Figure 9 **(A)** This patient has severe atrophy and weakness of the thenar muscles as well as the finger and wrist extensors. **(B)** A static wrist-extension splint with a thumb shell addition is coupled with a dynamic finger-extension device. **(C)** A complex but practical splint enables the patient to do certain (even fine) movements, such as writing with a pen.

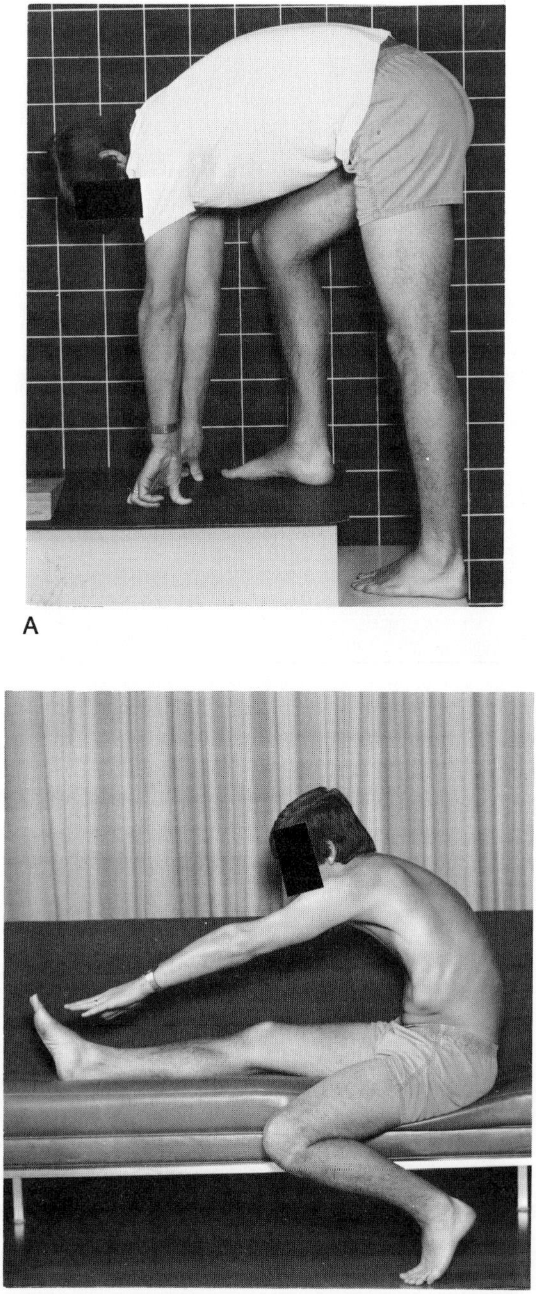

A

B

Figure 11 **(A)** Demonstration of maneuver for stretching the hamstring muscles. This figure shows stretching of the left hamstring. **(B)** Method of stretching the hamstrings while in the sitting position.

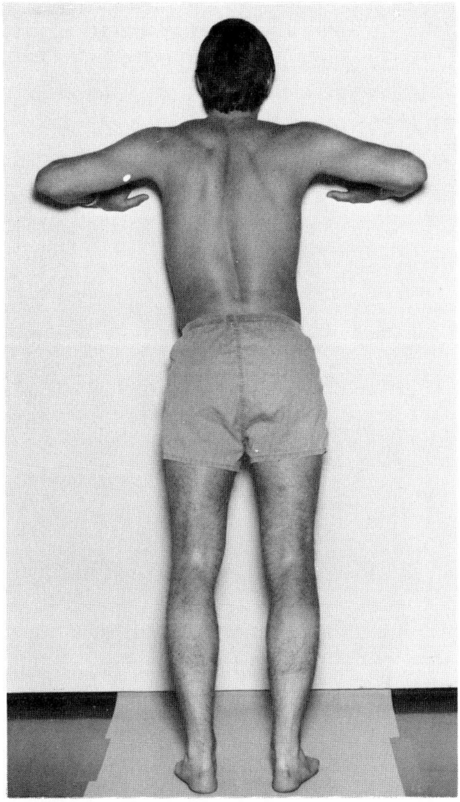

Figure 12 Maneuver for stretching both Achilles tendons as well as the hamstrings and pectoral muscles.

Triflo device (incentive deep-breathing exerciser) may help to maintain the functional capacity of the patient's lungs. If the patient's weakness is so great that walking any distance is difficult, a wheelchair should be used for long trips, for shopping, or for visiting outside the home.

Patients who have access to heated pools may do exercises in the water or may try walking in the water. Range of motion exercises for all the peripheral joints are easier in the water, and patients usually enjoy them more. Periarthritis of the shoulders secondary to muscular weakness and decrease in the range of motion of the joints are not uncommon. A trial of local heat and massage and pulley exercises is advisable. However, if the patient cannot do pulley exercises because of severe weakness, passive range-of-motion exercises, which can be applied by a member of the patient's family, should be considered. With advanced bilateral shoulder-girdle weakness, a characteristic appearance develops, with the patient's arms hanging limply from the sagging

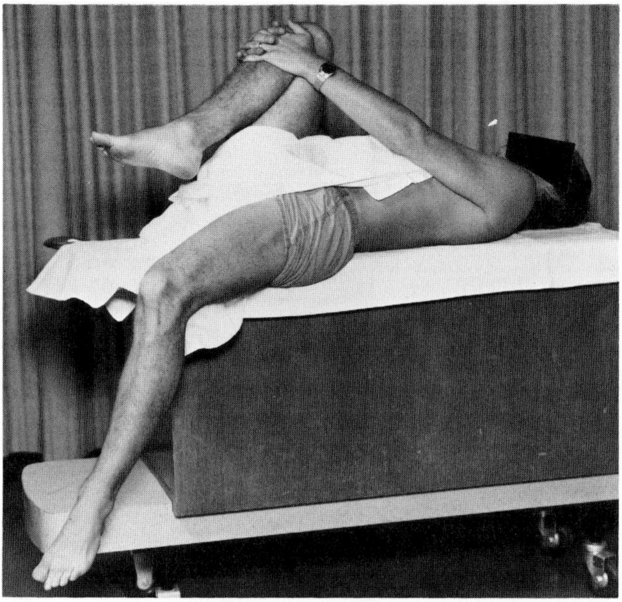

Figure 13 Method for stretching the left hip flexors. Right hip is flexed to prevent exaggerated lumbar lordosis, which otherwise would have been produced during the stretching maneuver.

shoulder girdles (Fig. 14), the so-called hanging-arm syndrome (5). In order to decrease the stretch on the shoulder ligaments, brachial plexus, and axillary vessels, a shoulder sling may be used (Fig. 15). A modified Bobath shoulder sling has been developed by our occupational therapy department for use in bilateral hanging-arm syndrome (Fig. 16).

Stage IV

By stage IV, the patient is confined to a wheelchair but remains almost independent. These patients have severe weakness of the lower extremities with mild involvement of the upper extremities. Such a patient can perform most activities of daily living from the wheelchair. Many patients prefer electrically powered chairs. However, a wheelchair should be ordered by the physician after consideration of all aspects of a patient's disability in order to obtain the most appropriate equipment for that patient. Many types of wheelchairs with various modifications are available to fit the patient's needs. At this stage, a patient may require an electrically powered wheelchair with power keys to provide propulsion and to turn the chair in different directions. Such wheelchairs are now available and can be conveniently transported. These wheelchairs allow the patient to maintain useful function for months or years.

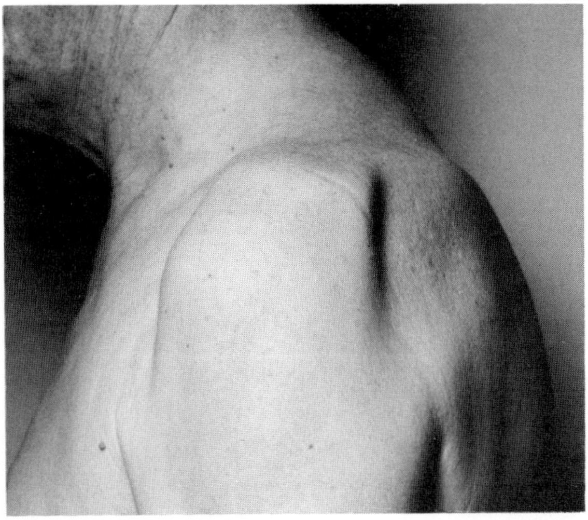

Figure 14 Patient with atrophy of left shoulder-girdle muscles. This patient had a sagging left shoulder.

Passive exercises are particularly important to prevent contractures and to retard the changes secondary to disuse. It is often necessary to instruct the family in the application of such exercise. The patients themselves often can participate actively in exercises for distal joints, elbows, wrists, and fingers, because the active exercises of such joints are not fatiguing. The physiatrist should review the uninvolved musculature of such patients to see whether there are muscles that these patients could strengthen to assist them in maintaining their independence.

Bathroom facilities need to be modified so the patient can continue to be as independent as possible. Use of a shower chair and a hand shower enable the patient to bathe with only minor assistance. Elevated toilet seats enable the patient to get on and off the seat more easily. Grab bars in appropriate areas of the bathroom facilitate the patient's ability to move independently. At this stage, if the patient cannot feed himself/herself because the shoulder abductors and elbow flexors are weak but the shoulder adductor muscles are strong (Fig. 17), he or she may be able to to feed himself/herself by using a ball-bearing feeder that can be attached to the wheelchair (Fig. 18). The patient and the family should be instructed in the proper methods of transferring the patient to and from the bed and chair.

Stage V

At stage V, the patient is in a wheelchair and is dependent. There is both pronounced weakness of the lower extremities and moderate or

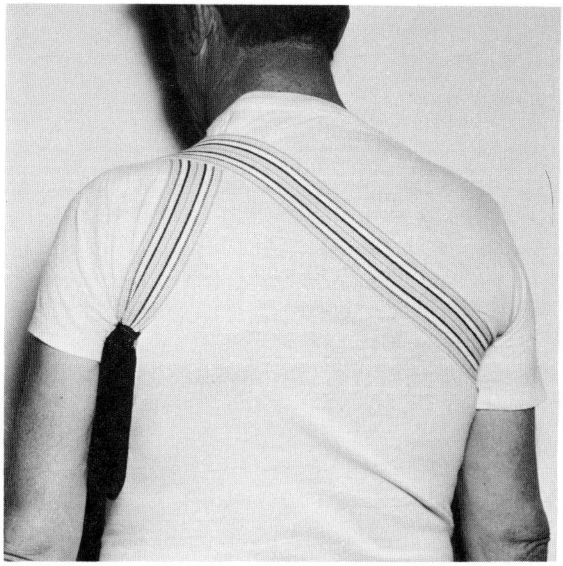

Figure 15 Application of a Bobath shoulder sling to decrease the sagging of the shoulder and to reduce the stretch on the brachial and axillary neurovascular bundle.

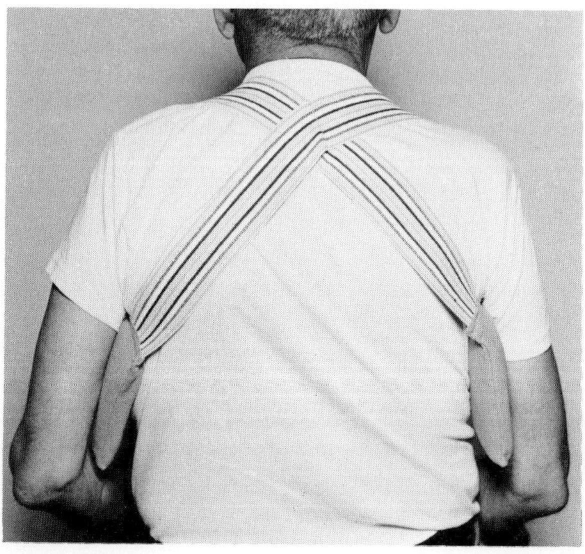

Figure 16 Demonstration of a modified Bobath sling. This sling is used for bilateral shoulder-girdle weakness, the so-called hanging-arm syndrome.

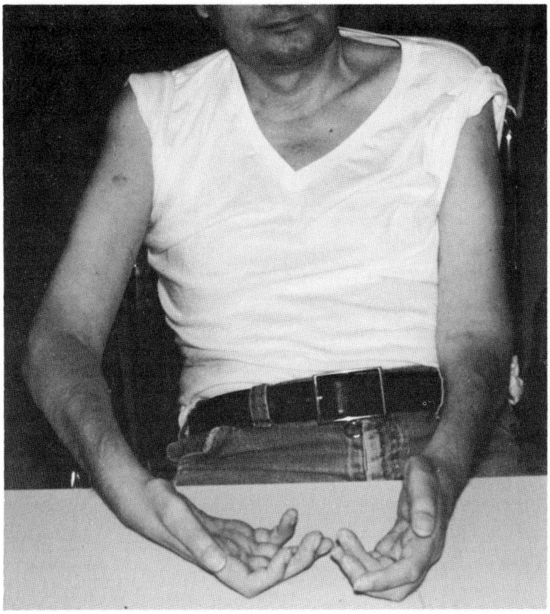

Figure 17 This patient has severe atrophy and weakness of the distal and proximal muscles of the upper extremities. However, his shoulder adductor muscles remain fairly strong.

pronounced weakness of some muscle groups of the upper extremities. The patient requires proper devices, such as a Hoyer lift, for transfer to and from the wheelchair. The family must be instructed in the technique of transferring the patient to and from the bed, so that the lift can be used with a wheeled shower chair. Many of these patients cannot rise from the sitting position and thus need proper support to prevent pressure sores over such areas as the ischial tuberosities.

By proper positioning and changing of the patient's position during the day every two hours and during sleep every four hours, one can decrease the pain that is caused by the patient's inability to change positions. Ankle-foot splints with proper paddings or a foot board with a pillow are useful for positioning the paralyzed lower extremities in bed (Fig. 19). The use of wheelchair cushions and water mattresses plus synthetic sheepskins not only contributes to proper skin care but also adds to the patient's comfort.

Patients in this stage of the disease often complain of pain on lying down and of being unable to move for hours while in bed. Therefore, the principles of proper positioning should be taught to increase

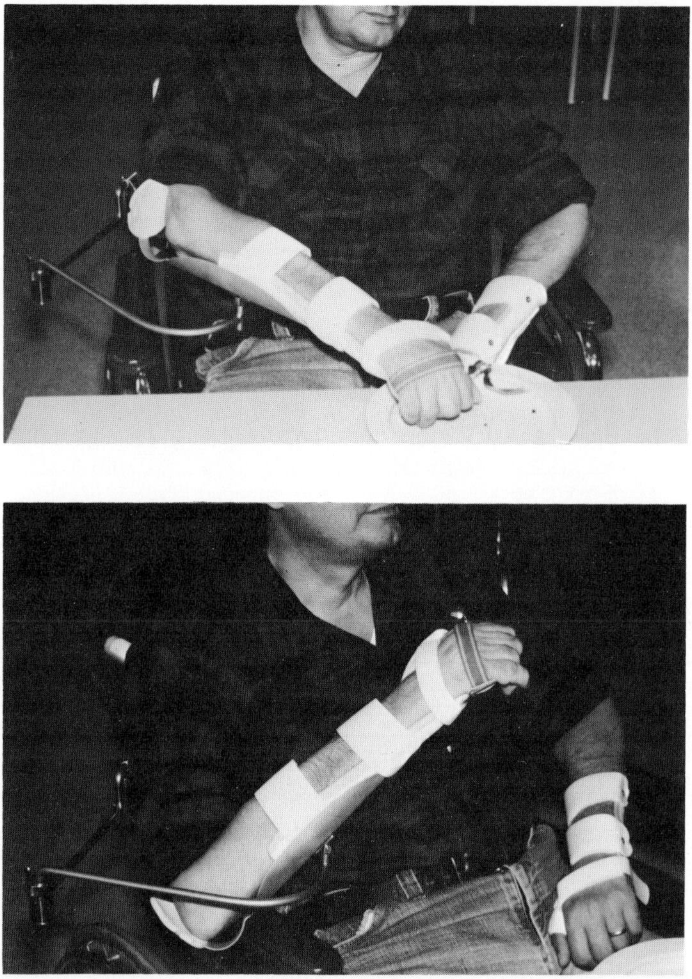

Figure 18 After application of a static wrist-extension thumb shell splint, a universal cuff (for holding fork, spoon, and so forth), and a ball-bearing feeder, the patient shown in Figure 17 can do certain activities of daily living, such as self-feeding.

the patient's comfort and to reduce the possibility of the development of contractures. Weakness of nuchal musculature may require the addition of a head-extension support to the wheelchair and the use of a cervical collar to prevent or decrease mechanical neck pain.

If the patient has weakness of the shoulder girdle muscles, the use of arm splints or a resting splint while the patient is in a wheelchair

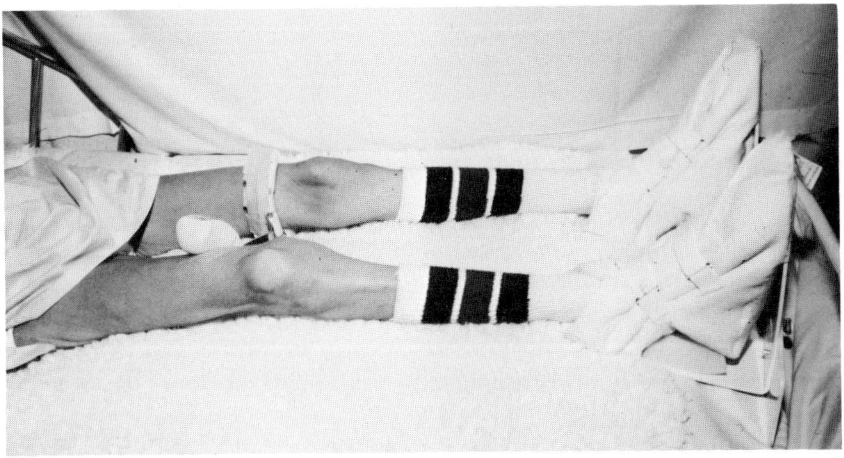

Figure 19 This patient has severe weakness and spasticity of the lower extremities. Proper positioning plus application of a knee-separator brace stretches the tight hip adductors, prevents injury to the lower extremities, and helps in hygiene and cleansing of the rectogenital area. Also, use of a foot board or application of an ankle-foot dorsiflexion-positioning splint would prevent or decrease the possibility of the development of contractures.

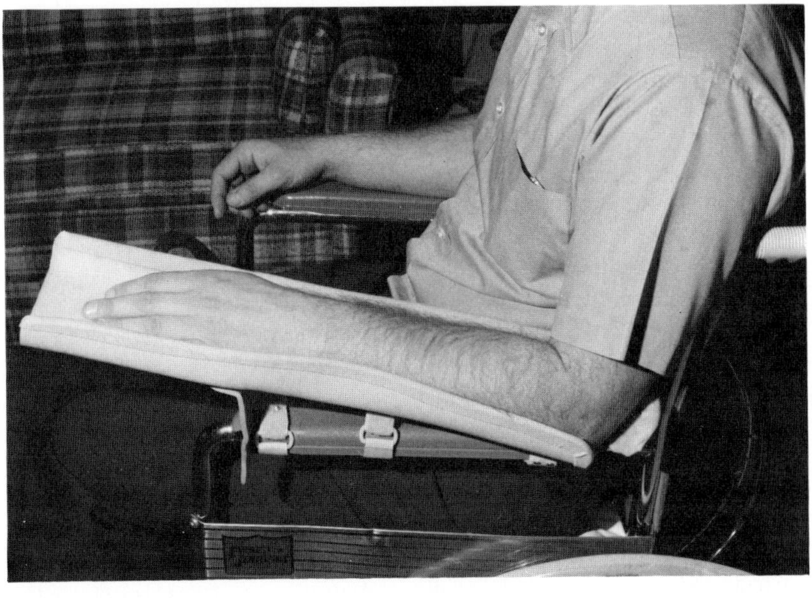

Figure 20 A gutter splint is applied to the arm rest of a wheelchair. Such supports prevent painful stretching of the brachioaxillary neurovascular bundle in wheelchair-bound patients with shoulder-girdle muscle weakness.

will decrease the painful stretch on the brachial plexus and add to the patient's comfort (Fig. 20).

Stage VI

In stage VI, the patient is bedridden. He or she is unable to perform any of the useful activities of daily living and needs maximal assistance. Proper mattresses and beds must be available, and the family must be assisted and instructed in the care of the patient. Often the most severe symptoms are due to bulbar involvement, but this is not necessarily true. If there is a problem with coughing up the usual overnight accumulation of respiratory secretions, the patient's family should be instructed in methods of postural drainage. The techniques used at this stage are similar to those that are essential for the care of any quadriplegic patient, except that the patient with ALS does not have bladder involvement or sensory deficits and rarely has bed sores.

In the advanced stages of the disease, the patient's bowel and bladder function may be affected by immobility. Urinary calcium excretion increases during prolonged bed rest (4), predisposing the patient to the development of urolithiasis. Urolithiasis may be prevented by increasing the patient's fluid intake to dilute the concentration of calcium in the urine. The patient's daily fluid intake should be kept at a minimum of 2 liters (about 10 glasses) of water or any kind of juice. This maintains an adequate urinary output and also helps to regulate the patient's bowels. Stool softeners, bulk formers, or laxatives may be used if indicated.

Patients who have paralysis of the lower extremities, especially of the flaccid type, may develop thrombophlebitis of the lower extremities, particularly when they are in dependent positions. Trauma during transfer activities also can induce phlebitis. Preventive measures such as application of elastic support hose and intermittent elevation of the lower extremities should be considered.

Proper diet is important at any stage. In a study of 110 patients with ALS at the Mayo Clinic, there was an increased incidence of obesity in patients with more advanced disease. Patients whose weights were 25% above the upper limit of their ideal weight were considered to be obese. In stages I and II, about 18% of the patients were obese, while in stages III to V, somewhat more than 50% of the patients were obese (Fig. 21). The obesity in these patients is presumed to be related to their lack of activity. Moreover, significant correlation existed between obesity and walking endurance. In a group of patients in stages I and II, more than 85% of the nonobese patients had no limitation in walking endurance, whereas fewer than 70% of the obese patients had no walking limitation (12) (Fig. 22).

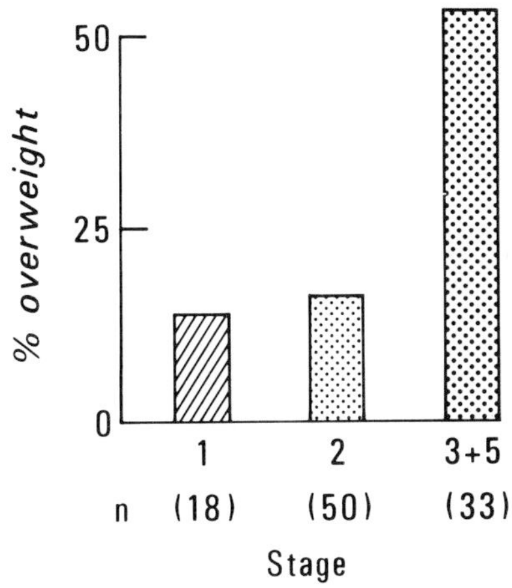

Figure 21 Relationship of stage of ALS and obesity.

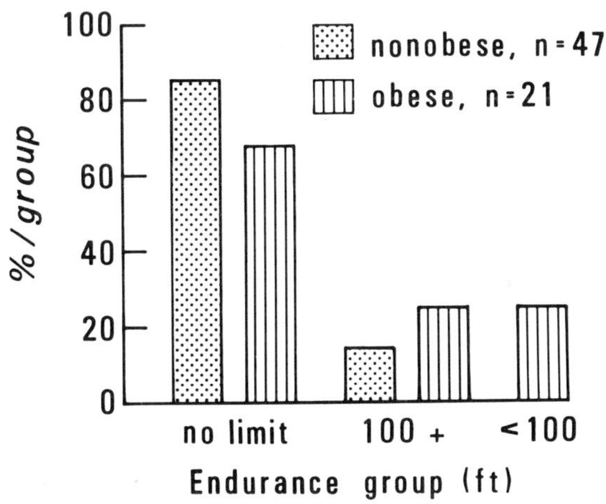

Figure 22 Relationship of endurance and obesity in patients with stages I and II ALS.

PYRAMIDAL INVOLVEMENT

Involvement of the pyramidal pathways results in hyperreflexia and spasticity. These symptoms usually do not constitute a major portion of the patient's complaints, if one excludes the spastic dysarthria that occurs with the involvement of the corticobulbar pathways. Antispasticity medications, such as baclofen, decrease the spasticity and improve the patient's ambulatory activities. In ambulatory patients, however, the spasticity of the lower extremities may serve as a splinting effect and may help the patient to walk better. Occasionally, ambulatory patients with spastic legs have more weakness and a greater decrease in ambulation endurance after the use of antispasticity medications. In these situations, either the medication should be stopped or smaller doses should be used.

BULBAR PARALYSIS

Involvement of the brainstem with so-called bulbar symptoms may occur at any stage in the clinical course of ALS. The symptoms of such involvement are usually prominent in the terminal stages of the disease, although their occurrence does not necessarily presage a brief clinical course. Because of the involvement of the bulbar musculature about the throat, the patient has difficulty in speaking and swallowing, and eventually respiration is compromised. The management of the various manifestations of bulbar palsy will be discussed in other chapters.

REFERENCES

1. Abramson AS: Atrophy of disuse: A definition. Arch Phys Med 29: 562–570, 1948

2. Asher RAJ: The dangers of going to bed. Br Med J 2:967–968, 1947

3. Brown WF: Functional compensation of human motor units in health and disease. J Neurol Sci 20:199–209, 1973

4. Donaldson CL, Hulley SB, Vogel JM, et al: Effect of prolonged bed rest on bone mineral. Metabolism 19:1071–1084, 1970

5. Eaton LM, Mulder DW, Miller RD, et al: Symposium on amyotrophic lateral sclerosis. Proc Staff Meet Mayo Clin 32:425–462, 1957

6. Krusen FH (Editor): *Handbook of Physical Medicine and Rehabilitation,* ed 2. Philadelphia, WB Saunders Co., 1971

7. Lenman JAR: A clinical and experimental study of the effects of exercise on motor weakness in neurological disease. J Neurol Neurosurg Psychiatry 22:182–194, 1959

8. Liberson WT, Asa MM: Further studies of brief isometric exercises. Arch Phys Med Rehabil 40:330–336, 1959

9. Mulder DW, Howard FM Jr: Patient resistance and prognosis in amyotrophic lateral sclerosis. Mayo Clin Proc 51:537–541, 1976

10. Müller EA: Influence of training and of inactivity on muscle strength. Arch Phys Med Rehabil 51:449–462, 1970

11. Norris FH Jr, Ü KS, Denys EH, et al: Amyotrophic lateral sclerosis (letter). Mayo Clin Proc 53:544, 1978

12. Sinaki M, Mulder DW: Amyotrophic lateral sclerosis: Functional staging and rehabilitation techniques with 110 patients (abstract). Arch Phys Med Rehabil 59:520, 1978

13. Sinaki M, Mulder DW: Rehabilitation techniques for patients with amyotrophic lateral sclerosis. Mayo Clin Proc 53:173–178, 1978

14. Smith RA, Norris FH Jr: Symptomatic care of patients with amyotrophic lateral sclerosis. JAMA 234:715–717, 1975

12 The Role of Exercise

Richard T. Moxley III

Very limited information exists describing the effects of either local muscle-strength training or endurance exercise in patients with amyotrophic lateral sclerosis. Only one study has examined the effect of training a specific muscle group. This study involved six ALS patients and confined its training program to the biceps and triceps (24). The program consisted of 11–21 daily sessions depending on the particular patient and muscle group. Each session consisted of 30 maximal isometric contractions carried out at 36–60-second intervals. The strength of the patient each day was taken as the mean of the first 5 contractions performed. Two patients showed strength improvement comparable to that of normal controls, but as a group the patients exhibited no significant increase in strength. Nevertheless, this investigation did report a definite decrease in spasticity as a result of isometric exercise training. A more recent evaluation of whole body exercise in ALS patients has found that a program of regular endurance exercises, primarily swimming, has beneficial effects (31). Neither this report nor the previously mentioned one described any deleterious side effects related to exercise training.

BENEFITS OF EXERCISE

Many factors influence the capacity for aerobic muscular activity (3), and regular involvement in a cardiorespiratory conditioning program has produced significant improvements in healthy subjects (11). The following physiologic changes accompany regular exercise training:

1. Decreased heart rate at rest and during submaximal exercise.

2. Increased maximum oxygen consumption.

3. Displacement of the oxygen-hemoglobin dissociation curve to the right.

4. Decrease in blood lactate content and lactate release from the exercising limbs during submaximal exercise.

5. Decreased respiratory quotient during submaximal exercise.

6. Decreased blood pressure during submaximal exercise using trained limb muscles.

Regular exercise promotes adaptive changes in respiratory enzyme activity in muscle and the composition of muscle mitochondria (20); it also causes a decrease in the muscle respiratory quotient (20) and retards muscle protein catabolism (17). Exercise in the trained or untrained state stimulates amino acid retention and glucose uptake without requiring elevated levels of insulin (1, 30, 42).

These attributes of regular physical activity support a recommendation of both cardiorespiratory and specific muscle-group exercises to patients with ALS. If these normal responses occur in patients with ALS, a carefully monitored, individualized exercise program may prevent or slow the development of rest atrophy during the course of the disease. Such an exercise program might thereby provide a higher degree of functional performance at any given stage of the patient's illness. Moreover, a regular exercise program might allow for greater bone mineralization and might decrease the tendency for fractures found among patients with ALS. These potential benefits, although not proven to occur after exercise in patients with ALS, seem worth pursuing. Physicians often counsel their patients to go home and rest to preserve their strength. This advice, although well intended, contradicts our current understanding of muscle training and may encourage the development of rest atrophy in the remaining muscle tissue these patients possess. A regular stimulus is required to maintain strength.

INDIVIDUALIZED EXERCISE PROGRAMS

The development of an individualized exercise program demands more than the difficult task of motivating the patient, it also requires specifically tailored exercise activities and a regular mechanism for monitoring the patient's participation. The ALS patients most able to perform endurance type training (whole body physical activity) are those in the early stages of illness; however, activities such as swimming or riding a stationary bicycle may be possible in the later stages. Training programs to develop local muscle strength are applicable at any stage of the illness and may be useful in combination with endurance training in early stages to attempt to strengthen focally weak muscles.

Before recommending a specific exercise program, the physician should explain to the patient that limited information is available about the effects of exercise in ALS. A monitored, individualized exercise program is necessary to avoid undesirable side effects such as excessive fatigue, muscle strain, or cramps. This program will require the patient's active assistance in identifying early side effects. It will demand the patient's help in tailoring the exercise sessions to meet not only his or her daily time availability, but also the varying degree of muscle strength as the underlying disease progresses.

Cardiorespiratory Exercise

Before undertaking vigorous cardiorespiratory exercise, a patient should receive not only a detailed medical and neurologic examination but also a resting 12-lead electrocardiogram and an exercise stress test (see Table 1) (19, 27). The use of an exercise stress test to develop a target heart rate as a goal for cardiorespiratory exercise is an important feature of a monitored exercise program, and detailed information concerning this approach is available (16, 19, 37–39). The exercise prescription that a patient receives should involve work at an intensity that does not elevate the heart rate above the level at which the patient has been tested (27). The type of exercise as well as its intensity, frequency, and duration should be carefully tailored to each patient's fitness and clinical status.

The cardiorespiratory training program should be developed with the patient's internist and, under optimal circumstances, a cardiovascular disease–oriented physiologist. A physical educator or someone similarly trained can recommend specific types of exercises as well as provide instruction for both exercise and calisthenic warm-up activities (see Appendix I for an example). Many medical centers have begun to acquire such personnel as members of their cardiology departments to assist with the development of exercise programs to prevent coronary artery disease.

Localized Muscle Training

Specific muscle group strength-training utilizing some modification of the DeLorme method (see Appendix II) can be instituted with the help of either a physical therapist or physical educator (6–9, 12–14, 16, 23, 33, 34, 36, 40). Rehabilitation medicine departments frequently use the

Table 1 Contraindications to Exercise Training and Conditions Requiring Special Precautions[a]

Absolute Contraindications	*Relative Contraindications*	*Conditions Requiring Special Consideration and/or Precautions*
Acute myocardial infarction	Repetitive or frequent ventricular ectopic activity	Controlled dysrhythmia
Manifest circulatory insufficiency (congestive heart failure)	Uncontrolled or high-rate supraventricular dysrhythmia	Conduction disturbance: complete atrioventricular block, left bundle branch block, Wolff-Parkinson-White syndrome
Rapidly increasing angina pectoris with effort	Ventricular aneurysm	Fixed-rate pacemaker
Dissecting aneurysm	Moderate aortic stenosis	Electrolyte disturbance
Ventricular tachycardia and other dangerous dysrhythmias	Severe myocardial obstructive syndromes (subaortic stenosis)	Certain medications: digitalis, β-blockers, and drugs of related action
Severe aortic stenosis	Untreated severe systemic or pulmonary hypertension	Angina pectoris and other manifestations of coronary insufficiency
Active myocarditis		
Recent embolism, either systemic or pulmonary	Marked cardiac enlargement	Cyanotic heart disease
Thrombophlebitis	Severe anemia	Intermittent or fixed right-to-left shunt
Acute infectious disease	Uncontrolled metabolic disease (diabetes, thyrotoxicosis, myxedema)	Marked obesity
	Neuromuscular, musculoskeletal, or arthritic disorders	Renal, hepatic, and other metabolic insufficiency
	Overt psychoneurotic disturbance requiring therapy	

[a] Reprinted with permission from Haskell WL: Design of a cardiac conditioning program. In *Exercise and the Heart.* Edited by NK Wenger. Philadelphia, FA Davis Co, 1978, p 95. Adapted from Fox SM, Naughton SP, Haskell WL: Physical activity and the prevention of coronary heart disease. Ann Clin Res 3:404, 1971.

DeLorme method of graduated resistance exercises, and these departments provide a useful resource in developing this type of training program for a patient. One recently published, updated rehabilitation medicine text has sections devoted to isometric and isotonic training by the DeLorme method and to exercise approaches for patients with lower motor neuron diseases (5).

Progress Reports

Whether the exercise training is cardiorespiratory or limited to selected muscle groups, weekly or every-other-week progress reports are necessary to assess the effectiveness of the training program, to evaluate the heart rate profile, and to minimize the occurrence of serious side effects such as those described in Table 2 (19, 27). These progress reports also provide an important stimulus to motivate the patient to continue the exercise program. One way to record this information is to use cards that indicate the number of days during a specific week on which the patient exercised, along with an outline of the type of exercise, its intensity (average heart rate before, during, and after), and duration.

Table 2 Indications of Overexertion During an Exercise Session[a,b]

Indications During or Immediately After Exercise	*Delayed Indications*
Anginal discomfort	Persistent tachycardia (heart rate should return to within 10 beats of preexercise rate within 10 minutes after exercise)
Dysrhythmia	
Inappropriate tachycardia	Chronic or prolonged fatigue (patient should not feel general fatigue on following day or any unusual muscle soreness)
Inappropriate bradycardia	
Severe leg pain (claudication)	Insomnia
Pallor or cyanosis	Weight gain due to fluid retention
Ataxia, lightheadedness, confusion	
Nausea, vomiting	
Dyspnea continuing for more than several minutes	

[a] Reprinted with permission from Haskell WL: Design of a cardiac conditioning program. In *Exercise and the Heart.* Edited by NK Wenger. Philadelphia, FA Davis Co, 1978, p 102.
[b] These indications mean that the intensity or duration of exercise should be reduced during subsequent sessions.

EXERCISES AND PRECAUTIONS

Several types of cardiorespiratory exercises are appropriate for a patient in the early stages of ALS, for example, walking, stationary or regular cycling, swimming, certain rhythmic continuous calisthenics, certain rhythmic household chores, and a limited number of occupational tasks. Activities such as jogging or rope jumping may need to be limited to the atypical cases with restricted weakness and a chronic course. As the disease progresses, activities requiring significant leg support may not be feasible. In these instances, various types of arm exercises along with other non-weight-bearing activities can be used for cardiorespiratory training.

In instances in which arm exercise constitutes the major stimulus to training, the heart rate elevation produced by the activity should be lower than that selected as a target using leg exercise. The reason for this difference resides in the pressor reflex that accompanies many types of arm exercise (15). Sustained forceful grip produces a disproportionate rise in arterial blood pressure and an increased myocardial oxygen consumption for a given heart rate compared to a comparable heart rate level stimulated by whole body or leg exercise.

If data from normal subjects are applicable to ALS patients, the content of the patient's diet and his or her acid-base status may influence physical conditioning and exercise capability. Consuming a meal relatively high in carbohydrate one to two hours after cardiorespiratory exercise appears to provide an additional training benefit beyond that produced by the exercise alone. Previous studies have suggested that the intramuscular store of glycogen increases in athletes consuming such a meal one to two hours after a vigorous exercise session and that this enhances their maximal exercise capacity (10). Whether such a response occurs in patients with a neuromuscular disease remains to be proven. As a related point, one recent investigation has demonstrated that acidosis decreases maximum exercise performance while alkalosis appears to increase cardiorespiratory capacity (22). Diets or medications that produce an acidotic state may be undesirable for anyone undergoing a training program and should, if possible, be avoided in physically active ALS patients.

The cardiorespiratory exercise training programs in use today usually assume normal vascular regulation and muscle metabolism. It is likely that there are derangements in both these areas in ALS patients. However, there are studies indicating that exercise may even improve these abnormalities in patients with selected diseases such as neurocirculatory asthenia, cerebral palsy, or spinal muscular atrophy. Thus, it is not totally speculative to suggest that exercise may improve ALS patients, since they share certain common clinical features with patients who have these selected diseases. A few reports have indicated that abnormalities in blood flow (29) and metabolic regulation (4, 18, 26, 29) may exist in patients with either primary anterior horn cell disease, ALS, or cortical spinal tract dysfunction. As Figure 1 indicates, resting forearm blood flow is normal in patients with wasting from myotonic dystrophy, but a broad range of blood flow values is found in denervated patients with anterior horn cell disease (29). Two of the patients with forearm muscle weakness and wasting from anterior horn cell disease (open circles in Fig. 1) showed significantly greater resting blood flows than did patients with myotonic dystrophy who had comparable wasting or patients with denervation who had less weakness and wasting. The cause of this elevated blood flow is unclear, but it may indicate autonomic dysfunction. Certain vasomotor disorders such as neurocirculatory asthenia require regular exercise training to reverse their symptoms (21, 41), and exercise in ALS patients having abnormal resting blood flow might possibly improve circulatory efficiency.

Defects in skeletal muscle metabolism and blood flow have been described in patients with various types of lesions of the upper motor neurons. One investigation of five patients with forearm muscle weakness secondary to a variety of upper motor neuron lesions demonstrated that electrically induced exercise lowers oxygen uptake and increases the

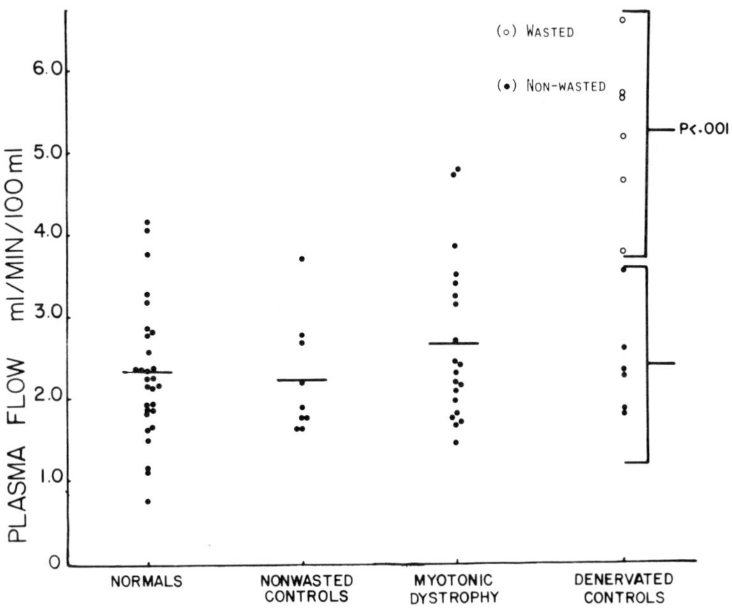

Figure 1 Resting plasma flow was measured three times using the Evans blue-dye continuous-infusion method in patients who had fasted overnight. (Reprinted with permission from Moxley RT, Griggs RC, Goldblatt D: Decreased insulin sensitivity of forearm muscle in myotonic dystrophy. J Clin Invest 62:857–867, 1978.)

proportion of lactate released in these patients as compared to similarly stimulated normal controls (18). However, whole body exercise training programs have increased cardiovascular performance and mobility in cerebral palsy patients, who presumably suffer from metabolic derangements similar to those noted previously (4, 18, 25, 26).

CASE REPORT

Figure 2 emphasizes the effects of cardiorespiratory training in a patient with anterior horn cell disease. It summarizes the progress produced by a regular swimming program over an eight-month period in a 36-year-old man with a 12-year history of a very slowly progressive form of spinal muscular atrophy. More clinical data along with the results of an investigation of forearm muscle metabolism in this patient have been reported previously (28). Before he developed symptoms of spinal muscular atrophy, the patient had been a competitive swimmer. Since the diag-

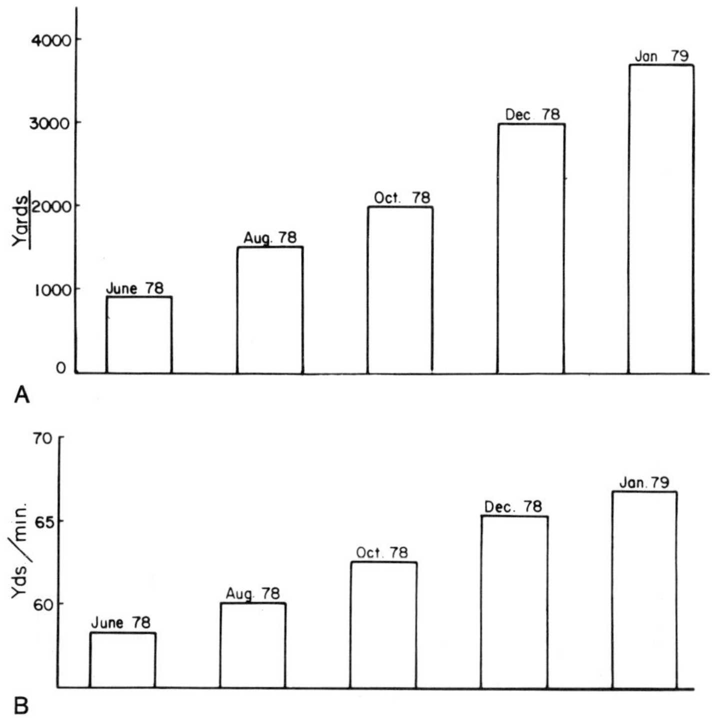

Figure 2 **(A)** Total yards swum during exercise sessions. **(B)** Velocity during 500-yard freestyle swimming sessions. The patient is a 36-year-old man with spinal muscular atrophy.

nosis of his disease, he has worked part time as a swimming coach. This patient has pursued an individualized exercise program that has required three to four swimming sessions per week. Exercise heart rate and muscular discomfort are monitored frequently throughout the course of each exercise session. The patient has exercised at an intensity not exceeding his target heart rate of 160 beats per minute. The duration of the sessions has gradually increased from an initial period of less than 30 minutes to a workout lasting approximately 90 minutes. The initial swimming workouts in June 1978 consisted of swimming 500 yards freestyle, a rest period, 200 yards breast stroke, a rest period, and 200 yards backstroke. His January 1979 exercise program is much more innovative and vigorous. It is summarized as follows:

1. 500 yards freestyle followed by a rest;
2. 500 yards freestyle, each 100 yards followed by a rest;
3. 400 yards backstroke, each 200 yards followed by a rest;
4. 400 yards backstroke, each 100 yards followed by a rest;
5. 400 yards breast stroke, each 200 yards followed by a rest;
6. 200 yards breast stroke, each 100 yards followed by a rest;
7. 600 yards prone kicking, each 200 yards followed by a rest;
8. 100 yards breast stroke followed by a rest;
9. 300 yards prone kicking, each 50 yards followed by a rest;
10. 200 yards freestyle, each 100 yards followed by a rest;
11. 150 yards prone and supine kicking, each 50 yards (or more often) followed by a rest.

During this eight-month period of cardiorespiratory training, the patient's resting heart rate declined from 68 beats per minute to 52 beats per minute. The patient states that he is now much less likely to become fatigued performing activities of daily living; for example, he was able to tolerate all-day Christmas shopping in December 1979, whereas in previous years he could tolerate only one to two hours of shopping at a time. The patient has been particularly cautious to avoid excessive fatigue and overdoing his exercise program. He has observed certain side effects during the course of his workouts. Cramps sometimes develop in the toes and arch of a foot but work themselves out without necessitating cessation of swimming activity. Cramps that develop in the calf and peroneal musculature are more significant and have caused him to rest at poolside before resuming exercise. Occasionally he has noted a twinge and muscle pull in the muscles of the upper back, particularly the upper portion of the trapezius. On one occasion, this required a two-week layoff to resolve the discomfort. The patient has discovered that by alternating the type of exercise, the duration of rest periods, and the intensity of his workouts, he can avoid serious muscle cramping and pulling. He has discovered that to maintain his level of fitness, he must swim at least three days a week. A layoff of several days requires a two-week period of makeup exercise to return him to the level he had achieved before layoff. This anecdotal case report supports the contention that regular physical activity may be helpful in selected patients with anterior horn cell disease and need not be associated with serious side effects.

SIDE EFFECTS

A note of caution is in order. The symptoms described in Table 2 serve as signals cautioning the physician that the patient has overdone his or her exercise. It is important to individualize the exercise program and to monitor it frequently to avoid undesirable side effects. Studies of swimming in rats have shown that significant myocardial damage occurs when the exercise load and duration of activity exceed their typical levels (2). Less specific deleterious side effects of exercise were reported in a few of the articles in the exercise symposium published in 1967 (35). One article describes the additive stress to normal individuals of high humidity and heavy work performed for several hours. Obviously, factors such as these would be particularly stressful to someone with a reduced total motor neuron pool. Patients with ALS have to be cautious in their physical activity programs.

SUMMARY

Individualized, monitored, cardiorespiratory and specific muscle-group exercise training may offer important functional benefits to patients with ALS. To achieve this goal requires the coordinated assistance of the patient's internist, a work physiologist or physical educator, a physical therapist, and the patient's neurologist. Frequent review of the patient's exercise progress on a weekly or every-other-week basis is necessary to tailor the program to the patient's neurologic state and to avoid unwanted side effects related to overexertion.

Acknowledgments

Thanks should be given to Dr. David Goldblatt, Professor of Neurology at The University of Rochester School of Medicine and Dentistry, for his guidance in preparing this manuscript. My appreciation also goes to Dr. Samuel Fox, Professor of Medicine at George Washington University School of Medicine, and to Dr. William L. Haskell, Clinical Associate Professor of Medicine and Co-Director of the Cardiac Rehabilitation Program at Stanford University School of Medicine, for their advice and instruction in exercise physiology and cardiology. My special gratitude goes to my wife, Joan Moxley, for the artwork in Figures 1 and 2.

APPENDIX I. WARM-UP EXERCISES

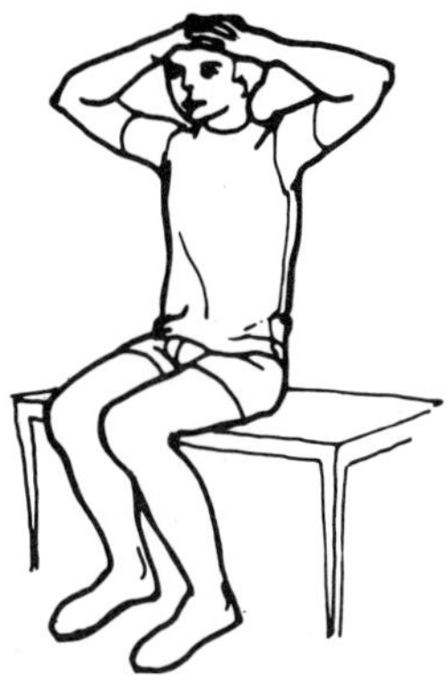

Warm-up: Deep Breathing

Directions: While in a sitting position, lock hands on top of head and extend elbows out to sides. Take slow deep breaths. Do *not* breathe rapidly or hold breath.
Number of times to perform exercise: starting number = 10 (3 times daily); increase per week = 0; maximum number = 10 (3 times daily).

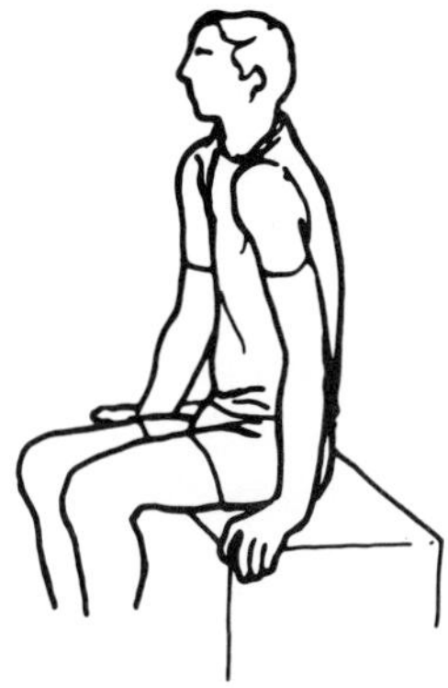

Adduction of Shoulders

Directions: In a sitting position, keep back straight and hold arms at sides of body. Pull shoulders forward and in toward midline of body. Relax. Do *not* hold shoulders forward for a prolonged period of time. Return to starting position and repeat.
Number of times to perform exercise: starting number = 5; increase per week = 5; maximum number = 30.

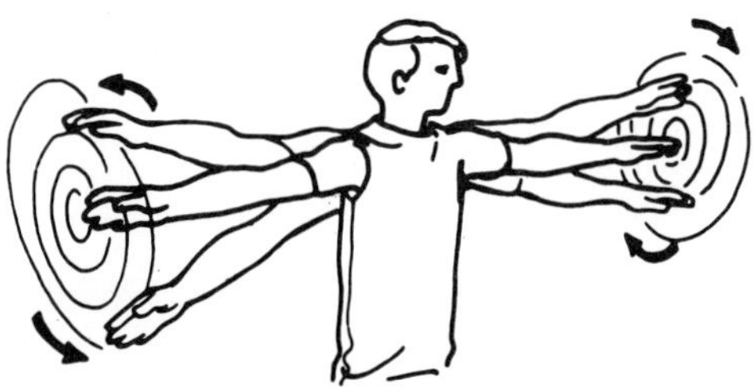

Arm Circles

Directions: Stand with arms extended out to sides at shoulder level. Make small circles and gradually increase their size. Reverse direction.
Number of times to perform exercise: starting number = 5; increase per week = 5; maximum number = 30.

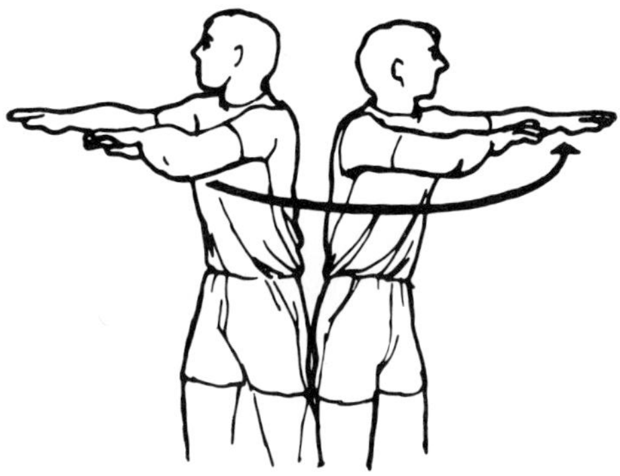

Trunk Twisters

Directions: Stand with arms extended out to sides at shoulder level. Swing arms horizontally at shoulder level while rotating at waist, left to right and right to left. Allow arms to bend at end of swing. Return to starting position and repeat.
Number of times to perform exercise: starting number = 5; increase per week = 5; maximum number = 30.

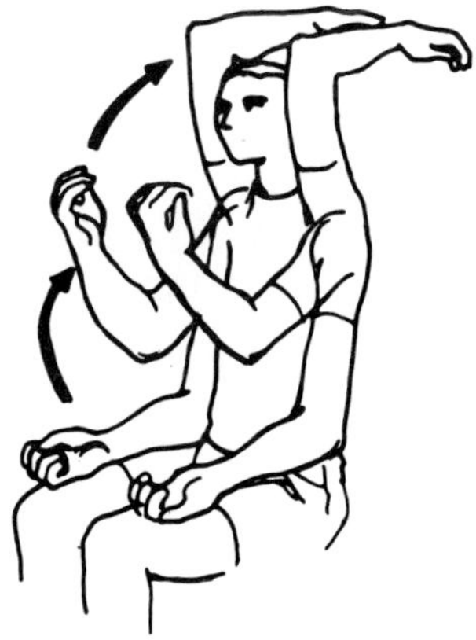

Raising Bent Arms

Directions: In a sitting position, keep back straight. Place hands, palms up, loosely closed, on lap. Keeping arms in this bent position, raise arms up and back until upper arms are in line with ears. Return to starting position and repeat.
Number of times to perform exercise: starting number = 5; increase per week = 5; maximum number = 30.

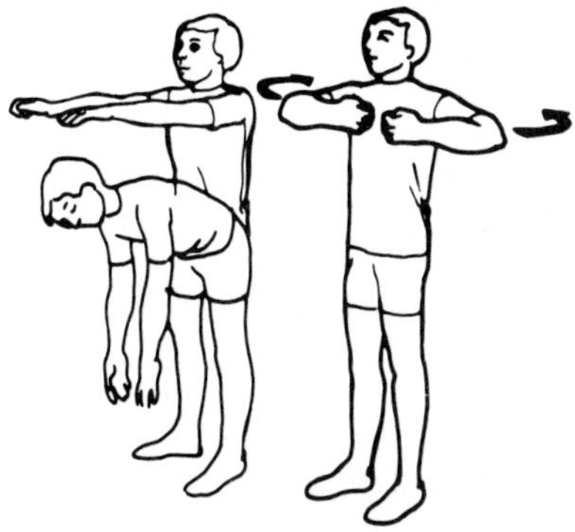

Toe Touches

Directions: Stand with feet spread shoulder width and arms extended out in front of body; slowly bend forward at waist and reach for toes. Return to starting position with arms extended at chest level in front of body. Bend arms at elbows and touch fists near but not touching shoulders. Return to starting position and repeat.
Number of times to perform exercise: starting number = 3; increase per week = 3; maximum number = 18.

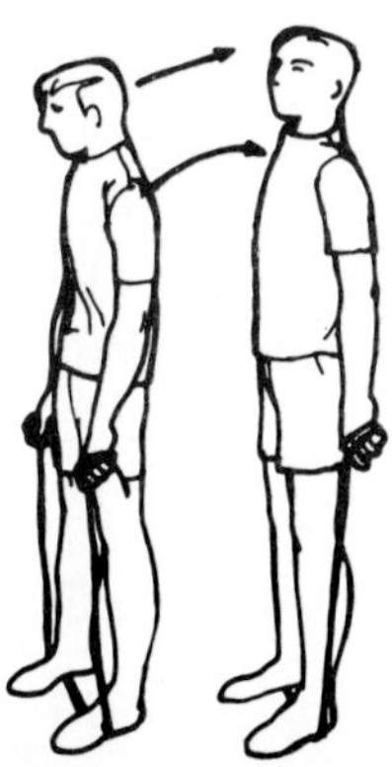

Shoulder Shrug with Rope

Directions: Stand, holding one end of a cotton rope in each hand, as if about to jump rope. Stand on loop of rope. Arms should be straight and shoulders relaxed. Adjust grasp on rope so that rope is straight but not taut or tight. Slowly stand fully upright. Hold head high and in line with back and shoulders. Rope will now be taut. Return to starting position and repeat.
Number of times to perform exercise: starting number = 5; increase per week = 5; maximum number = 30.

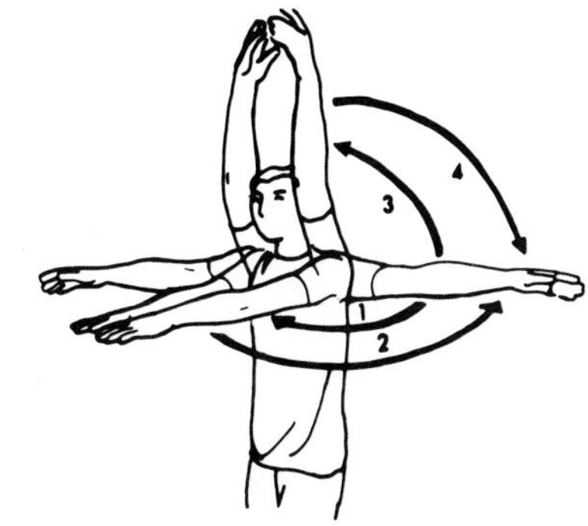

Arm Lifts

Directions: Stand with feet spread shoulder width, extend arms out to sides at shoulder level. Bring hands together in front of chest. Return to starting position. Raise arms above head until elbows are close to ears. Return to starting position and repeat.
Number of times to perform exercise: starting number = 3; increase per week = 3; maximum number = 18.

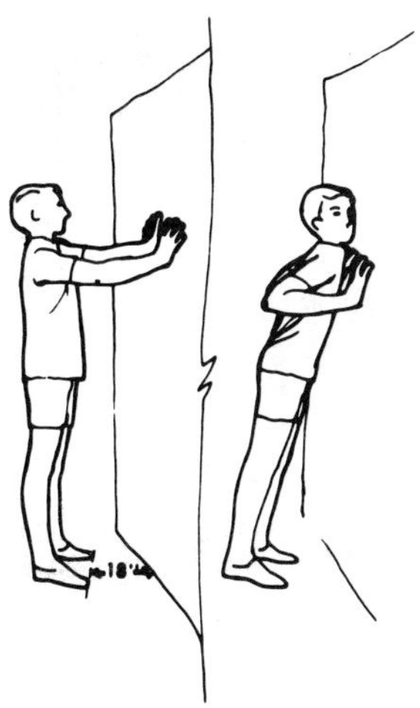

Wall Pushups

Directions: Face a wall and stand 18 inches from it. Raise arms to shoulder level and place palms of hands on wall. Slowly lower body until chest is within an inch of wall. Press away from wall and return to starting position. If you have to strain to push away from wall, move closer to it. Repeat.
Number of times to perform exercise: starting number = 3; increase per week = 3; maximum number = 18.

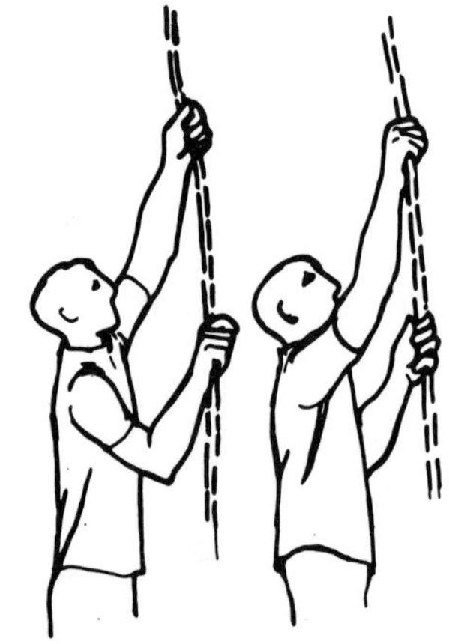

Imaginary Rope Climb

Directions: Reach one hand above head as if grasping a rope. Lower hand as you raise other hand to grasp rope. Continue alternating hands as if pulling yourself up a rope.
Number of times to perform exercise: starting number = 5; increase per week = 5; maximum number = 30.

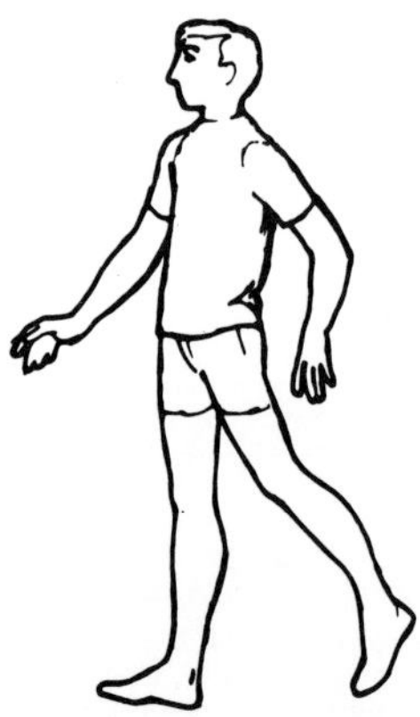

Cool-Down: Walking

Directions: Walk for 10 minutes while swinging arms.

APPENDIX II. MODIFIED DELORME METHOD

Exercise Format for Muscle-Group Training

1. Perform 5 or 10 repetitions at a resistance approximately 50% of the maximum for that week.

2. After a 1–2-minute rest, perform 5 or 10 repetitions at a resistance about 75% of maximum.

3. After another 1–2-minute rest, perform 5 or 10 repetitions at 100% of the maximum determined at the start of the week.

Specific Muscle-Group Exercise Program

1. Use *isotonic* rather than *isometric* exercise.

2. Determine the 5- or 10-repetition resistance maximum once every 1 or 2 weeks (e.g., the maximum amount of weight that can be lifted consecutively 5 or 10 times).

REFERENCES

1. Ahlborg G, Felig P, Hagenfeldt HR, et al: Substrate turnover during prolonged exercise in man. Splanchnic and leg metabolism of glucose, free fatty acids, and amino acids. J Clin Invest 53:1080–1090, 1974

2. Arcos JC, Sohal RS, Sun SC, et al: Changes in ultrastructure and respiratory control in mitochondria of rat heart hypertrophied by exercise. Exp Mol Pathol 8:49–65, 1968

3. Astrand P: Aerobic work capacity during maximal performance under various conditions. Circ Res 20-21(Suppl 1):202–210, 1967

4. Bar-or O, Inbar O, Spira R: Physiological effects of a sports rehabilitation program on cerebral palsied and post-poliomyelitic adolescents. Med Sci Sports 8:157–161, 1976

5. Basmajian JV (Editor): *Therapeutic Exercise,* ed 3. Baltimore, Williams & Wilkins Co, 1978

6. Belka DE: Comparison of dynamic, static, and combination training on dominant wrist flexor muscles. Res Q 39:244–250, 1966

7. Berger R: Effect of varied weight training programs on strength. Res Q 33:168–181, 1961

8. Berger RA: Comparative effects of three weight training programs. Res Q 34:396–398, 1963

9. Berger RA: Comparison of the effect of various weight training loads on strength. Res Q 36:141–146, 1964

10. Bergstrom J: Local changes of ATP and phosphorylcreatine in human muscle tissue in connection with exercise. Circ Res 20–21(Suppl 1): 91–98, 1967

11. Clausen JP: Circulatory adjustments to dynamic exercise and effect of physical training in normal subjects and in patients with coronary artery disease. Prog Cardiovasc Dis 18:459–495, 1976

12. DeLateur BJ, Lehmann JF, Fordyce WE: A test of the DeLorme axiom. Arch Phys Med Rehabil 49:245–248, 1968

13. DeLorme TL: Heavy resistance exercises. Arch Phys Med 27:607–630, 1946

14. DeLorme TL, Walkins AL: Techniques of progressive resistance exercise. Arch Phys Med 29:263–273, 1948

15. Donald KW, Lind AR, McNicol GW, et al: Cardiovascular response to sustained (static) contractions. Circ Res 20-21(Suppl 1):15–32, 1967

16. Fox SM, Naughton JP, Gorman PA: Physical activity and cardiovascular health, Parts I, II, III. Mod Concepts Cardiovasc Dis 41:17–30, 1972

17. Goldberg A: Protein turnover in skeletal muscle. J Biol Chem 244: 3217–3222, 1968

18. Hagenfeldt L, Landin S, Wahren J: Substrate utilization in paretic human forearm muscle during electrically induced exercise. Clin Sci 41:361, 1971

19. Haskell WL: Design of a cardiac conditioning program. Cardiovasc Clin 9:93–106, 1978

20. Holloszy J, Rennie M, Hickson R, et al: Physiological consequences of the biochemical and adaptations to endurance exercise. Ann NY Acad Sci 301:440–450, 1977

21. Holmgren A: Vasoregulatory asthenia. Can Med Assoc J 96:904–907, 1967

22. Jones NL, Sutton JR, Taylor R, et al: Effect of pH on cardiorespiratory and metabolic responses to exercise. J Appl Physiol 43:959–964, 1977

23. Knowlton GC, Bennett RL: Overwork. Arch Phys Med 38:18–20, 1957

24. Lenman J: A clinical and experimental study of the effects of exer-

cise on motor weakness in neurological disease. J Neurol Neurosurg Psychiatry 22:182–194, 1959

25. Lundberg A: Oxygen consumption in relation to work load in students with cerebral palsy. J Appl Physiol 40:873–875, 1976

26. Lundberg A, Pernow B: The effect of physical training on oxygen utilization and lactate formation in the exercising muscle of adolescents with motor handicaps. Scand J Clin Lab Invest 26:89–96, 1970

27. Merriman JE: Exercise prescription for apparently healthy individuals and for cardiac patients. Cardiovascular Clin 9:81–92, 1978

28. Moxley RT, Griggs RC, Goldblatt D: Decreased insulin sensitivity of forearm muscle in myotonic dystrophy. J Clin Invest 62:857–867, 1978

29. Moxley RT, Griggs RC, VanGelder V, et al: Effects of denervation and wasting on skeletal muscle blood flow in man. Neurology 28:400, 1978

30. Moxley RT, Pozefsky T: Metabolic changes accompanying skeletal muscle hypertrophy. Clin Res 24:366A, 1976

31. Norris FH Jr, Ü KS, Denys EH, et al: Amyotrophic lateral sclerosis. Mayo Clin Proc 53:544, 1978

32. Oberman A, Kouchoukos NT: Role of exercise after coronary artery bypass surgery. Cardiovasc Clin 9:155–172, 1978

33. O'Shea P: Effects of selected weight training programs on the development of strength and muscle hypertrophy. Res Q 37:95–102, 1963

34. Petersen FB: Muscle training by static, concentric and eccentric contractions. Acta Physiol Scand 48:406–416, 1960

35. Physical activity and the heart: Symposium. Can Med Assoc J 96: 1967

36. Pollock M, Wilmore J, Fox SM: *Health and Fitness Through Physical Activity*. New York, Wiley, 1978

37. Prog Cardiovasc Dis (Exercise I) 18:421–506, 1976

38. Prog Cardiovasc Dis (Exercise II) 19:1–90, 1976

39. Prog Cardiovasc Dis (Exercise III) 19:91–106, 1976

40. Rasch PJ, Morehouse LE: Effect of static and dynamic exercises on muscular strength and hypertrophy. J Appl Physiol 11:29–34, 1956

41. Schoenfeld Y, Shapiro Y, Drory Y, et al: Rehabilitation of patients

with NCA (neurocirculatory asthenia) through a short term training program. Am J Phys Med 57:1–8, 1978

42. Wahren J, Felig P, Hendler R, et al: Glucose and amino acid metabolism during recovery after exercise. J Appl Physiol 34:838–845, 1973

Commentary

Katharine M. Donohoe

I want to make a concrete suggestion about where to find assistive devices in the community. In addition to consultation with an occupational therapist, physical therapist, and physiatrist, the patient may wish to review publications that visually present occupational aids that he or she can use at home. One is the catalogue from Fred Sammons Inc., *The BEOK Self-Help Aids* [P.O. Box 1586, Winter Park, FL 32790; telephone: (305)628-0545]. Another is the *Green Pages Rehab Source Book* [Fred Sammons Inc., P.O. Box 32, Brookfield, IL 60513; telephone: (800)323-7305]. Our patients have felt that being able to see the different assistive devices, from built-up spoons to special knives and scrub brushes, has been an asset. They particularly like the kitchen and homemaking aids, which are quite inexpensive.

Theodore L. Munsat

Just like everyone else, I frequently recommend exercise for ALS patients. I think it is important to give them something active to do to prevent contractures and, especially, shoulder problems as well as to preserve whatever function they still have. However, I think we have to be cautious about excessive exercise, as there is evidence that it can be harmful. Healthy persons, especially those who have not been trained, who are pushed beyond a certain limit can develop muscle fiber breakdown and myoglobinuria. It is clear in Duchenne dystrophy that even minimal exercise can raise serum enzyme creatine phosphokinase (CPK) significantly for about 24 hours. Whether this is harmful or not has not been proven, but the rise in CPK may indicate additional damage. There is also experimental evidence from animal studies suggesting that, if the supply of anterior horn cells is depleted, any excessive metabolic demand will accelerate the breakdown of the anterior horn cells that remain. Conceivably, there is a level beyond which those anterior horn cells cannot be pushed, and I think it might be a mistake to push ALS patients too hard. I think we have to keep an eye on that, particularly in a disease that progresses.

Forbes H. Norris, Jr

I have no hard data, merely favorable clinical experience with exercise programs, which, as Dr. Moxley states in his chapter, have not appeared to harm ALS patients when judiciously ordered and performed. I particularly favor pool therapy. Many of our patients were told that there was nothing to be done, so they gave up hope, went home and to bed. Most people are too sensible to do that, but some poor souls do become despondent, do give up hope and take to bed, and those are the worst cases I see. Not only do they have multiple contractures and painfully frozen shoulders, but also they have profound disuse atrophy compounding the ALS weakness.

They are also depressed; the concerned physician has only to show a little interest to produce an increase in the patient's strength. Perhaps the important point here is that the treatment of morale is as important as any somatic treatment we can offer. The maintenance of hope and the promotion, for as long as possible, of the ability to do at least simple self-care activities have crucial roles in supporting morale.

In my experience, the main problem with exercises is persuading patients to undertake and actually perform them on a daily basis; we live in a sedentary society. An important reason for frequent but less strenuous exercise sessions is the avoidance of fatigue, which is not only bad for morale but also potentially productive of injury in certain circumstances, e.g., falling when running. If the treatment prescribed is exhausting or debilitating, the patient may well conclude either that the prescription is misdirected or that he ought to see another physician or pursue some other course. It is very important that the patient's fatigue be taken into account when any exercise program is given. Several brief periods of exercise during the day are safer and easier than a single prolonged exercise session, though the latter is preferable to two or three even greater efforts per week.

I should mention that in most cases ALS patients are very sensitive to chilling; pool exercise, for example, must be done in a warm pool. We have had several patients who lost a dangerous amount of strength because they became chilled and then much more fatigued. Dr. Denys has recently published findings on the effects of cooling of the muscles in ALS patients (1).

The basic question is: is exercise truly helpful, or does it merely reduce disuse atrophy? I do not know the answer. The approach suggested by Dr. Moxley ought to be pursued; it at least gives an objective measure for this problem. One reason we at Pacific Medical Center have not developed a scientific study of the role of active exercise in patients with ALS is that we have been unable to develop a series of control patients who will give informed consent to such a trial.

I have been actively discouraging patients from jogging and running. Most patients with ALS have flaccid arm weakness and spastic leg weakness. The legs are apt to weaken or the feet to stumble, precipitating a fall in which the weakened arms cannot play the normal protective role. We have had several dozen ALS patients who have fallen and suffered fractures, dislocations, or severe sprains while jogging.

REFERENCE

1. Denys EH, Norris FH: Amyotrophic lateral sclerosis impairment of neuromuscular transmission. Arch Neurol 36:202–205, 1979

13 Definition and Scope of the Communication Disorder

Arnold E. Aronson

Bulbar amyotrophic lateral sclerosis eventually destroys speech altogether without appreciably impairing language, intellect, reason, or emotion. The patient's speech declines relentlessly from normal articulation to subhuman grunting and groaning. The disorder is technically a dysarthria, ultimately an anarthria. Defined as a speech disorder from central nervous system or peripheral nervous system disease (or both), dysarthria is characterized by loss of speech muscle strength or coordination. In ALS it is actually a mixture of two pure forms: flaccid (or lower motor neuron) dysarthria and spastic (or bilateral upper motor neuron) dysarthria. The proportion of spasticity and flaccidity varies within and among individuals, depending in part on the chronology of the disease. Flaccidity may be more prominent at one point, spasticity at another, or there may be an equal mixture of the two.

PHYSIOLOGIC CHANGES RESULTING IN DYSARTHRIA

Classification of the speech musculature into functional units permits more careful analysis of the physiologic changes resulting in dysarthria (Fig. 1).

Respiration

Normal speech requires approximately 500 ml of tidal air volume. Patients with ALS who have atrophy and paresis or paralysis of the inter-

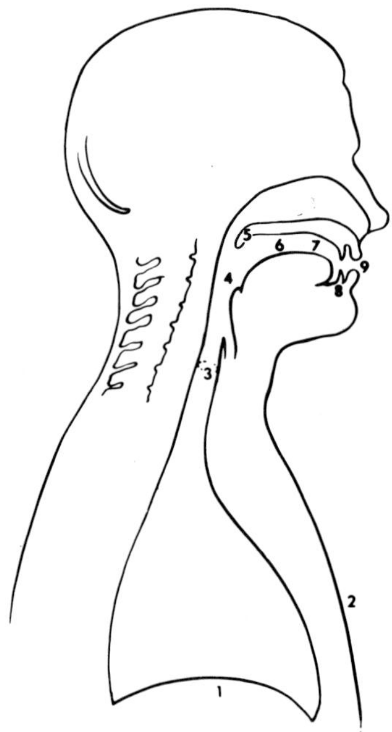

Figure 1 Schematic diagram indicating speech musculature commonly impaired in patients with ALS. 1. Abdominal muscles and diaphragm. 2. Thoracic muscles. 3. Laryngeal muscles. 4. Pharyngeal muscles. 5. Velopharyngeal muscles. 6, 7. Tongue muscles. 8. Mandibular muscles. 9. Facial muscles. (Adapted with permission from Netsell R: A developing framework for research in speech production. Progress Report No. 1. Madison, Speech Research Laboratory, Neurological and Rehabilitation Hospital, University of Wisconsin, June 1971.)

costal and diaphragmatic musculature and of the secondary muscles of respiration demonstrate reduced length of utterance and increased frequency of inhalation as a result of inadequate exhalatory air volume. They are incapable of producing a normally loud voice because of inadequate infraglottal air pressure.

Phonation

If spasticity is predominant, hyperadduction of the true and false vocal folds, technically a pseudobulbar dysphonia, will require that the exhaled air be forced through a constricted glottis. Such elevated laryngeal resistance to the exhaled air stream, coupled with a reduced exhalatory force, decreases the volume of voice in addition to producing a strained hoarseness or harshness because of abnormal vocal-fold vibration. A greater flaccid (lower motor neuron) component produces adductor vocal-fold weakness, literally a unilateral or bilateral vocal-fold paresis or paralysis. An excess volume/velocity of unphonated air produces extreme breathiness and reduces loudness. Secondary problems from such weakness are inhalatory stridor, dyspnea, and dysphagia. Pooling of saliva in the pyriform sinuses of the larynx adds to the dysphonia a telltale wet, gurgly component. Rapid voice tremor or flutter, particularly on vowel prolongation, signifies the flaccid component.

Resonation

Essential to intelligible speech is the ability to seal the velopharyngeal port by soft palate and pharyngeal sphincter action. Paresis or paralysis preventing velopharyngeal closure permits exhaled air to escape through the nasal passages and out the nares during speech—in effect stealing intraoral pressure and thus diminishing fricative and plosive consonant force. These sounds, therefore, lose their identity; intelligibility is reduced, and we hear hypernasality and nasal emission of the airstream.

Articulation

Articulation determines the intelligibility of speech more than any other factor. The speedy and highly targeted action of the tongue, lips, cheeks, and mandible shapes the phonated and resonated air stream from lungs, larynx, and pharynx.

Tongue

The tongue is responsible for all speech sounds except /p/, /b/, /m/, /f/, and /v/. In patients with ALS, the tongue is weak, atrophied, and subject to fasciculations. Reduction of tongue strength and speed may reveal early ALS through distortion of consonants, as the tongue is no longer able to make firm contact with the teeth and hard palate. A study of tongue strength by Dworkin et al. showed that, whereas healthy men could protrude the tongue anteriorly with an average force of 2086 g, men with ALS were able to press the tongue only 1129 g (4). Healthy women could press the tongue 1965 g, whereas women with ALS could press it only 957 g. Carrow et al. found tongue atrophy and dysphagia to be the two most prevalent neurologic signs in ALS patients with severely reduced speech intelligibility, and 83% of their patients who had severe loss of intelligibility also had tongue atrophy (2). Another characteristic change of the tongue musculature in patients with ALS is slowness of movement, as evidenced by a reduced rate of alternate motion and slow contextual speech. Dworkin et al. found that, whereas healthy adults can repeat syllables at an average of six syllables per second, patients with ALS had a maximum of four syllables per second (4).

Also interfering with articulation is the intraoral accumulation of saliva. It blocks transmission of sound and forces the patient to articulate with the jaws occluded to prevent drooling.

Lips

For normal speech, the lips must be capable of compression, one against the other or the lower lip against the upper incisor teeth. They must be able to retract for certain vowel sounds and become rounded for others. The cheeks must be compressible so that intraoral pressure can be maintained. When the circumoral musculature is weakened, bilabial sounds are either distorted because the lips give way, releasing air prematurely on plosive sounds, or omitted because the lips cannot be approximated at all.

Mandible

Neither the tongue nor the lips can perform their assigned articulatory tasks unless the mandible can be elevated close to the maxilla, where it serves as a platform for tongue and lip movements. Masseter and temporalis muscle weakness prevent such elevation, and this compounds articulatory defects derived from lip and tongue weakness.

QUALITY OF SPEECH IN ALS

The question, "What is the speech of ALS like?" can be answered only as follows: "It depends on when in the course of the disease the speech is assayed." The difference between speech samples of early and late dysarthria in ALS is so considerable that it is difficult to conceive of them as coming from the same source. The first insidious sign of onset may be only a nondescript hoarseness or articulatory imprecision that is unnoticed by the patient, although others may be sensitive to the change. When the disease begins with the bulbar speech musculature, the otolaryngologist is often the first physician consulted. However, because the speech signs are mild, an erroneous diagnosis of functional voice or speech disorder is common. As the dysarthria progresses and dysphagia and other neurologic signs develop, the organic etiology becomes apparent.

The physical causes of the noticeable speech defects are difficult or impossible to see in the early stages. Listening, however, often provides clues to neurogenicity. The following signs are typical:

1. While the patient utters a prolonged vowel sound, the clinician listens for *strained, harsh voice quality* and *flutter or tremor of voice.* The patient may also have a *weak cough.*

2. While the patient pronounces a sentence devoid of nasal sounds, the clinician listens for *hypernasality* and feels the bridge of the nose or holds a mirror under the nares to look for *abnormal air leakage* and *nasal emission of air.*

3. As the patient repeats the syllables /pa/, /ta/, and /ka/ as rapidly and evenly as possible, the examiner listens for abnormally *slow and laborious movement.*

4. The tongue is examined for *weakness, atrophy, and fasciculations.*

5. The patient is questioned concerning *reduced threshold for crying or laughter.*

The pseudobulbar cry or laugh is a telltale diagnostic sign and a serious social and psychologic burden. Often in response to relatively innocuous comments by others, the patient erupts into uncontrollable wailing—embarrassing, distracting, and interfering with speech at the moment.

The essential features of pseudobulbar laughter and crying have been described by Kreindler and Pruskauer-Apostol (6). Pseudobulbar laughter and crying seem to occur without adequate cause, often in response to nonspecific stimuli, and are usually triggered by human interaction. The patient may be quiescent for a relatively long time until someone speaks to him or her, at which point the patient may begin to laugh or cry spasmodically after a short latency. Incongruity between the level of internal emotion and the external appearance of joy or melancholy is presumed. The laughter or crying occurs abruptly without the normal graded approach of a smile or frown, and, consequently, such outbursts take on a stereotyped automatic and paroxysmal quality. The cry or laugh is impossible to interrupt or modify because it is involuntary. Facial, thoracic, and abdominal muscle contractions are incongruously excessive in comparison with the audible signs of crying, laughter, or tears. The cry is usually a long wail rising in pitch and often reaching falsetto levels. Sometimes the cry occurs without a voiced air stream; this is aptly described as "mute grimacing." The patient may switch from crying to laughter without an apparent reason, giving the erroneous impression of emotional lability. The locations of lesions producing pathologic laughter extend beyond the corticobulbar tracts. Involuntary laughter has been reported to occur in patients with brainstem and hypothalamic tumors; it may result from stimulation of the floor of the third ventricle or from temporal lobe infarction. Some studies implicate the internal capsule and surrounding basal ganglia (1, 5).

The most deviant speech dimensions in patients with ALS are, according to a study of 30 patients by Darley et al., imprecise consonants, hypernasality, harsh voice quality, slow rate, monopitch, short phrases, distorted vowels, low pitch, monoloudness, excess and equal stress on all syllables of a word, prolonged intervals between words and syllables, reduced stress on syllables and words, prolonged phonemes, strained/strangled voice quality, breathy voice quality, audible inhalation or stridor, inappropriate silences, and nasal emission (3).

CASE STUDY

Nine months before coming to the Mayo Clinic, a 61-year-old man noticed a change in his voice which he thought was due to a throat infection. At first his hoarseness varied from day to day—sometimes it was better, sometimes it was worse—until finally it was present most of the time. Next, he noticed that he had begun to talk through his nose and had difficulty whistling. He began to have frequent episodes of hiccups and became aware of an uncomfortable sensation in the region of his larynx; he began to choke often on both solids and liquids. He noticed an increase in emotionality. On retiring to bed, he experienced choking, coughing, and momentary difficulties in breathing, which he had to sit up to alleviate.

Neurologic examination showed hyperactive deep reflexes bilaterally, although the electromyogram was normal. Speech pathology examination revealed a strained/strangled hoarseness, a rapid tremor or flutter of the voice on vowel prolongation, a wet or gurgly component to the voice, hypernasality and nasal emission, articulatory imprecision, and abnormally slow rate.

Before the patient came to the Mayo Clinic he had been given a palatal lift prosthesis in an attempt to alleviate the velopharyngeal insufficiency. However, we found that it provided little help. The main source of his poor speech intelligibility was extreme weakness of the tongue and inability to elevate the mandible.

We began a regimen of tongue-strengthening exercises on an experimental basis consisting of two daily sessions of approximately one-half hour each over a five-day period. The patient started out with a maximum anterior tongue force of 202 g (normal is 2086 g). By the end of the week, his tongue force had improved to an average of 331 g; however, this amount of improvement had no effect on his speech. We also attempted to elevate the mandible in a splint in order to approximate the jaws to facilitate articulation; however, this, too, proved to be unsuccessful.

This patient's history illustrates the typical obstacles that confront the clinician who attempts to treat the speech disorders of such patients. Overcoming basic articulatory muscle weakness either by muscle-strengthening regimens or by other kinds of compensation remains the chief key to improving speech intelligibility. Techniques for overcoming these obstacles must be acquired if we are to prolong the quality of the patient's life through preservation of communication.

REFERENCES

1. Aschari AN, Colover J: Posterior fossa tumors with pathological laughter. JAMA 235:1469–1471, 1976

2. Carrow E, Rivera V, Mauldin M, et al: Deviant speech characteristics in motor neuron disease. Arch Otolaryngol 100:212–218, 1974

3. Darley FL, Aronson AE, Brown JR: *Motor Speech Disorders.* Philadelphia, WB Saunders Co, 1975

4. Dworkin JP, Aronson AE, Mulder DW: Tongue force in normals and in dysarthric patients with amyotrophic lateral sclerosis. J Speech Hear Disord, in press

5. Haymaker W, Kuhlenbeck H: Pathologic laughter and crying. In *Clinical Neurology.* Edited by AE Baker, LH Baker. Hagerstown, Harper and Row, 1976

6. Kreindler A, Pruskauer-Apostol B: Neurologic and psychopathologic aspects of compulsive crying and laughter in pseudo-bulbar palsy patients. Revue Roumaine de Neurologie 8:125–139, 1971

14 Treatment of Communication Disorders

Janice L. Elliott

Arthur J. Hudson

As Dr. Aronson pointed out in the previous chapter, the individual with amyotrophic lateral sclerosis who is losing normal speech is also becoming imprisoned with unfulfilled needs, unresolved questions, and, at times, extreme anxieties that need expression. Thus, improvement of communication becomes necessary for ordinary living and peace of mind and may be lifesaving with the critically ill patient. In the following discussion, we shall deal with the various means available to facilitate communication for ALS patients with varying degrees of dysarthria.

SPEECH THERAPY TECHNIQUES

The goals of speech therapy for ALS patients with dysarthria are to improve and maintain speech intelligibility. Darley et al. have outlined several general principles of speech treatment that apply to the patient with ALS (5). In general, patients are encouraged to compensate for deficits in speech by making the most effective use of the remaining level of function of the speech musculature. As the disease progresses, there will be a greater need to use the compensatory skills learned earlier in the course of the disease.

Normally, speech production is a highly automatic behavior. The patient with ALS must learn to monitor and to exert voluntary control over speech in order to make changes in the speech pattern. The concentration and effort required to monitor and modify speech in ALS is fatiguing, and therefore a noticeable deterioration in speech can develop when the patient is tired, particularly in the more advanced stages of dysarthria. The very nature of ALS causes patients to become depressed and discouraged, and, therefore, they may not be interested in contributing the required effort. Patients in whom the disease initially involves the bulbar musculature often put forth a better effort to improve their speech than do those in whom the disease is well advanced before bulbar impairment is evident. As the patient's speech deteriorates, frequent monitoring and encouragement are needed to help him or her maintain compensatory speech skills. It is important to remember that a patient with adequate speech production one month may need additional instruction to maintain intelligibility in the next month.

Speech therapy should commence with the first sign of dysarthria, while the patient still retains a good deal of control over the speech musculature. It is valuable, even before any speech impairment is apparent, to introduce the speech pathologist to the patient along with the physiotherapist and other health professionals who will attend him or her. Early attention of this kind by the speech therapist enables the neurologist to have a more precise evaluation of bulbar function and provides a baseline appraisal for the speech pathologist in future assessments.

The speech assessment will reveal what characteristic of the patient's speech interferes most with intelligibility. Once a change in the patient's speech pattern is evident, specific instruction can be given on how to change the manner of speaking to improve or maintain intelligibility. Darley et al. have organized the most extensive outline of speech therapy procedures to improve articulation, resonance, phonation, and prosody in dysarthric patients (5). These techniques are described here in relation to the ALS patient.

Articulation

Slowing the Rate of Speech

Imprecise articulation can be improved by slowing the rate of speech. This is accomplished by breaking polysyllabic words into syllables, such as "el-e-phant," prolonging vowel sounds, and increasing the length of interword pauses. However, slowness is a predominant characteristic of speech in the ALS patient, and it may be unnecessary to teach this strategy.

Exaggerated Articulation

Exaggerated articulation can also result in clearer speech production. This strategy involves voluntarily extending the range of motion of the lips, tongue, and jaw and increasing the effort made to produce each sound. This technique is tiring, and the ALS patient is often not able to speak in this manner for more than a few minutes. However, it does improve intelligibility until the patient fatigues.

Sound Drills

Consonant sounds that require elevation of the tip of the tongue such as /t/, /d/, /l/, /n/, /s/, /z/ or the back of the tongue such as /k/ or /g/ are particularly difficult for the patient with ALS to produce correctly. These patients are frequently receptive to drills in making these sounds.

Alternative Speech Movements

Patients with ALS may be unable to make a certain sound in the usual manner. In such cases, they must be taught alternative means to accomplish the target sound. For example, if lip closure is not possible, a close approximation of /b/ can be made through contact of the upper front teeth with the lower lip instead of through the usual bilabial place of articulation.

Resonance

Reducing Hypernasal Resonance

Other common characteristics of speech in ALS patients that can interfere greatly with intelligibility are hypernasal resonance and nasal emission of air due to impaired palatopharyngeal closure. In the early stages of the disease, the patient can be trained to monitor hypernasality. A more open mouth posture during speech facilitates oral versus nasal emission of air. Moncur and Brackett have outlined some drills to develop self-monitoring of nasality during speech production (7).

Palatopharyngeal Prosthesis

As the disease develops, it may be worthwhile to employ a palatal lift prosthesis to restore palatopharyngeal closure. Other procedures may be useful such as an injection of Teflon into the nasopharyngeal tissues to produce a swelling that permits better apposition of the nasopharynx with the soft palate (3).

Phonation

Voice Quality

Patients with a strained or a hoarse quality to the voice can be taught to initiate phonation with a sigh or a hum. Speaking in a more relaxed, slightly breathy manner can also result in a clearer voice. An overly breathy voice can be improved by initiating speech with a hard glottal attack.

Pitch

Patients with ALS may acquire an abnormally low-pitched voice. In the initial stages of the disease a more optimal pitch can be identified, and the patient can be encouraged to raise the pitch through practice and monitoring.

Loudness

A patient who cannot achieve adequate loudness can compensate for this disability initially by speaking at a slower rate and articulating as clearly as possible. In some cases electrical amplification may be required. Boone (4) and Moncur and Brackett (7) give drills and suggestions for the remediation of voice disorders.

Prosody

Changes in prosody such as monopitch and monoloudness are frequently apparent in the speech of the ALS patient. These disorders can be improved through practice in producing sentences with a variety of intonation patterns to make differences in meaning. However, it may be preferable to sacrifice prosody for intelligibility, as occurs when the patient speaks at a slow rate.

PHYSIOTHERAPY TECHNIQUES

Respiratory difficulties can be minimized through maintenance of erect posture of the trunk while the patient is sitting and periodic postural drainage with suctioning to remove excess secretions in the trachea and bronchi. The manual procedures developed by Dr. Margaret Rood that are based on stimulation of cutaneous and musculotendinous receptors such as brushing and stretching do not appear to have been tested in patients with ALS, although they are claimed to be of benefit in facilitating respiration in patients with other conditions (1). For patients who are dependent on a communication device, it is important to ensure the optimal function of the limbs used to operate the device. This would be a part of the routine physical and occupational therapy management of patients with ALS.

CONTROL OF SALIVA

Slowing the rate of speech allows the patient to swallow between sentences to control salivation. Atropine and related belladonna alkaloids can be helpful in controlling salivation in patients who cannot properly swallow their saliva. The dose of atropine should commence at 250 to 500 μg orally four times a day and be increased gradually until the desired effect is obtained. Other medications that produce dryness of the mouth as a side effect are used, such as clonidine hydrochloride. However, their primary or other side effects may be a disadvantage.

COMMUNICATION DEVICES

Patients with Some Usable Speech

Patients with ALS who have fairly good articulation and resonance but poor phonotory and respiratory function have difficulty achieving adequate loudness levels, especially in a group situation or over the telephone. A small voice amplifier, with either a hand-held or around-the-neck microphone, is helpful for these patients, and an amplifier can be installed in the telephone to increase the loudness level of the patient's voice over the telephone. An electrolarynx can be used by patients who articulate clearly but cannot phonate or who phonate very softly. An electrolarynx is a battery-operated electrical vibratory sound source. The patient holds the electrolarynx against his or her throat or, in some models, the sound is presented through a plastic tube into the patient's mouth. The patient then articulates the sound into words.

Buekelman and Yorkston described a method whereby a patient with severe dysarthria but an intact language system can point on an alphabet board to the initial letter of the word that he or she is speaking (2). This can be faster than spelling out the whole word and significantly increases the intelligibility of the dysarthric patient.

In the future, automatic speech recognition by computers may become sensitive enough to decipher severely dysarthric speech that is unintelligible to the human listener. The patient's utterance could then be presented to the listener by computer through synthetic speech (10).

Patients without Vocal Communication

Patients with ALS whose speech is totally unintelligible require an alternative communication system. Such systems have major limitations since most were not designed specifically for ALS patients and, therefore, do not meet all of their requirements. The most common problem is that they do not permit communication to occur as quickly as natural speech, and therefore more attention and patience are required from the listener. Hagen found that, unless a patient can complete a message in less than three minutes with no more than five corrected errors, the average listener will not attempt to communicate with the patient (6). This situation is often observed with the ALS patient. Other problems encountered with some of the more elaborate communication devices are lack of easy and logical operation, unreliable performance, excessive bulk and weight, and considerable cost to the patient for short-term benefit. Often, by the time a patient with ALS has learned to use one of the available instruments, his or her physical skills have declined such that a new device and new skills are needed. Thus, in obtaining these instruments some thought must be given to their practicality and the future needs of the patient.

The type of communication device that is most appropriate for a given patient depends on the kind and degree of deterioration from ALS, the particular communication needs, emotional state, and educational level of the patient. The most severely limiting factor is the level of motor function. The physical and the occupational therapists' assessments of the patient's motor function are important in deciding on which device would be appropriate for a given patient at a particular time. The social worker's input is helpful in evaluating the patient's communication needs and emotional state at home or at work.

Communication systems are most easily designed for patients with unimpaired or minimally impaired hand function. The fine motor control and speed of movement of the hand are well suited for nonvocal communication. Communication systems that utilize movements of other parts of the body, such as the legs and feet, must be more sophisticated.

A wide variety of communication aids are available for the patient with no usable speech but only mildly impaired hand function. Writing by hand is the simplest way for these patients to communicate. A typewriter is faster than writing but is less portable. The following devices offer increased portability: the Phonic Mirror Handi-Voice (HC Electronics Inc., Mill Valley, CA), the Canon Communicator (Telesensory Systems Inc., Palo Alto, CA), and the Elkomi II (Prentke Romich Co., Shreve, OH). The Phonic Mirror Handi-Voice HC110 is a battery-operated voice system consisting of a manually operated keyboard that is connected to an electronic voice box and speaker; it has a vocabulary of approximately 500 words. The Canon Communicator is a portable tape typewriter. The Elkomi II resembles a hand-held calculator and has a visual word display. These devices and a complete catalogue of other communication aids can be found in the *Non-vocal Communication Resource Book* edited by Gregg C. Vanderheiden (11).

Patients with Arm Weakness and No Speech

A patient whose hand function has deteriorated to a moderate degree will require a communication device that does not demand much accuracy and strength of hand movement to operate. Many simple systems can be developed for these patients such as an alphabet board, a board on which words and sentences are written, or cards with written words and sentences or pictures. The cards could be attached to a bracelet. The range of arm movements across a board or page can be reduced by using a pointer. Depending on the patient's emotional state, he or she may or may not desire a more sophisticated communication system.

The Paralyzed Patient

For the more seriously paralyzed patient, a more complex, modular communication system with interchangeable component parts is required (Fig. 1). It should be adaptable to the patient's reduced level of motor function. The selection of an operative switch or "input interface" is crucial. It must have adequate sensitivity to accept the most feeble input by the patient with a minimum of unintentional signals. Examples of input interfaces are pointing with a finger or use of a joy stick, tilt switch, or foot trolley.

The most feasible input interface for the severely paralyzed patient is the ocular transducer, which monitors eye movement. The ocular transducer developed by Rinard can be mounted on conventional eyeglasses and used effectively with the Etran Communicator (8, 9). The modified Etran display provides 64 characters for use by the patient (Fig. 2). For example, to specify the letter "N" the eye starts from the center point, moves left center to indicate the box, then left top to indicate the area on the board corresponding to the position of the letter in the box, and finally returns to the center position.

Typical output interfaces are a typewriter, television monitor, and light-emitting diode. A speech synthesizer currently undergoing evaluation has shown promising results (12). A modular communication system offers the capacity for modification and expansion to provide additional services such as the display of reading material, adjustment of an electric bed, and control of a nurse call switch.

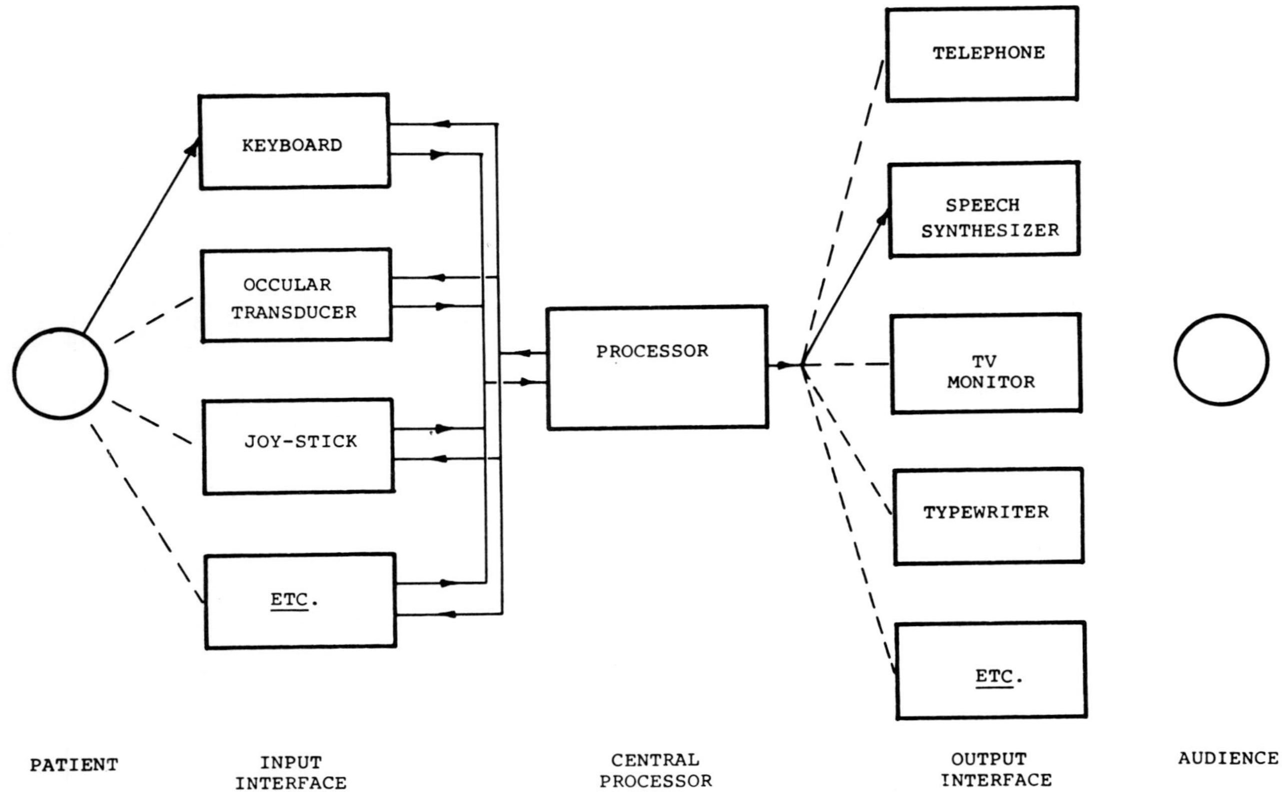

Figure 1 Schematic block diagram of modular communication systems.

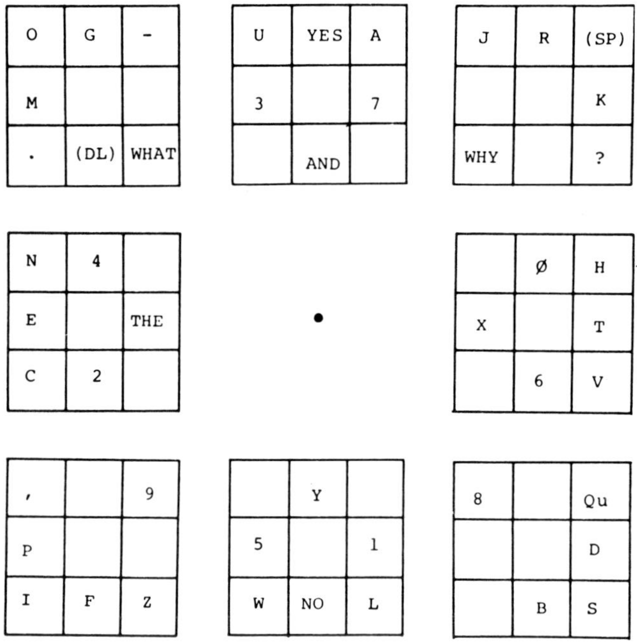

Figure 2 Modified Etran display (see text for description.)

SUMMARY

Although speech therapy and physiotherapy will not reverse or retard the progressive loss of motor function in patients with ALS, there is no doubt that the dysarthria can be much improved in patients who do not have very severe bulbar or respiratory muscle weakness. For the patient with such weakness, a large variety of communication aids are available, and a number of electronic devices have been developed for the more profoundly paralyzed individual.

Apart from breathing difficulties, loss of the ability to communicate is probably the most devastating functional deprivation that an ALS patient must endure. Thus, attempts to improve the dysarthria or to teach the patient how to use a communication device can be of immense value.

Acknowledgments

The authors are grateful to Gordon Campbell for his advice on the engineering aspects of communication devices and to Delva Bethune for her counsel on physiotherapy techniques.

REFERENCES

1. Bethune D: Neurophysiological facilitation of respiration in the unconscious adult patient. Physiotherapy Canada 27:241–245, 1975

2. Beukelman DR, Yorkston K: A communication system for the severely dysarthric speaker with an intact language system. J Speech Hear Disord 42:265–270, 1970

3. Bluestone CD, Musgrave RH, McWilliams BJ, et al: Teflon injection pharyngoplasty. Cleft Palate J 5:19–22, 1968

4. Boone DR: *The Voice and Voice Therapy.* Englewood Cliffs, NJ, Prentice-Hall, 1971

5. Darley FL, Aronson AE, Brown JR: *Motor Speech Disorders.* Toronto, WB Saunders Co, 1975

6. Hagen C: Assistive communication systems for the anarthric and severe dysarthric patient: A rationale for their use and criterion for their selection. Scand J Rehabil Med 10:163–168, 1978

7. Moncur JP, Brackett IP: *Modifying Vocal Behavior.* New York, Harper and Row, 1974

8. *Participants Resource Book.* National Workshop on Non-Vocal Communication Techniques and Aids, University of Wisconsin, 1975

9. Rinard G, Rugg D: An ocular control device for use by the severely handicapped. Presented at the Conference on Systems and Devices for the Disabled, Boston, MA, June 1976

10. Robinson AL: Research news. More people are talking to computers as speech recognition enters the real world. Science 203:634–638, 1979

11. Vanderheiden GC: *Non-vocal Communication Resource Book.* Baltimore, University Park Press, 1978

12. Warrick A, Nelson P, Cossalter J, et al: Synthesized speech as an aid to communication and learning for the non-verbal. Proceedings of the Workshop on Communication Aids for the Non-verbal Physically Handicapped. Ottawa, June 1977

15 Living without Speech

Eric H. Denys

The prospect of a permanent disability from any illness has a profound impact on physical and psychologic coping mechanisms. The patient who is willing to expend the effort, however, can usually make accommodations that enable him or her to lead a useful and rewarding life, as is frequently seen in blind or quadriplegic individuals. This is equally true for victims of ALS, but the challenge is greater.

The usual progression of motor impairment in ALS results in a changing and increasing disability that requires constant adjustment. The patient's ability to communicate erodes, but the mind remains intact. Thus, he or she must experience the additional psychologic anguish of increasing isolation from family and friends. The retention of mental capabilities, however, also holds hope for ALS patients in that even the most severely paralyzed patient has the potential to continue meaningful relationships if a means of communication can be developed.

Fortunately, many patients retain the ability to speak when their hands become paralyzed or continue to communicate with written messages when their voice becomes unintelligible. There is, however, no easy solution when speech is unintelligible and the hands and feet are unable to write, point, or serve any useful function.

While the search for a cause and cure of ALS continues, the need to alleviate immediate suffering remains pressing. The mechanisms of speech and their malfunctions are discussed elsewhere in this volume, as are the aids available for the speech handicapped. This chapter emphasizes the needs of the most severely paralyzed patients, those who are deprived of all means of communication and who are truly "locked in." These patients no doubt deserve our greatest attention, for any remedy to free them from their totally dependent isolation would be enormously gratifying.

It cannot be stressed enough that with rare exceptions the communication devices currently available were not designed for ALS patients and therefore may not meet their specific needs. Voice amplifiers increase only volume, not intelligibility. The electrolarynx (a sound emitter that is placed against the larynx) requires manipulation of the sound by the patient's lips and tongue, which are usually no longer functional by the time the ALS patient requires this kind of help.

Problems of increasing paralysis may limit the useful life of any one device and make it impractical for the amount of time, money, and effort required. For instance, the Elkomi II, the Phonic Mirror Handi-Voice Model HC110, and the Canon Communicator require finger dexterity, which may deteriorate over time. The Auto-Com requires less finger movement, but the patient must be able to move a magnetic pointer over a lap board. (The names, addresses, and telephone numbers of the manufacturers of these devices are listed in Appendix I.) Home-made devices carry the same risk, especially when progression of the disease is not anticipated or not taken into account at the time the device is built. For example, a light source attached to the forehead enables the patient to trigger an array of light-sensitive switches. These switches can activate solenoids, which in turn depress the keys of an electric typewriter. Progressive weakness of the neck muscles (a very common problem in ALS), however, will limit its usefulness.

Several factors should be considered before one selects a communication aid for a patient with ALS.

EXPENSE VERSUS USEFUL LIFE

A simple device that is inexpensive but effective should be used regardless of its lifespan. For example, a built-up foam mantle around a pen offers a firmer grip and is easily obtained. A magic erase board, with its light weight and firm background, is far superior to a piece of paper. Alphabet boards can be made easily from cardboard. It has been my experience that once a patient becomes unable to hold a pen the next step is to have him or her point at letters, words, or symbols on an alphabet board; not only the hands but also the feet can serve as pointers, if necessary with a rod or pencil attached to them.

More sophisticated communication devices are often activated by means of one or more fingers; an electric typewriter is the prototype. An electric typewriter is bulkier than some of the devices mentioned previously, but they all share a major limitation: they do not take into account the predominantly distal weakness of the patient with ALS. Two commercially available push-button devices have an additional restriction in that they lack a permanent record. The Elkomi II can display only a few words at a time which parade by like the stock market ticker tape. The Handi-Voice emits a computer voice but does not leave a record. This limitation should be considered against the significant cost of such devices when thought is given to their purchase. Prices now range from a few hundred to a few thousand dollars.

FUNCTIONAL INDEPENDENCE

The necessity of having a relative or attendant present to receive or record the message is an important factor to consider in choosing an assistive device. The advantage of personal contact can be overshadowed by the absolute dependence of the patient in this type of situation. Therefore, a communicator that can display a message or make a permanent record should be considered.

The Canon Communicator offers some advantage (as long as sufficient finger dexterity is present) because it is fairly small, the size of a calculator, and makes a record of the letters by printing them on a narrow strip of paper. The Auto-Com is a lapboard with a display of words and letters selected by means of a pointer magnet; the selection appears on a LED display, which can store some 30 characters, and is printed on a narrow strip of paper.

The Tufts Interactive Communicator (T.I.C.) has a matrix display of eight rows of eight letters. A light moves stepwise on the vertical axis, and when the desired row is reached the patient activates a switch that changes the light's direction of travel to the horizontal plane. When the desired letter is reached, another selection is necessary to store the letter on a small (5 × 5-inch) display. The message can also be printed, either simultaneously or later, on a narrow strip of paper. Such devices are called strip printers; they are somewhat inconvenient because the long narrow strips of paper make the message difficult to read. The trigger can be any mechanical switch that can be activated by the patient, for example, a micro switch or a breath switch (also called a pneumatic or puff-sip switch). According to the latest information this device is no longer made, but some may still be available.

Videocom II was developed initially for a severely paralyzed ALS patient at the Institute of Medical Sciences in San Francisco. It consists of a relatively small unit containing electronic parts and a fairly large monitor screen (7 × 7 inches) that offers good visibility of the message from a distance. Messages consisting of 12 lines of 32 characters each can be displayed. To make up a message, the patient uses a switch to select letters and symbols as they appear temporarily at the bottom of the screen. The sequence in which these letters are shown is determined by one of four different programs that can be interchanged easily by the manufacturer. Of the two most efficient programs, one presents the letters in the order of statistical frequence of use (scanning); the other uses a matrix similar to the one in the T.I.C. (encoding). If the patient is able to control an additional switch (accelerator), he or she can temporarily speed up the scanning to reach the desired symbol faster. An electronic memory bank can store the contents of one screen page while another is being printed. There is a built-in nurse call and additional power outlets for other devices such as a page turner, radio, or television. Because the entire message first appears on the screen, errors can be corrected. Once the message is considered complete, it can be transferred to a printer, which comes as a separate unit. The printed message appears on a conventional four-inch-wide roll of paper similar to that used in a cash register. The type of trigger switch again will depend on the patient's physical handicap.

THE PATIENT'S DISABILITY

There is a pressing need for a universally applicable switch that can be used with a minimum of adjustments by ALS patients with advanced weakness. The only limitations on the technologic capabilities and possibilities of communicators are those of cost and the patient's disability.

A flicker of movement in a hand can be amplified by suspending the hand in a rubber band and allowing gravity to assist the patient's movement. If the patient can rotate the head, he or she might be able to use a cheek switch consisting of a tiny rod extending upward from a switch mounted on the chest. Personal experience with an ordinary dime store balloon (they come in all sizes and shapes) connected by means of plastic tubing to a pneumatic switch has been very encouraging. (Information on such devices is available through Micro Communications Devices, Inc. Address is given in Appendix I.) The necessary to and fro movement is minimal, and the balloon can be placed anywhere close to a moving part of the body. A regular problem encountered in fitting switches is that active movement is necessary not only to engage the switch but also to reverse the direction of movement and prepare for the next selection.

Breath switches are usually not applicable to patients with ALS because of the facial weakness associated with speech impairment. Because of the capriciousness of the disease, any muscle may be spared for long periods of time and should therefore be evaluated in terms of its potential for communication. Eye blinking, for example, is always preserved and in rare cases may be the only way for the patient to signal messages of yes and no to an attendant pointing at an alphabet board. The feasibility of an eye-blink trigger for ALS patients is currently under investigation at Micro Communication Devices. The major drawback at present seems to be the inability of some patients to open the eyelids fully because of forehead weakness. Other manufacturers are experimenting with direct selection of letters by means of an infrared light beam reflected off the eyes. Additional work is needed before devices using this principle will be commercially available and affordable.

MOTIVATION AND LEARNING

Learning is part of growing up, and when disability occurs at a young age the extra time and effort required to master a complex device is a small price to pay if it speeds up the acquisition of knowledge and communication skills. However, the prospective is different in patients with ALS. Here, the emphasis is on immediate substitution of a lost skill. It may come as a surprise that even the reward of improved communication does not always seem to provide the necessary drive to spend time learning a new skill. Experience with Videocom II has shown that, of the different programs available, patients have repeatedly preferred a slower program that does not require learning (scanning) to a program that requires only a minimal degree of learning (encoding).

Relatives of patients who are no longer able to communicate verbally or by writing often have great hopes that an electronic communication device will provide a solution, if the cost can be absorbed. Their enthusiasm, however, may be greater than that of the patient, and it is therefore highly recommended that the patient's motivation be assessed before an expensive device is purchased. It is fair to say that if the patient has sufficient perseverance to spell letter by letter and is willing to expend effort to communicate through eye blinking, an electronic communication device will change his or her life tremendously. Occasionally, a patient will enjoy the presence of his or her loved ones, will listen with great interest to their stories, and will enjoy watching television. But, aside from signaling their basic needs, some patients seem to resign entirely from active communication.

CHANGING PATTERN OF LIFE

Our daily activities and plans for the future are made with the assumption of uninterrupted good health. When illness strikes, finding us unprepared, we inevitably accomplish less by our usual standards, and our expectations have to be adjusted. Amyotrophic lateral sclerosis is a striking example: physical handicap, financial hardship, and emotional pain face an intact mind. Advancing paralysis will impose a slower pace of life; interests will change, and quality will be appreciated more than quantity. The same applies to speech, for, in the presence of severe paralysis, it is a most valuable basic human need. To lose speech, or in a broader sense communication, means to become isolated, locked in. Any improvement or substitute for unintelligible speech will therefore open up the patient's world. Concerns for form and speed give way to the essential, concern for what is said. It is therefore necessary to respect the patient's tempo, and to avoid pressuring him or her to respond quickly. To extract information by guessing is often tedious and frustrating; it only reminds the patient of the handicap. What seems slow to us may be satisfactory to the patient. Moreover, access to a communication device with a message display and printing capability will greatly enhance independent activity. It will be slow, but time is one thing the patient has. Patience is what we can offer in our effort to improve communication.

APPENDIX I. DEVICES AND MANUFACTURERS

Auto-Com: Trace Center, University of Wisconsin, 922 ERB, 1500 Johnson Drive, Madison, WI 53706; telephone: (608)262-6966.

Canon Communicator: Telesensory Systems, Inc., 3408 Hillview Avenue, Palo Alto, CA 94304; telephone: (415)493-2626.

Elkomi II: Prentke Romich Co., Shreve, OH 44676; telephone: (216)567-2906.

Phonic Mirror Handi-Voice, Model HC110: HC Electronics, Inc., 250 Camino Alto, Mill Valley, CA 94941; telephone: (415)383-4000.

T.I.C. (Tufts Interactive Communicator): Tufts New England Medical Center, Box 372, 171 Harrison Avenue, Boston, MA 02111; telephone: (617)956-5000.

Videocom II: Micro Communications Devices, Inc., 12388 Priscilla Lane, Los Altos Hills, CA 94022; telephone: (415)981-5588, (408)941-8035.

16 Pharmacologic and Surgical Modalities

Richard A. Smith

Arthur Dawson

Parvis Foroozan

Those of us who have chosen to work with patients who have amyotrophic lateral sclerosis have no miracles with which to treat them, but we have learned through close observation that some of these patients live truly miraculous lives. Patients who were told they had three years to live are still walking and talking many years after diagnosis, and patients who have undergone respiratory arrest are back at the office with the aid of a respirator. As early as the 1960s, data had accumulated suggesting that the course of ALS varies widely. More recently, a concept of host resistance has been offered to explain this variation. The central question is whether variation in the course of ALS is ordained by factors beyond the reach of patient or physician, or whether such factors as hope and medical care can materially benefit these patients. Although no data are available regarding these points, it is our belief that patient care is one of the variables of "host resistance," and that both subjective and objective values of this treatment can be expressed in the form of prolonged patient survival.

The day-to-day reality that a patient with ALS must face helps to make it understandable that both the patient and the physician may have ambivalent feelings regarding the symptomatic treatment of ALS. The medical literature reveals that there was little interest in the chronic care of ALS until 25 years ago. Subsequent investigation of ALS-related problems by physicians in medical and surgical specialties has expanded our knowledge of ALS and has provided information as to the nature of the symptoms that might respond to treatment. Contributions to the medical and surgical management of ALS are not well chronicled in the medical literature. It is possible that tracheostomy and feeding gastrostomy have long been used to manage respiratory and alimentary complications of ALS. Similarly, muscle relaxants, quinine, and phenytoin (Dilantin) were probably used by unheralded practitioners for treatment of cramps and muscle spasms due to the disease. No doubt these therapies were considered unremarkable and thus were not recorded. There are specific historic landmarks that remind us that knowledge of the clinical syndrome of ALS has been slow to accrue. In the 1950s, Smith, Mulder, and Code drew attention to the disorder of esophageal function (46), and Mulder, Lambert, and Eaton described the myasthenic syndrome of ALS (36). In the same period, Miller, Mulder, and colleagues at the Mayo Clinic (Rochester, Minnesota) described alveolar hypoventilation as a rare presenting symptom of ALS (29). Advances in the sixties included Bosma and Brodie's description of disabled pharyngeal function in ALS (2) and Mill's description of the use of cricopharyngeal myotomy for treatment of dysphagia secondary to bulbar palsy (30). In 1966, Mulder wrote "Treatment of anterior horn cell disease" (33). The seventies have seen further interest in the clinical features of ALS. The pathophysiology of dyspnea, dysarthria, and sialorrhea have been examined (8, 15, 18) and the psychiatric aspects of ALS have been studied (20). In addition, two extensive reviews on the treatment of ALS have been published (17, 48).

DYSPHAGIA

Pathophysiology

Eating is a complex phenomenon that involves intimate interaction between volitional and reflex activity. After food has been introduced into the mouth and chewed, swallowing is initiated by the tongue, which pushes the food bolus posteriorly into the oral pharynx. The tongue then lifts and seals the nasopharynx, and the larynx rises to assist with closure of the supraglottis. Synchronous with contraction of the pharyngeal constrictor muscles, which move food into the esophagus, the upper esophageal sphincter relaxes. In the esophagus, swallowing evokes a peristaltic wave that helps to move the food bolus.

Problems with eating are a major concern for the ALS patient. With use of cineradiography, Bosma and Brodie have demonstrated several kinds of pharyngeal dysfunction in ALS patients (2). The most serious of these disabilities is laryngeal penetration of the food bolus. Such penetration occurs during swallowing or, more commonly, after resumption of respiration after swallowing. Some ALS patients with pharyngeal dysfunction have demonstrated extraordinary pharyngeal motor capacities. The palatopharyngeal isthmus, which remains open during speech, may be adequately sealed during swallowing by action of both the soft palate, which may displace beyond its normal range, and the pharyngeal constrictor. As swallowing progresses, closure of the lower pharynx may be accomplished by exceptional displacement of the constrictor walls.

Esophageal motility has been examined by measurement of intraluminal pressure using catheters connected to pressure transducers. This technique allows determination of the integrity of both the pharyngeal and esophageal sphincters and the esophagus. Smith, Mulder, and Code reported that, of 19 ALS patients studied, most had abnormalities of the middle and lower esophagus (46). Peristaltic contraction was often feeble in these patients; in some, the esophagus failed to respond to swallowing, and in others, peristaltic contraction was supplanted by simultaneous contraction of large esophageal segments. Two of the 19 patients had normal esophageal motility, and 3 patients had disturbance of either the pharyngealesophageal or lower esophageal sphincters. Sphincteric abnormalities consisted of low resting pressure associated with feeble contraction of the sphincter upon swallowing. These abnormalities have been attributed to involvement of the dorsal motor nucleus of the vagus nerve. That some of these abnormalities may be a result of the myasthenic syndrome is demonstrated by improvement of the condition after administration of anticholinesterase. A study of 10 ALS patients at the Scripps Clinic and Research Foundation, using an open-tip perfused catheter technique, revealed that the low resting pressure seen in the upper esophageal sphincter could be augmented by administration of edrophonium chloride (Tensilon) (Fig. 1), resulting in a

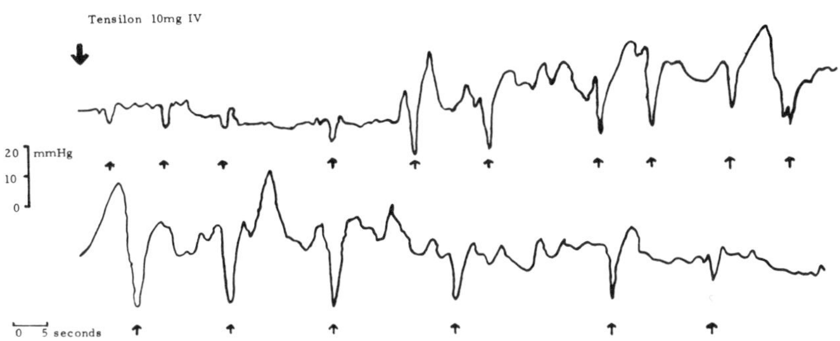

Figure 1 Results of esophageal motility study with an open-tip catheter in the upper esophageal sphincter. Arrows indicate a dry swallow. Significant improvement can be seen in the amplitude of sphincter pressure and relaxation after intravenous administration of 10 mg of edrophonium chloride (Tensilon). Improvement occurs promptly and lasts for 10–12 minutes.

sensation of improved swallowing function by the patient. Esophageal complexes showed nonspecific abnormality in most patients. Lower esophageal sphincter pressure was generally normal.

Motility studies of upper esophageal sphincter function have been hampered by technical difficulties. Perfused catheters are not tolerated well because of aspiration of fluid, and the nonperfused catheter technique is unsatisfactory because of technical limitations. More recently, miniature transducers have been used, which seem to be both accurate and free of the problems associated with perfused catheters. However, because of both the semicircular shape of the sphincter anteriorly and a rigid posterior wall, use of numerous catheters with sensitive transducers may be necessary to assess sphincteric function accurately.

In addition to mechanical disruption of swallowing, attention has been directed to possible abnormality of the digestive process in patients with ALS. Quick and Greer reported disturbance in pancreatic exocrine function in ALS patients, manifested by poor absorption of triolein I 131 and abnormal secretin test (41). These results have not been confirmed by subsequent investigators (28, 52).

Therapy

Sensory cuing can be used to aid swallowing. Adjustments in the taste, texture, and temperature of food often make it possible for patients with advanced disease to continue to swallow. This is illustrated by the ability of patients who expectorate water to swallow ice chips or to swallow a pill with applesauce.

Some patients with predominantly bulbar symptoms can be taught to place a small polyethylene tube into the pharynx via the mouth.

Surgery is an effective remedy for dysphagia that results from bulbar palsy. There are several treatment alternatives. Lebo and Norris have reported improvement in swallowing after cricopharyngeal myotomy (26). However, although the cricopharyngeal muscle is thought to act as an obstacle to swallowing in some ALS patients, Bosma and Brodie found no evidence of a cricopharyngeal bar abnormality in six ALS patients (2).

A feeding gastrostomy or jejunostomy has been used for patients with chronic central nervous system disease (7, 42). However, these feeding procedures have been frequently associated with complications when used to maintain the nutritional status of comatose patients. Feedings must be carefully managed in order to minimize diarrhea and discomfort due to excess osmotic load. These problems can limit the usefulness of these therapies.

The most satisfactory surgical method for supplementing food intake is cervical esophagostomy. This procedure can be performed un-

Table 1 Effect of Cervical Esophagostomy on the Weight of a Patient with ALS

Weight (pounds)	*Date*
145	11/72
137.5	1/73
129	3/73
114.5[a]	6/73
113	8/73
114	10/73
113	1/74

[a] At time of surgery.

der local anesthesia with minimal risk of side effects, which include cellulitis and recurrent laryngeal palsy (40). The operation is best performed on the left side of the neck, since the esophagus is situated to the left of the midline. The cutaneoesophageal fistula heals within two to three weeks, leaving a small opening through which the catheter can be easily changed. Fluids can be introduced via a feeding syringe, and puréed food can be placed in a feeding bag and allowed to flow by the force of gravity. It is our preference to feed patients food that has been prepared at home in a blender rather than feed them a food formula. After the esophagostomy, the patient's weight stabilizes; Table 1 illustrates the results of esophagostomy in one patient.

Based on the observation that weight usually stabilizes after cervical esophagostomy, it is reasonable to conclude that weight loss in the late stages of ALS is due primarily to diminished food intake. Weight loss early in the disease is probably due to loss of muscle mass.

SIALORRHEA

Pathophysiology

Most salivary secretions are contributed by three paired glands: the parotid, the submandibular, and the sublingual. Saliva is secreted at a rate of 0.5–2.0 ml/minute unless increased secretion occurs in response to a provocative stimulus. As far as is known, secretion of saliva is normal in patients with ALS. When drooling occurs as a symptom of ALS, it is due to either impairment of swallowing or a weakness of facial muscles involving the lower lip.

Therapy

A number of therapeutic strategies are available for control of sialorrhea (47). Theoretically, an anticholinergic drug that affects the parasympathetic nervous system should control sialorrhea; however, no drug is entirely adequate in this respect. Atropine given orally may be helpful for a limited time. Empirically, amitriptyline has been found to be effective in some patients over a relatively prolonged period. Its mode of action is presumably due to a central anticholinergic effect.

It is technically feasible to reduce salivary secretion by ligation of the salivary ducts, by removal of the sublingual glands, or by irradiation of the salivary glands, but these therapeutic modalities are not usually justified. Occasionally, transtympanic neurectomy is a useful therapeutic adjunct. Surgery is based on the fortuitous anatomic localization of the chorda tympani and tympanic plexus in the middle ear, thus affording the surgeon easy access to the principal nerves innervating the salivary glands. The relationship of these structures is shown in Figure 2. The submandibular and sublingual glands receive parasympathetic innervation primarily via the chorda tympani, whereas the parotid glands are innervated via Jacobson's plexus. However, variations in neural innervation may exist. These additional pathways may account for failure to completely denervate the salivary glands in some patients. Denervation markedly affects the salivary glands. They are rendered unable to adjust to functional demand, and, as first observed experimentally by Claude

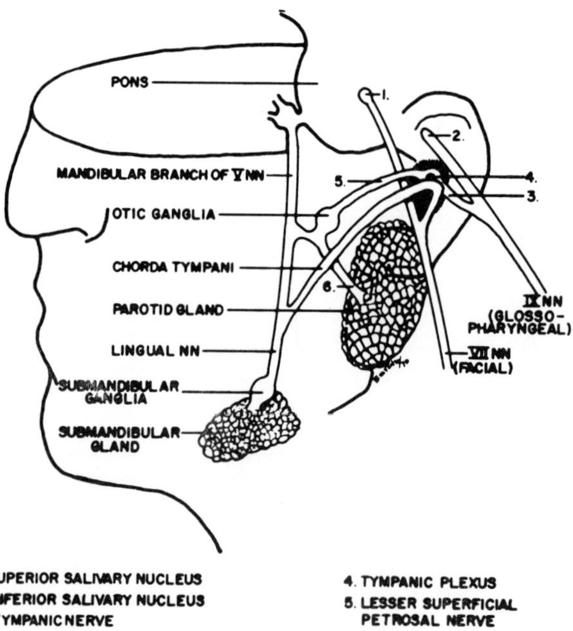

Figure 2 Innervation of the salivary glands.

Bernard in 1864, the denervated glands may atrophy as much as 30% within a few weeks after surgery (3). Wallenborn noted that marked atrophy of the rabbit parotid gland occurred 29 weeks after denervation by tympanic neurectomy (3). Emmelin et al. noted that denervated gland regained its original weight after reinnervation (14). Although chronic atropinization experimentally induces histologic changes similar to those that result from denervation, it does not produce atrophy (13). Denervation hypersensitivity, as can be expected by Cannon's law, is observed, but it is not pronounced in humans after section of the chorda tympani, possibly because such surgery does not completely denervate the submaxillary and sublingual glands. After unilateral denervation, unaltered glands may increase in size. The following case illustrates the result.

A 56-year-old man with bulbar ALS of two years' duration presented with dysphagia and drooling (resting secretion, 1.5 cc/3 minutes). A tympanic neurectomy was performed on the left side and subsequently on the right side. Drooling was alleviated. Follow-up studies at six months showed a significant reduction of resting salivary secretion (0.3 cc/3 minutes).

The risk of overtreatment of sialorrhea appears to be small. None of our patients has complained of excessive dryness. Many of our patients had observable hypertrophy of the minor salivary glands about the palate. Transtympanic neurectomy does not denervate these glands. The secretions that remain appear to be more viscid than those observed before treatment. It should be remembered that regeneration of the sectioned nerves can occur; this regeneration may account for the return of symptoms in some patients. Recurrence of drooling may also reflect progression of the disease. If dysphagia increases in severity, drooling may recur; tracheostomy also may aggravate drooling because of reduced evaporation of fluid from the mouth.

DYSPNEA

Pathophysiology

During quiet breathing the diaphragm is the principal muscle of inspiration, while expiration is accomplished mainly by energy stored during inspiration in elastic elements of the lungs and chest wall. The intercostal and accessory muscles contribute to stabilization of the chest wall during quiet breathing, but during the hyperpnea of exercise, with added respiratory loads and probably with assumption of the supine posture, the relative contributions of the muscles of the chest wall progressively increase (10). Although which respiratory muscles are most affected in ALS depends on the distribution of the motor neuron disease, generally the diaphragm is involved earlier than the chest wall, since the upper and midthoracic spinal segments are basically spared (35). For a time, the intercostal and accessory muscles can compensate for weakness of the diaphragm, but progressive hypoventilation and respiratory failure eventually develop.

Although the progression of respiratory symptoms is usually orderly and is most pronounced with advanced disease, a variety of clinical presentations can be seen. Instances have been described in which alveolar hypoventilation was the presenting manifestation or in which the diagnosis was recognized only when the patient could not be weaned from mechanical ventilatory support (16, 45). In some cases shortness of breath is an omen of rapid respiratory failure leading to death, whereas in others it may persist for some months without obvious progression.

Most patients with ALS ultimately die of the respiratory complications associated with their disease. These complications are of three main types: (*a*) weakness of the muscles of inspiration, leading to dyspnea and, later, hypoventilation and chronic respiratory failure; (*b*) motor dysfunction of the pharynx, glottis, and larynx, leading to impairment of mechanisms that protect the lower respiratory tract from aspiration of food, saliva, and upper airway secretions; and (*c*) weakness or incoordination of the larynx, glottis, and expiratory muscles, leading to impaired cough and inability to clear the lower airways.

Lung function tests may be of great assistance in recognition and assessment of the progress of respiratory muscle weakness. These measurements are more readily quantified than most other methods of evaluating muscle function, and, apart from their prognostic significance, they may be useful for the assessment of new drugs or other treatments (35). Nakano and associates performed serial tests of lung function in a group of 25 patients with ALS and showed that pulmonary function tended to deteriorate with time. Tests that help to assess voluntary respiratory muscle function (e.g., spirometry, maximum voluntary ventilation, and maximum inspiratory and expiratory pressure) correlate best with the progression of the disease and have the advantages of being inexpensive and readily available. Figure 3 shows the flow–volume loop of one of 16 patients studied at the Scripps Clinic before and after intravenous administration of a 10-mg bolus of edrophonium hydrochloride. Vital capacity and peak inspiratory and expiratory flows improved significantly after the drug was given. This response was observed in 5 of the 16 patients tested.

Therapy

In the early stages of ALS, patients benefit from instruction regarding pulmonary toilet. Emphasis is placed on avoiding aspiration. Specific therapeutic measures are usually limited to the administration of Pneumovax, a vaccine recently developed for prophylaxis against *Pneumo-*

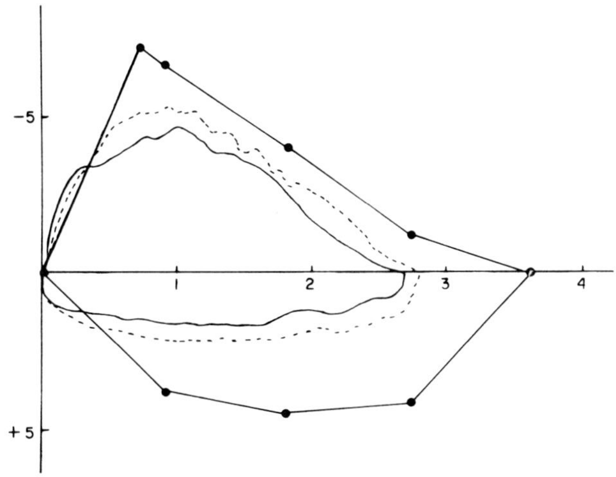

Figure 3 Flow–volume loop before and after administration of edrophonium hydrochloride. The x axis represents volume (in liters) expired, as measured from full lung inflation. The y axis represents flow in liters/second (negative represents expiratory-positive inspiration). Straight solid lines represent predicted values based on age, sex, and height.

coccus, and the administration of flu vaccine. In some cases it is important to treat intercurrent respiratory infections vigorously. It is our practice to hospitalize ALS patients who develop bronchitis or pneumonia after an upper respiratory infection.

The management of aspiration is critical because patients may die suddenly as a result of choking or gradually as a result of aspiration pneumonia. By giving careful attention to chewing and swallowing, most ALS patients can avoid aspiration, but once the patient loses the ability to take food or drink without the constant threat of choking it is important to recommend tube feeding or cervical esophagostomy. If aspiration continues as a result of pooling of saliva, the physician has several therapeutic choices: (*a*) reduction of salivary secretions; (*b*) tracheostomy (if secretions are not adequately reduced); or (*c*) surgical closure of the larynx (32). The last technique is simple and effective. Unfortunately, this procedure eliminates any remaining speech, but with advanced disease most persons with ALS have already lost useful speech.

If hypoventilation progresses to the point where there is troublesome carbon dioxide retention or severe dyspnea during rest, the physician must decide whether to offer or withhold a life-support device. In making this decision, the physician should be aware that some remarkable patients continue to live useful and complete lives with the help of a respirator and electric wheelchair. In the author's opinion, candidates for such treatment should have audible speech and retain the use of at least one arm.

DYSPHONIA

Pathophysiology

Speech is made possible by modulation of the breath by a series of musculoskeletal valves. This occurs by coordinated action of the vocal cords, palate, tongue, and lips, each of which contributes to the repertoire of speech. Understandably, disruption of speech is among the cruelest of the non–life-threatening symptoms of ALS.

Amyotrophic lateral sclerosis results in a mixed dysarthria because of the admixture of bulbar and pseudobulbar features. Darley et al. studied 30 ALS patients and found speech to be severely affected in all (9). Speech was slow and monotonous and often unintelligible due to poor articulation of both vowels and consonants. As a result of malfunction of the palatopharyngeal valve, speech was commonly hypernasal.

Therapy

At present there is little documentation to support the use of pharmacologic or surgical treatment of dysphonia due to ALS. Injection of Teflon or silicone into the nasopharynx might favorably affect the hypernasal speech of ALS. However, there are no published data on use of this technique in ALS patients, although it is now standard treatment for a variety of other speech disorders (27). In cases in which speech is lost due to alveolar hyperventilation, I have observed patients speaking after tracheostomy and use of artificial ventilation. In such cases, mechanical ventilation restores speech by giving patients the breath to activate the speech mechanisms that remain relatively intact. Use of the Pitt tracheostomy tube has enhanced speech rehabilitation in patients with tracheostomies.

WEAKNESS, SPASTICITY, CRAMPS, AND PAIN

Pathophysiology

Weakness is the final common path by which the pathologic process of ALS expresses itself. The limbs are usually involved and early weakness is commonly asymmetric. Bulbar weakness is manifested by dysphagia or dysphonia. In "pure form," ALS may be evidenced by muscular atrophy or spasticity, but in most cases symptoms result from an admixture of upper and lower motor neuron signs. Pathologically, the principal substrate for weakness is injury to the anterior horn cell and/or the corticospinal tracts. Abnormal fatigability in ALS apparently was recognized by Aran as early as 1850 (38).

Lambert and Mulder elaborated the electromyographic and clinical features of the myasthenic syndrome in ALS (34). They found that the myasthenic syndrome was best demonstrated in muscles that were most affected by the disease process. They observed both variability of motor unit potentials in approximately 50% of ALS patients and decay of the evoked action potential similar to that seen in myasthenia gravis. Further proof of the presence of a neuromuscular block was provided by the fact that ALS patients were found to be exquisitely sensitive to d-tubocurarine.

In addition to weakness, ALS is manifested by alteration of muscle tone and by cramps. Patients complain of muscular stiffness; muscular rigidity and spasticity are easily demonstrated. The neurophysiologic basis for these phenomena is thought to result from interference of the normal synergistic action of the alpha motoneuron with the fusimotor system. The nature of the supersegmental pathways that influence spinal segments are not well defined, but there is evidence that at least some of these fiber tracts are adrenergic or GABAergic in character (4).

Cramps, which may be the harbinger of ALS, are often extremely painful. Fortunately, they usually subside as the disease progresses. The origin of cramps is not known for sure (25); the neural discharge responsible for cramps may originate in the peripheral nerves or in the spinal cord. Norris et al. postulate that increased activity of normal spinal motor mechanisms may account for cramps (36). However, Lambert found that repetitive nerve stimulations distal to the site of an anesthetic block could induce a cramp (22).

Therapy

Mulder and Lambert reported observable clinical improvement of cramps in ALS patients given an anticholinesterase (34). Temporary improvement in strength was noted after administration of pyridostigmine bromide. Unfortunately, this mode of therapy is usually ineffective within several weeks. Guanidine, a drug known to affect synthesis of acetylcholine, might benefit ALS patients with a myasthenic syndrome (37). However, this has not been convincingly demonstrated. Because of the presence of a defect in neuromuscular transmission in some ALS patients, caution must be exercised in administering nondepolarizing drugs, such as d-tubocurarine, to ALS patients during anesthesia (44, 54). As a rule, depolarizing muscle relaxants (e.g., succinylcholine) should also be avoided. These drugs could cause hyperkalemia when administered to patients with neuromuscular disease (6, 51) and, as a result, could cause cardiac arrest (49).

Cramps usually respond to treatment with phenytoin (Dilantin, 100–200 mg/day) or quinine sulfate (180–300 mg/day). These medications may be given in one daily dose. Their mechanism of action is presumed to be due to their effect on muscle membrane (19). Spasticity may respond to administration of muscle relaxants. There are several classes of these drugs. The centrally acting agents, of which mephenesin is the prototype, are thought to exert their effect by suppression of spinal polysynaptic reflexes. Agents such as diazepam and meprobamate, which have psychotropic effects, are also prescribed as muscle relaxants. These drugs have sedative effects that may indirectly account for their usefulness as muscle relaxants. However, the therapeutic effect of these drugs is not restricted to their effect on arousal. For example, diazepam also inhibits polysynaptic spinal reflexes and fusimotor activity and may inhibit brain stem–activating systems (4). A newer agent, dantrolene sodium, exerts its effect on muscle by direct action on excitation–contraction coupling, possibly by effecting release of calcium from the sarcoplasmic reticulum (12).

Although muscle relaxants might in theory offer considerable advantage in the symptomatic treatment of ALS, in practice they often prove to be of limited use and in some instances have adverse effects. Landau concluded that spasticity is not the primary cause of motor disability in patients with spasticity (24). With use of spinal anesthesia, which preferentially blocks small fusimotor fibers, Landau et al. found that motor activities such as walking might not improve in patients in whom spasticity has temporarily been alleviated (23). In fact, rather than hinder the patient, spasticity may serve a useful function by producing a splinting effect.

Rivera et al. recently reported a small group of ALS patients in whom dantrolene sodium was poorly tolerated (3). Severe muscular weakness was seen in four patients on a daily dose of 75 mg of the drug. Sialorrhea and dysphagia were noted in five patients, and in one patient respiratory failure developed within 12 hours of administration of dantrolene. Pazzaglia reported success in relieving spasticity in five ALS patients who were treated with baclofen (39), and Castaneda has reported similar results (5). Side effects, particularly gastrointestinal complaints, somnolence, and depression, were common.

Pain secondary to soft tissue injury may complicate ALS. The shoulder joint appears to be especially vulnerable. Chronic subluxation of the shoulder is usually asymptomatic, but after a fall it may be necessary to hospitalize patients for treatment of severe shoulder pain. Usually these acute problems respond favorably to treatment with heat, massage, and physical therapy, but a chronic pain syndrome may result, and the patient may develop a typical shoulder–hand syndrome. A rare patient may complain of muscle aching and muscle pain, usually in the legs. These complaints are as yet poorly defined in the ALS literature, although the occurrence of pain in diseases related to ALS has received recent attention. Hudson et al. have reported on a group of patients with fasciculation and pain (21), and Snider et al. have described the occurrence of muscular complaints in patients with Parkinson's disease (50). Injury to sensory neurons may be the basis for sensory symptoms in ALS (11).

While the notion that ALS is a painless affliction may need to be reassessed in light of these atypical cases, it is essential to exclude the more mundane causes of pain in patients with unexplained weakness and pain.

DEPRESSION

Depression frequently occurs in the setting of medical illness. The more severe the illness, the more common the occurrence of depression. Patients with pain, who are confined to bed, or who have decreased alertness are most likely to exhibit changes in affect (31). Houpt et al. found the pattern of depression in a population of ALS patients to be similar to that seen in inpatients on a general medical ward (20). Approximately 32% of ALS patients were moderately depressed and 2.5% were severely depressed. About 10% of patients exhibited early morning awakening, diurnal variation, or psychomotor retardation; on the basis of the psychiatric literature, these symptoms may indicate a role for tricyclic antidepressants in treatment of ALS (1).

CONCLUSION

This review has emphasized some of the treatment strategies that may be employed in the care of patients with ALS. Effective treatment of ALS patients requires close liaison with colleagues in both medical and surgical fields. At all times, consideration must be given to the ease, comfort, benefit, and cost of the recommended treatment. As a rule, the least therapy is the best therapy. In our institution, a minority rather than a majority of patients undergo surgical treatment, and administration of drugs is minimized.

Our goal has been to seek a rational basis for therapy. By expanding our basic knowledge of the disease process, it may be possible to develop better treatment methods, even before definitive treatment is available.

By analogy with myasthenia gravis—in which drugs with anticholinesterase aid but do not cure—and with Parkinson's disease—in which L-dopa may modify symptoms but does not arrest the disease—we must continue to search for clues as to the pathophysiology of ALS with the hope that such clues will lead to discoveries in therapy of ALS. The insight gained from the study of axonal transport, neurotrophic substance, or animal models of ALS may or may not solve the riddle of this disease, but research certainly will brighten the future for treatment.

REFERENCES

1. Bielski RJ, Friedel RO: Prediction of tricyclic antidepressant response. Arch Gen Psychiatry 33:1479–1489, 1976

2. Bosma JF, Brodie DR: Disabilities of the pharynx in amyotrophic lateral sclerosis as demonstrated by cineradiography. Radiology 92:97–103, 1969

3. Burgen ASV, Emmelin NG: *Physiology of the Salivary Glands.* Monographs of the Physiological Society, No. 8. London, Edward Arnold Ltd, 1961, pp 103–104

4. Calne B: *Therapeutics in Neurology.* Oxford, Blackwell Scientific Publication, 1975, pp 222–229

5. Castaneda C: Investigation of CIBA 34, 647-Ba in neurological spastic syndromes. Arch Sem Med Mex 54:13–16, 1967

6. Cooperman LH: Succinylcholine-induced hyperkalemia in neuromuscular disease. JAMA 213:1867–1871, 1970

7. Dalessio DJ, Pittman FE, Wolff HG: Gastrostomy in the management of myasthenia gravis. Arch Neurol 5:18–20, 1961

8. Darley FL, Aronson AE, Brown JR: Differential diagnostic patterns of dysarthria. Speech Hearing Res 12:246–269, 1969

9. Darley FL, Aronson AE, Brown R: Mixed dysarthrias. Disorders of multiple motor systems. In *Motor Speech Disorders.* Philadelphia, WB Saunders, 1975, pp 229–235

10. Derenne J-Ph, Macklem PT, Roussos C: The respiratory muscles: Mechanics, control and pathophysiology. Am Rev Resp Dis 118:373–390, 1978

11. Dyck PJ, Stevens JC, Mulder DW, et al: Frequency of nerve fiber degeneration of peripheral motor and sensory neurons in amyotrophic lateral sclerosis. Neurology 25:781–785, 1975

12. Dykes MHM: Evaluation of a muscle relaxant: Dantrolene sodium (Dantrium). JAMA 231:862–864, 1975

13. Emmelin N, Jacobsohn D, Muren A: Effects of prolonged administration of atropine and pilocarpine on the submaxillary gland of the cat. Acta Physiol Scand 24:128–143, 1951

14. Emmelin N, Muren A, Stromblad R: Effect of anastomosis between the hypoglossal and sympathetic nerves on the supersensitivity of the denervated submaxillary gland. Acta Physiol Scand 41:35–48, 1957

15. Fallat RJ, Jewitt B, Bass M, et al: Spirometry in amyotrophic lateral sclerosis. Arch Neurol 36:74–80, 1979

16. Geoffrey RP, Appenzeller O: Dyspnea as the presenting symptom in amyotrophic lateral sclerosis. Dis Chest 42:558–562, 1962

17. Goldblatt D: Treatment of amyotrophic lateral sclerosis. Adv Neurol 17:265–283, 1977

18. Goode RL, Smith RA: The surgical management of sialorrhea. Laryngoscope 80:1078–1089, 1970

19. Hoffmann WW, Smith RA: Hypokalaemic periodic paralysis studied in vitro. Brain 93:445–474, 1970

20. Houpt JL, Gould BS, Norris FH: Psychological characteristics of patients with amyotrophic lateral sclerosis (ALS). Psychosom Med 39:299–303, 1977

21. Hudson AJ, Brown WF, Gilbert JJ: The muscular pain–fasciculation syndrome. Neurology 28:1105–1109, 1978

22. Lambert EH: Electromyography in amyotrophic lateral sclerosis. In *Motor Neuron Diseases. Research on Amyotrophic Lateral Sclerosis and Related Disorders.* Edited by FH Norris Jr, LT Kurland. New York, Grune and Stratton, 1969, pp 135–153

23. Landau WM, Weaver RA, Hornbein TF: Fusimotor nerve function in man. Arch Neurol 3:217–219, 1960

24. Landau WM: Spasticity: The fable of a neurological demon and the Emperor's new therapy. Arch Neurol 31:217–219, 1974

25. Layzer RB, Rowland LP: Cramps. N Engl J Med 285:31–40, 1971

26. Lebo CP, Ü KS, Norris FH Jr: Cricopharyngeal myotomy in amyotrophic lateral sclerosis. Laryngoscope 86:862–868, 1976

27. Lewy P, Cole R, Wepman J: Teflon injection in the correction of velopharyngeal insufficiency. Ann Otol Rhinol Laryngol 74:874–879, 1965

28. McEwan AG, Hightower NC, Carney LR, et al: Exocrine pancreatic function in patients with amyotrophic lateral sclerosis. Am J Dig Dis 16:107–110, 1971

29. Miller RD: Pulmonary disability as a symptom of amyotrophic lateral sclerosis. Proc Staff Meet Mayo Clin 32:436–437, 1957

30. Mills CP: Dysphagia in progressive bulbar palsy relieved by division of the cricopharyngeus. J Laryngol Otol 78:963–964, 1964

31. Moffic HS, Paykel ES: Depression in medical in-patients. Br J Psychiatry 126:346–353, 1975

32. Montgomery WA: Surgical laryngeal closure to eliminate chronic aspiration. N Engl J Med 292:1390–1391, 1975

33. Mulder DW: Treatment of anterior horn cell disease. Mod Treatment 3:243–249, 1966

34. Mulder DW, Lambert EH, Eaton LM: Myasthenic syndrome in patients with amyotrophic lateral sclerosis. Neurology 9:627–631, 1959

35. Nakano K, Bass H, Tyler HR, et al: Amyotrophic lateral sclerosis: a study of pulmonary function. Dis Nerv Syst 37:32–35, 1976

36. Norris FH Jr, Gasteiger EL, Chatfield PO: An electromyographic study of induced and spontaneous muscle cramps. Electroencephalogr Clin Neurophysiol 9:139–147, 1957

37. Norris FH Jr, Fallat RJ, Calanchini PR: Increased paralysis induced by guanidine in motor neuron disease. Neurology 24:135–137, 1974

38. Norris FH Jr: Systems disorders and atrophies. In *Handbook of Clinical Neurology*. Vol. 22, Part 2. Edited by JM DeJong, HL Klawans. New York, American Elsevier, 1975

39. Pazzaglia P: The muscle-relaxant of a GABA derivative (CIBA 34-647-Ba). Rivista Sperimentale di Freniatria e Medicina Legale delle Alienazioni Mentali 95:3–10, 1971

40. Pezow FM: Complication of cervical esophagostomy. Arch Otolaryngol 90:171–172, 1969

41. Quick DT, Greer M: Pancreatic dysfunction in patients with amyotrophic lateral sclerosis. Neurology 17:112–116, 1967

42. Redo SF, Barnes WA: A new method for establishing a gastrostomy or jejunostomy with evaluation in 26 patients. Surg Gynecol Obstet 110: 193–196, 1960

43. Rivera VM, Breitbach WB, Swanke L: Dantrolene in amyotrophic lateral sclerosis. JAMA 233:863–864, 1975

44. Rosenbaum KJ, Neigh JL, Strobel GE: Sensitivity to nondepolarizing muscle relaxants in amyotrophic lateral sclerosis: report of two cases. Anesthesiology 35:638–641, 1971

45. Serpick AA, Baker EL, Woodward TE: Motor system disease. Review and discussion of a case presenting with alveolar hypertension. Arch Intern Med 115:192–197, 1965

46. Smith AWM, Mulder DW, Code CF: Esophageal motility in amyotrophic lateral sclerosis. Staff Meet Mayo Clin 32:438–440, 1957

47. Smith RA, Goode RL: Sialorrhea. N Engl J Med 283:917–918, 1970

48. Smith RA, Norris FH: Symptomatic care of patients with amyotrophic lateral sclerosis. JAMA 234:715–717, 1975

49. Smith RB: Hyperkalaemia following succinylcholine administration in neurological disorders. A review. Can Anaesth Soc J 199–201, 1971

50. Snider SR, Fahn S, Isgreen WP, et al: Primary sensory symptoms in parkinsonism. Neurology 26:423–429, 1976

51. Tobey RE, Jacobsen PM, Kahle CT, et al: The serum potassium response to muscle relaxants in neural injury. Anesthesiology 37:332–336, 1972

52. Utterback RA, Cummins AJ, Cape CA, et al: Pancreatic function in amyotrophic lateral sclerosis. J Neurol Neurosurg Psychiatry 33:544–547, 1970

53. Wallenborn WM: Parotid gland atrophy produced by transtympanic destruction of tympanic plexus. Laryngoscope 78:132–144, 1968

54. Wise RP: Muscle disorders and the relaxants. Br J Anaesth 35:558–563, 1963

Commentary

Victor M. Rivera

Dr. Smith and his associates have outlined the techniques of giving symptomatic management to patients with ALS.

It is known that 20% of ALS patients tend to have a prolonged spontaneous stabilization, as indicated by the retrospective studies of Mulder and Howard (2). Murray Sanders (6), as noted by Tyler in his report of recent double-blind studies (7), has observed partial and temporary improvement of ALS patients in his uncontrolled series, changes that have not been stressed in the literature. Whether these are spontaneous remissions or changes favored by the drug he used remains controversial. However, we cannot realistically wait and hope for those spontaneous periods of stabilization to occur; rather, active and sometimes aggressive measures, such as Dr. Smith describes, remain the core of the only acceptable treatment we can offer to our patients (Table 1).

Dr. Smith referred to the use of pyridostigmine bromide (Mestinon) and neostigmine bromide (Prostigmin) in selected patients with dysphagia and pulmonary insufficiency due to ALS. In our experience, these pharmacologic agents have provided very limited results. In fact, as a word of warning, one of the common side effects of pyridostigmine—increased salivation—may aggravate the existing problem of sialorrhea and thus provoke aspiration of saliva due to massive accumulation of secretions. An important consideration when prescribing cholinesterase inhibitors for patients with ALS is an awareness of their muscarinic effects.

For the management of sialorrhea, we have found the use of trihexyphenidyl hydrochloride (Artane), 2–4 mg three times a day to be effective (4). This anticholinergic drug, which is commonly used in the management of Parkinson syndrome, is well tolerated by ALS patients and does not produce the undesired effects of other agents, such as amitriptyline hydrochloride (Elavil). In 1977, we initiated the use of clonidine to control drooling in these patients (5). Clonidine, a central alpha-adrenergic stimulator, is widely used as an antihypertensive agent and probably decreases the sympathetic outflow from the brain; it has been shown to decrease salivation in experimental animals. The most common side reaction in humans is dry mouth. Provided that the medication is initiated cautiously in small but increasing amounts to reach an individual dose, blood pressure levels in normotensive individuals usually remain unaltered. At an oral dose of 0.5–1.0 mg of clonidine twice daily, the desired result of decreased salivation has been remarkable in most cases. In view of the danger of serious reactions due to abrupt discontinuation of the drug, the patient is instructed in gradual withdrawal.

Table 1 Symptomatic Management of ALS

Symptom	*Treatment*
Muscle weakness	Physical therapy Orthotic device Pyridostigmine bromide (Mestinon),[a] neostigmine bromide (Prostigmin),[a] or guanidine HCl [a]
Muscle spasticity	Diazepam (Valium)[b] Dantrolene sodium (Dantrium)[b] Baclofen (Lioresal)[b]
Muscle cramps	Trial of phenytoin, quinidine, or procainamide
Speech disorders	Speech therapy Microphones and amplifiers Alphabet charts Computerized sound apparatus with prerecorded phrases
Dysphagia	Puréed or ground food "Chicken swallow" techniques Feeding tubes Gastrostomy or esophagostomy Cricopharyngomyotomy
Sialorrhea	Amitriptyline HCl (Elavil)[b] Trihexyphenidyl HCl (Artane)[b] Clonidine Surgical denervation or extirpation of salivary glands Irradiation of salivary glands
Respiratory insufficiency	Pulmonary toilet Incentive spirometer Tracheostomy Automated ventilation

[a] In very selected cases.
[b] Individually titrated.

We have not observed any other effects from clonidine in any of our patients with ALS. I should mention, however, that we tried clonidine in a patient with slight sialorrhea and without dysphagia. This patient complained of extreme dry mouth to the point that we had to discontinue the medication. Again, we have to be selective of the patient who is going to use the medication; nevertheless, no observable change in fasciculations has been noted with this drug.

Effective management of spasticity may provide substantial comfort and relief in the affected ALS patients. While methocarbamol and diazepam

(Valium) in the usual dosages are ineffective, dantrolene sodium (Dantrium) can be dangerous because of the low tolerance that ALS patients exhibit to this drug. Patients taking dantrolene sodium also exhibit increasing weakness, de novo appearance of dysphagia and sialorrhea, and, in certain cases, respiratory difficulties (3). Any antispasticity agent might increase the preexisting weakness of the ALS patient.

Baclofen (Lioresal), in individually titrated doses, can be helpful in selected cases with marked spasticity, jaw-jerk clonus, and painful spasms (Table 1).

Dr. Smith mentioned the use of cricopharyngomyotomy, a procedure we feel has great potential for temporarily but substantially alleviating dysphagia in certain ALS patients. In our experience, with the use of pre- and postoperative videotape esophagograms, it seems that patients who preserve tongue motion but experience more difficulty in initiating the swallowing process tend to improve more consistently and for a longer period.

Dr. Fallat and Dr. Griggs have reviewed the topic of pulmonary dysfunction elsewhere in this volume. I shall mention only that, according to our own observations, persistent higher total lung capacity indicates better prognosis for survival, whereas arterial–alveolar gradients and $PaCO_2$ are usually preserved until late stages of the illness (1). The small, plastic, disposable incentive spirometer is a simple device that actually performs the role of a home respiratory therapist, provides physical therapy to the accessory chest muscles and diaphragm, keeps the patient interested with breathing exercises, prevents atelectasis and infection, and performs other functions.

It is our belief that the patient with ALS can be aided simply by treating his or her symptoms (Table 1). The patient can then live with the disease with more hope and comfort and avoid the prevalent attitude of hopelessness. Further, the physician's symptomatic therapy will encourage the patient to continue life with dignity and to fight the disease; this encouragement alone may be of considerable therapeutic benefit to patient and family.

REFERENCES

1. Alvarez A, Calderon M, Griffin BT, et al: Pulmonary function abnormalities in ALS (abstract). In *Proceedings of the 11th International Congress of Neurology.* Excerpta Medica ICS #427:46, 1977

2. Mulder DW, Howard FM: Patient resistance and prognosis in ALS. Mayo Clin Proc 51:537–541, 1976

3. Rivera VM: Symptomatic care of patients with amyotrophic lateral sclerosis. JAMA 235:2584–2585, 1976

4. Rivera VM: Amyotrophic lateral sclerosis: management and symptomatic treatment. Ann Med Ctr del Oro 2:78–88, 1979

5. Rivera VM, Breitbach W, Swanke L: Dantrolene in amyotrophic lateral sclerosis. JAMA 233:863–864, 1975

6. Sanders M, Fellowes ON: Use of detoxified snake neurotoxin as a partial treatment for amyotrophic lateral sclerosis. Cancer Cytology 15:26–30, 1975

7. Tyler HR: Double-blind study of modified neurotoxin in motor neuron disease. Neurology 29:77–81, 1979

Forbes H. Norris, Jr

Some ALS patients develop a peculiar, rigid state in which they become as stiff as boards. It may take several individuals to turn the patient over in bed. In such cases, reduction of rigidity can substantially alleviate nursing care problems. I agree with Dr. Rivera and infrequently administer dantrolene to ALS patients because of the drug's side effects. Baclofen has occasionally been very useful in these patients (4) and seems to have less potential for sedative side effects than diazepam; no major side effects of baclofen have occurred.

I would like to cite meperidine as being of benefit for dysphagia and the related problems of pseudobulbar palsy. I first administered meperidine in ALS some eight years ago for purely humanistic reasons to a patient with far-advanced and what I judged to be terminal ALS. He was aspirating his own saliva every few seconds and was in a desperate state. Much to my astonishment, with 50 mg of meperidine the patient began to handle his secretions better, was swallowing food better, and even regained some ability to manage solid food. He maintained this small but significant improvement on the same dose of meperidine for the next six months. Since then, I have been using it rather generously in patients with advanced ALS. It continues to give benefit, which I cannot explain by a simple narcotic effect. Two other patients benefited from meperidine in doses of 25–50 mg, 15 to 20 minutes before mealtime, for periods of 18 to 20 months, respectively. The drug's mode of action under these circumstances is obscure. It is possible that hyperactive pharyngeal-laryngeal reflexes in ALS interfere with function, and meperidine reduces such undesirable reflex activity. Other drugs, such as baclofen, should but do not have a similar effect.

Our experience with adverse effects of succinylcholine in patients with ALS has been reported previously (2, 5). We did not undertake any further trials with succinylcholine and cannot say whether the cardiac complication is the same as that reported by others (1).

Dr. Smith mentioned the glottic closure procedure drawn to our attention by Montgomery in 1975 (3). My associate in surgery, Dr. Charles Lebo, and I proposed this procedure to four patients, who blew out the subglottic suture line postoperatively, thus leading to much more severe difficulty than existed before. This area is prone to infection and we no longer recommend glottic closure unless, in carefully selected cases, laryngectomy and permanent tracheostomy are also performed.

REFERENCES

1. Cooperman LH: Succinylcholine-induced hyperkalemia in neuromuscular disease. JAMA 213:1867–1871, 1970

2. Lebo CP, Ü KS, Norris FH: Cricopharyngeal myotomy in amyotrophic lateral sclerosis. Laryngoscope 86:862–868, 1976

3. Montgomery WA: Surgical laryngeal closure to eliminate chronic aspiration. N Engl J Med 292:1390–1391, 1975

4. Norris FH, Ü KS, Sachais B, et al: Trial of baclofen in amyotrophic lateral sclerosis. Arch Neurol, in press

5. Ü KS, Norris FH, Denys EH, et al: Surgery in patients with amyotrophic lateral sclerosis (abstract). In *Proceedings of the 11th World Congress of Neurology.* Excerpta Medica ICS #427:45, 1977

W. King Engel

Dr. Smith and Dr. Rivera report that patients with ALS improve after administration of edrophonium or pyridostigmine. We have tried pyridostigmine on the basis of what the Mayo Clinic group previously reported, but we have been very disappointed because of the minimal benefit to the patient's weakness and the excessive fasciculations and salivation it creates (except in one atypical progressive muscular atrophy [PMA]–type ALS patient with preexisting diabetes mellitus, who benefited significantly) (2). I am also concerned about the use of placebo control in the respiratory tests Dr. Smith reports. The question I would like to ask is, Which ALS patients really derive clinical benefit from the anticholinesterase drugs, what percentage, and to what degree?

My second concern is with regard to the use of d-tubocurarine (curare). Dr. Smith and Dr. Rivera report that ALS patients are particularly susceptible to the effects of curare, but at what dose? At 5/80 or 8/80 of a curarizing dose? What percentage of ALS patients are susceptible? In our studies of myasthenia gravis and other neuromuscular diseases, we follow the curare-test incrementing-dose procedure summarized by Rowland et al. (3). Do ALS patients really have significant weakness at, say, 5/80 or less of a curarizing dose, which is the level I use as an indication of abnormal susceptibility? In addition, Dr. Smith and Dr. Rivera mentioned that d-tubocurarine and succinylcholine can be dangerous during surgery. At first I thought the concern was about an excessive junctional effect in the disease, but that really would not be an important consideration because the action of the drug would be offset very quickly after the surgery. However, the loss of potassium leads to the topic of malignant hyperthermia (a reaction that is provoked by these drugs in susceptible persons), but I have never seen or heard of malignant hyperthermia in an ALS patient (1). I would like more information regarding significant elevation of serum potassium (presumably due to loss from skeletal muscle), a reaction that these drugs can cause in any patient. I wonder whether there is a greater elevation of potassium and a greater incidence of cardiac arrest in ALS patients taking these drugs who undergo surgery. I have never warned a patient or a surgeon about the danger of these two drugs in ALS patients, and I wonder if I should.

REFERENCES

1. Eng GD, Epstein BS, Engel WK, et al: Malignant hyperthermia and central core disease in a child with congenital dislocating hips. Arch Neurol 35:189–197, 1978

2. Mulder DW, Lambert EH, Eaton LM: Myasthenic syndrome in patients with amyotrophic lateral sclerosis. Neurology 9:627–631, 1959

3. Rowland LP, Aranow H Jr, Hoefer PFA: Observations on the curare test in the differential diagnosis of myasthenia gravis. In *Proceedings of the Second International Symposium on Myasthenia Gravis.* Edited by HR Viets. Springfield, IL, Charles C Thomas, 1961, pp 411–434

Eric H. Denys

I think that there is a fairly simple explanation of why anticholinesterase medication, such as pyridostigmine bromide (Mestinon), may not work in ALS patients, or at least is not as beneficial as one might want it to be.

Decremental responses to repetitive stimulation have been shown in patients with ALS (2, 3, 4). In a recent study of 55 patients, we have shown that decremental responses are found more frequently when there is atrophy and that the magnitude of the decrement correlates with the degree of atrophy (1). We have also found larger decrements in muscles showing abundant fasciculations. Decremental responses were never very large (mostly $<10\%$, rarely $>20\%$). This can be explained on the basis that probably only a small pool of neurons is in a transient stage of neuromuscular transmission failure at a particular time. Edrophonium chloride (Tensilon) reduced the decrement. It should be emphasized, however, that the findings described only reflect the state of neuromuscular transmission in the particular muscle under study. Amyotrophic lateral sclerosis is a disease in which different muscle groups can be involved to various degrees; therefore, the effect of anticholinesterase medication will depend on both the number of muscles showing synaptic failure and the degree of decrement present in any one muscle. This explains why, in most cases, the benefit derived from this medication is minimal or mild.

REFERENCES

1. Denys EH, Norris FH: Amyotrophic lateral sclerosis impairment of neuromuscular transmission. Arch Neurol 36:202–205, 1979

2. Lambert EH, Mulder DW: Electromyographic studies in amyotrophic lateral sclerosis. Proc Staff Meet Mayo Clin 32:441–446, 1957

3. Mulder DW, Lambert EH, Eaton LM: Myasthenic syndrome in patients with amyotrophic lateral sclerosis. Neurology 9:627–631, 1959

4. Norris FH: Nerve stimulation studies in amyotrophic lateral sclerosis (abstract). In *Fourth International Congress on Electromyography,* Brussels, Belgium, 1971, pp 106–107

Richard A. Smith

As was discussed earlier, the clinical benefit of pyridostigmine bromide (Mestinon) is limited. It may, however, be useful in specific circumstances. For example, it may temporarily improve swallowing for several days, during which time the patient can be scheduled for elective esophagostomy. Prolonged administration of an anticholinesterase inhibitor to ALS patients is not advised and, on theoretical grounds, might even be deleterious.

With regard to succinylcholine, there is a body of medical literature, as referred to by Dr. Norris, suggesting that administration of succinylcholine to patients with neuromuscular disease may subject these patients to the risk of cardiac arrest (1, 2, 3). Dr. Norris has mentioned to me that he witnessed such an occurrence in at least one ALS patient. Until the matter is better studied, it seems reasonable to be cautious about the administration of succinylcholine to ALS patients.

REFERENCES

1. Cooperman LH: Succinylcholine-induced hyperkalemia in neuromuscular disease. JAMA 213:1867–1871, 1970

2. Lebo CP, Ü KS, Norris FH: Cricopharyngeal myotomy in amyotrophic lateral sclerosis. Laryngoscope 86:862–868, 1976

3. Ü KS, Norris FH, Denys EH, et al: Surgery in patients with amyotrophic lateral sclerosis (abstract). In *Proceedings of the 11th World Congress of Neurology.* Excerpta Medica ICS #427:45, 1977

Donald W. Mulder

In our experience, a neuromuscular conduction defect similar to that seen in myasthenia gravis occurs frequently in patients who have ALS (1). Muscle examination in these patients reveals increased muscle fatigability that is relieved by rest. The myasthenic symptoms are most apparent in muscles seriously affected by this disease of the anterior horn cells, and, perhaps for this reason, the response to neostigmine and related drugs is not as dramatic as it is in myasthenia gravis. However, in selected patients with ALS, the use of neostigmine is of distinct benefit. We have observed that patients taking this drug have had less difficulty in swallowing and talking. Some have been able to better use their upper extremities and have been able to maintain their head erect for the first time.

Unfortunately, the use of neostigmine does not alter the course of the disease, and the patient frequently notes an alarming increase in fasciculations and a distressing increase in salivation. Further, it may be possible to accentuate the weakness of extremely weak muscles with an overdose of neostigmine or similar drugs. We have previously reported on four patients, all of whom had an increased sensitivity to d-tubocurarine and increased weakness after an intravenous injection of this drug, with restoration of their

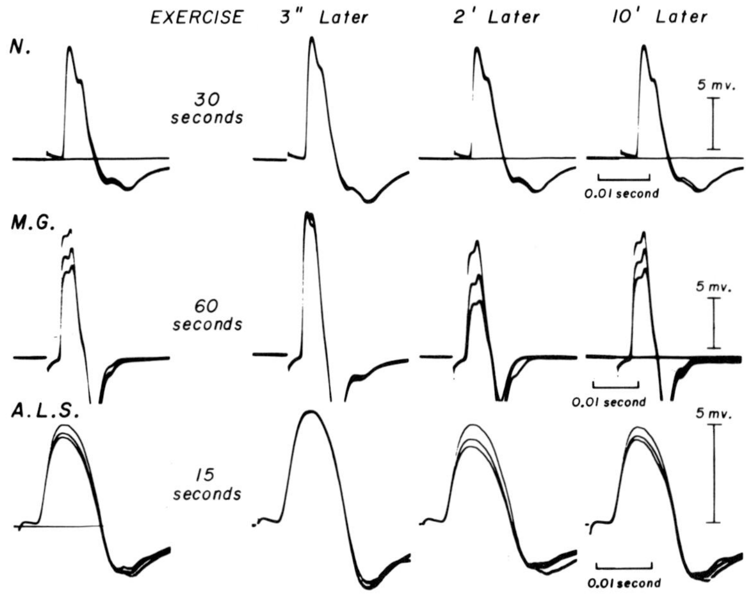

Figure 1 Responses of muscle to maximal stimulation of motor nerve at a rate of three shocks per second, before and after a brief period of voluntary muscle contraction. N. = normal person, showing the action potential of the hypothenar muscle in response to stimulation of the ulnar nerve. The responses were nearly exactly superimposed. M. G. = myasthenia gravis, showing the action potential of the hypothenar muscle in response to stimulation of the ulnar nerve. Before voluntary exercise of the muscle, the three responses declined progressively in amplitude. Three seconds after exercise, this defect was repaired and the initial amplitude was greater; two minutes later, the defect was more pronounced than it was before exercise; 10 minutes later, the defect was nearly as it was before exercise. A. L. S. = amyotrophic lateral sclerosis, showing the action potential of the biceps brachii in response to stimulation of the musculocutaneous nerve. The sequence of events was similar to that seen in myasthenia gravis. (Reprinted from Mulder DW, Lambert EH, Eaton LM: Myasthenic syndrome in patients with amyotrophic lateral sclerosis. Neurology 9:630, 1959.)

original strength after an intravenous injection of edrophonium chloride (1). For example, in one patient with ALS, injection of one-tenth the curarizing dose of d-tubocurarine (0.135 mg/kg of body weight) was followed by an increase in weakness; the strength of the right biceps muscle decreased from 36 to 9 units, and the grip of the right hand decreased in strength from 30 to 13 units. The left hand showed no appreciable changes. Intravenous injection of 10 mg of edrophonium chloride (Tensilon) restored the patient's strength to its previous level. In addition, in this patient and others, electromyographic studies revealed abnormalities suggesting the presence of a defect in neuromuscular conduction similar to that seen in myasthenia gravis. Since this report, we have seen many other ALS patients who have had a similar defect that was present on both clinical examination and in the patient's electromyographic examinations, including single-fiber studies (Fig. 1) (1).

The differentiation of myasthenia gravis from ALS usually can be made without difficulty, but, as Dr. Tyler suggests, such differentiation can be problematic. The muscular atrophy, fasciculations, hyperreflexia, and relentless progression of ALS are usually sufficient to differentiate the two conditions. The pattern of electromyographic abnormalities in ALS, including evidence of denervation, fasciculation, increased size, and reduced number of motor unit potentials, is also an aid in diagnosis. Ptosis and diplopia, which are among the commonest of symptoms in myasthenia gravis, are not features of the myasthenic syndrome associated with ALS. However, difficulty in talking and in swallowing is common in both diseases and may lead to confusion in diagnosis.

REFERENCE

1. Mulder DW, Lambert EH, Eaton LM: Myasthenic syndrome in patients with amyotrophic lateral sclerosis. Neurology 9:627–631, 1959

17 Nutritional Management

Richard T. Moxley III

Claudia Kempf

Meeting the nutritional requirements of patients with amyotrophic lateral sclerosis poses challenges to the physician and dietitian. As the disease progresses, several problems arise that affect nutrition. Difficulties with mastication and swallowing often appear. Alterations in gastrointestinal function and motility, usually related to decreased physical activity, cause constipation and, occasionally, impaction. These problems frequently impair nutrient intake and limit effective digestion. Obesity, hypocalcemia, or vitamin-deficiency states may develop and require early diagnosis to avoid treatment failures. To meet the caloric demand and other nutritional needs of a patient with ALS, the physician or dietitian must monitor dietary intake patterns and change the types of foods as well as their consistency as the need arises. Optimal management of the nutritional problems associated with ALS depends on a precise understanding of the significant differences in dietary requirements present among these patients. Unfortunately, there is a dearth of specific information on the caloric, nutrient, and fluid requirements of patients with ALS and other muscle-wasting diseases. This information shortage represents the major challenge to both the physician and dietitian in the development of an effective nutritional management program for the patient with ALS.

Table 1 lists five factors ordinarily operative in normal individuals to provide good nutrition. These are contrasted with various problems that occur in patients with ALS. The remainder of this chapter discusses these problems and provides guidelines that should aid the

Table 1 Nutritional Factors in Healthy Individuals and Corresponding Nutritional Problems in Patients with ALS

Nutritional Factors in Healthy Individuals	*Corresponding Problems in Patients with ALS*
Adequate diet	Obesity, malnutrition, vitamin and mineral deficiency, decreased fluid intake, decreased fiber
Normal mastication and swallowing	Bulbar symptoms
Normal gastric emptying	Gastric retention
Normal intestinal motility and absorption	Abnormal motility, exocrine pancreatic dysfunction
Normal hormonal regulation during meals	Altered insulin release

physician in correcting or minimizing some of these nutrition-related difficulties.

If a patient with ALS obviously suffers from some degree of obesity, or is suspected of having malnutrition, or a vitamin or mineral deficiency, the first step in management is to assess his or her dietary intake and to compare that with the presumed dietary needs (1, 33). One helpful method to acquire information about the patient's nutritional status is a self-administered three-day diet history. Although this approach depends on the patient's reliability, conscientious patients usually provide very accurate data. The patient maintains a diary of all intake on two typical weekdays and a typical weekend day. Before actually writing the diary, the patient should receive specific instructions from a clinical dietitian to ensure that there will be a complete and accurate food record. Dietitians place particular emphasis on an accurate estimation of the size of portions along with a complete description of the food items including brand names. Often the patient is shown food models that allow him or her to equate size of serving with a particular number of ounces. After completion of the three-day diet history, the patient needs to review the results with the dietitian. At this time, the dietitian may wish to obtain an additional 24-hour dietary recall, which provides an indication of the reliability of the three-day diet record.

If access to a dietitian is limited, a rough approximation of the adequacy of the patient's intake can be determined by a quick review of the patient's consumption of items from the basic four food groups: milk, meat, vegetables and fruits, and breads and cereals. The recommended intakes of items from the basic four food groups are available in standard nutrition texts (18). Another source of normative nutritional data is the Government Printing Office, which every four to six years publishes an updated text prepared by the National Research Council on the recommended daily dietary needs of normal men and women (33). Despite these sources of nutritional information, no long-term dietary studies of patients with ALS or other neuromuscular diseases are available to indicate whether significant differences exist between their minimum daily dietary needs and those cited in the various texts for normal individuals.

One simple method for estimating a patient's daily caloric requirements is that originally recommended by a joint committee of the American Diabetes Association and the American Dietetic Association. This method is outlined in Table 2.

To assist in determining whether a patient is performing very light, moderate, or very heavy exercise, it may be helpful to consult a detailed energy-cost table such as that available in the *Bioastronautics Data Book* (37). Most healthy adults spend their day performing tasks that are described as very light or light activity. For example, slow walking or ironing requires energy at a rate of approximately 4 kcal/minute. A cookie containing 200 calories would require 50 minutes of slow walking or ironing to burn off. Moderate activity such as slow swimming, gardening, or tennis expends approximately 6.5 kcal/minute, and such activities would have to be performed for 30 minutes to burn the calories provided by the 200-calorie cookie. Familiarity with the various oxygen costs of different levels of activity is important in redetermining the appropriate daily caloric requirements as ALS progresses. When patients become limited to a bed-and-wheelchair existence, their caloric demands may approximate those accounted for by their basal oxygen consumption. This marked decline in caloric need must be anticipated to avoid excessive caloric intake and obesity.

If a patient's dietary history confirms the clinical suspicion that he or she is malnourished and also may suffer from protein deficiency, it may be helpful to obtain certain laboratory tests. In severe protein-calorie malnutrition, there may be a decrease in plasma total protein, serum albumin, transferrin levels, and total lymphocyte count along with a decreased or absent delayed-hypersensitivity response (2, 9). However, such alterations are uncommon in patients with neuromuscular disease and should not be expected with mild degrees of protein-calorie malnutrition.

Vitamin deficiency states must be suspected frequently in patients with ALS, especially those undergoing phases of rapid weight loss, marked variations in dietary intake, or significant bouts of gastrointestinal dysfunction. Blood levels of specific vitamins should be measured and replacement therapy instituted as needed. Mineral deficiency, especially hypocalcemia, occurs commonly in ALS and requires intermittent laboratory evaluation (28, 30). Periodic checks of urine specific gravity may be helpful in monitoring hydration of debilitated patients. This

Table 2 Determining Individual Daily Caloric Requirements

STEP 1.	Determining standard weight from height	
	Women: Allow 100 lb for the first 5 ft of height. Add 5 lb for each additional inch	100 + (5 × No. inches) = _____
	Men: Allow 106 lb for the first 5 ft of height. Add 6 lb for each additional inch	106 + (6 × No. inches) = _____
	Small frame or build: Subtract 10% from weight determined above	No. lb − 10% = _____
	Large build: Add 10% to weight determined above	No. lb + 10% = _____
	Standard body weight	= _____
STEP 2.	Determining caloric needs	
	Basal calories	Standard body weight × 10 = _____
	Activity calories	
	Moderate to heavy activity	Standard body weight × 5 = _____
	Very light to light activity	Standard body weight × 3 = _____
	Very heavy to extreme activity	Standard body weight × 10 = _____
	Daily caloric need (basal calories + activity calories)	= _____
STEP 3.	Controlling weight	
	For weight loss of 1 lb/week: Subtract 500 calories from daily caloric needs	
	For weight gain of 1 lb/week: Add 500 calories to daily caloric needs	
STEP 4.	Estimating weight change	
	Percentage of weight change can be determined and classified as follows:	

$$\%\ \text{weight change} = \frac{(\text{usual weight} - \text{actual weight})}{\text{usual weight}} \times 100$$

1 week:	Significant weight change = more than 2% weight change
1 month:	Significant weight change = more than 5% weight change
3 months:	Significant weight change = more than 7.5% weight change
6 months:	Significant weight change = more than 10% weight change

measurement is most meaningful when taken on urine collected at home and can be performed by the visiting nurse or family members. A more accurate assessment of the patient's typical state of hydration is obtained in this way and not complicated by the atypical intake pattern often associated with a trip to see the doctor. The urine specific gravity and the diet history provide useful information concerning the adequacy of the patient's fluid intake.

The significantly obese patient with ALS poses a major treatment problem. Successful reversal of obesity most often depends on early detection; this is particularly critical in patients with muscle-wasting diseases. Figure 1 demonstrates this point by contrasting the effects of three weight-losing regimens in six obese patients (40). Starvation produced the most dramatic and rapid decline in body weight. On the basis of this criterion, starvation appears to be an optimal way to obtain weight loss. However, starvation dramatically increases urinary nitrogen loss, which reflects an associated loss in lean muscle mass. For this reason, starvation is not a desirable means for achieving even moderate weight loss in patients with an already decreased muscle mass. A more desirable regimen uses diets that are hypocaloric and contain either a normal proportion of carbohydrate and fat (CHO 50%, fat 35%) or contain a relatively high proportion of fat (5–7, 27, 36, 40). Figure 1 shows the relatively mild nitrogen loss that accompanies hypocaloric

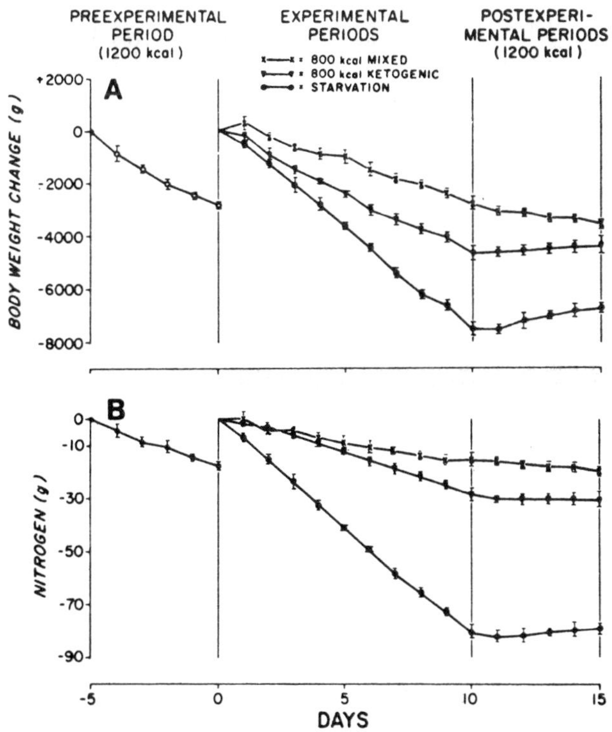

Figure 1 Effect of various weight-reduction regimens on **(A)** daily changes in body weight (mean ± SE) and **(B)** daily nitrogen balances (mean ± SE) of six obese subjects. Values are plotted cumulatively. (Reprinted with permission from Yang M, Van Itallie T: Composition of weight lost during short-term weight reduction. J Clin Invest 58:722–730, 1976.)

diets in contrast to total starvation. Both of the hypocaloric regimens (normal proportion = mixed, high fat = ketogenic) in Figure 1 allow for weight reduction with much less nitrogen loss. A comparison of these two diets reveals that the high-fat diet produces a significantly greater water loss than the diet with normal proportions of carbohydrate, protein, and fat. The return to a weight-stabilizing diet was accompanied by a phase of transient weight gain in patients who consumed the high-fat diet because of the additional water loss that occurred in these patients. In contrast, patients who consumed the hypocaloric diet of normal proportions failed to demonstrate the rebound weight gain after returning to a weight-stabilizing diet.

Treatment of mildly obese patients with ALS should be initiated early in the course of the disease and should utilize a weight-losing diet that is hypocaloric with the normal proportions of carbohydrate (50%), protein (15%), and fat (35%). After a return to a weight-stabilizing diet, careful serial follow-up assessments of body weight and diet composition are necessary to avoid the recurrence of obesity.

As ALS progresses, it is increasingly difficult to determine the appropriate target standard weight for a given patient. As weakness increases and muscle mass is lost, the relative proportion of muscle to fat declines. Use of a standard body-weight table may prove deceptive in some patients because total body weight may remain in the normal range despite a relative excess of adipose tissue (24). Table 3 presents data on the height, weight, and lean body mass of five patients with ALS. These data demonstrate the variable correlation that exists between the calculated standard body weight and the actual lean body muscle mass of a particular patient as determined by total body potassium counting. The first three patients in the table show reasonable correlations between their actual body weight and muscle mass and the standard or expected body weight and lean muscle mass values. However, patient 4 shows the disparity that can exist. Her actual weight is almost normal according

Table 3 Data from Five Patients with ALS

Patient No.	*Age (yr)*	*Height (cm)*	*Weight (kg)*	*Percentage of Ideal Weight*	*Lean Body Mass[a] (% of normal)*
1	29	166	45.0	74	80
2	56	170	56.0	88	86
3	73	182	68.9	94	84
4	49	165	52.0	93	56
5	69	164	62.0	111	81

[a] Determined by ^{40}K counting.

to the standard weight for height table adopted from the 1959 Metropolitan Life Insurance statistics. However, her lean muscle mass shows a much greater percentage decline from the normal standard than does her total body weight. This suggests a relative excess of adipose tissue in this patient.

There is no readily available, convenient way to measure lean muscle mass in patients with ALS, and this makes it almost impossible to quantitate the amounts of adipose and muscle tissue in a given patient. At the very least, serial weight measurements are necessary to monitor these patients. Some investigators have suggested using the ratio of a patient's 24-hour urinary creatinine excretion to an idealized 24-hour urinary creatinine excretion for healthy volunteers of that height and weight. This crude estimate of lean body mass has been based on a limited number of studies of healthy men and women, and has been used primarily in evaluations of malnourished and obese patients rather than in evaluations of patients suffering from various neuromuscular diseases. There is no totally satisfying, uniformly practical way to assess lean muscle mass in patients with ALS. As the clinical condition deteriorates and muscle wasting and weakness ensue, it seems inevitable that a certain amount of weight loss must be allowed to prevent a relative excess of adipose tissue. An exact figure is difficult to pinpoint, but a range of 5% to 15% below standard body weight is probably a reasonable target.

Bulbar weakness in ALS requires careful dietary management and often in its early stages requires a combination of liquid supplements and a regular diet of softened foods. As symptoms progress, the patient will eventually need a completely liquid diet plus vitamin and fiber supplements and then either a feeding esophagostomy, gastrostomy, or regular tube feedings. Table 4 lists some of the oral supplements that are available to these patients.

In prescribing various liquid diets or foods to be prepared at home in a blender, physicians as well as dietitians need to be sensitive to the patient's practical concerns. Whether the physician recommends a diet combining commercial and homemade foods or relies exclusively on one feeding method depends on the patient and his or her home situation. The following are some of the positive features of commercially available preparations:

1. Decreased labor and ease of use (important when the patient lives alone, travels, or has a disabled spouse).

2. Decreased bacterial contamination.

3. Increased control over dietary osmolarity.

4. Large selection to meet the needs of patients with digestive and absorptive insufficiencies.

Table 4 Commercially Prepared Foods That Are Suitable for Patients with ALS[a]

Product	*Brief Description*	*Comment*	*Solute Load*
Selected Oral Supplements			
Citrotein (Doyle)	Protein, vitamin, mineral supplement; orange flavor; powder; 12 1.18-oz pkg/box; $8.86	Lactose- and gluten-free	Low residue, 496 mOsm/kg water
Carnation Instant Breakfast	Complete food; multiple flavors; powder; 6 pkg/box; $1.20	Contains milk	Medium residue
Portagen (Mead-Johnson)	Medium chain triglycerides (MTC), corn oil; powder; one-lb can; $6.32	Lactose-free	Low residue
Sustacal Pudding (Mead-Johnson)	Milk, soy oil, food starch; Flavors: vanilla, chocolate, butterscotch; 4 5-oz tins/carton; $2.94	Contains milk	Medium residue
Preparations Useful for Oral Supplements and Complete Tube Feeding			
Ensure (Ross)	14% protein, 31.5% fat, 54.5% CHO; Flavors: vanilla, black walnut; 8-oz can; $0.65	Lactose-free	Well texturized, medium residue, 374 mOsm/kg water
Flexical (Mead-Johnson)	Protein hydrolysate, free amino acids, sucrose, dextrin, tapioca starch, MCT, corn oil; 8 2-oz tins/pkg; $15.32	Lactose-free	Medium residue, 800 mOsm/kg water
Isocal (Mead-Johnson)	Caseinates, soy protein, MCT, soy oil, corn syrup; 3.4% protein, 4.4% fat, 13.2% CHO; 8-oz can; $0.92	Lactose-free	Low residue, 350 mOsm/kg water
Meritene (Doyle)	Milk, caseinates, sugar, maltodextrin, corn syrup; Flavors: plain, chocolate, eggnog; one-lb can of	Contains milk	Medium residue, 640 mOsm/kg water

(Syntex)	5.5% fat, 10.1% CHO; 24 10-oz cans/case; $19.15		water
Precision LR (Doyle)	Egg protein, vegetable oil, maltodextrin; 8.8% protein, 0.3% fat, 84% CHO; Flavors: cherry, lemon, lime, orange; 36 3-oz pkg/case; $53.44	Lactose-free	Low residue, 525 mOsm/kg water
Sustacal (Mead-Johnson)	24% protein, 21% fat, 55% CHO; 12-oz can; $1.18	Contains lactose, gluten-free	Medium residue, 625 mOsm/kg water
Vivonex-Std (Eaton)	Balanced element diet; powder; crystalline amino acids, safflower oil, glucose, glucose oligosaccharides; 6 80-g pkg/box; $11.50; Flavor pkg, 60 2-g pkg/box; $6.30	Lactose-free	Low residue, 500 mOsm/kg water
Vivonex-High Nitrogen	Elemental diet; powder; unflavored; 10 80-g pkg/box; $39.43	Lactose-free	Low residue, 844 mOsm/kg water
Primary Tube Feeding Preparation			
Complete B (Doyle)	Balanced isotonic diet; 4% protein, 4% fat, 12% CHO; meat, milk, pureed fruit; 13.6-oz can; $1.94 (1979)	Contains milk	Low residue, 517 mOsm/kg water

[a] All prices quoted are 1979 retail prices.

Despite these advantages of commercially available preparations, diets prepared at home in a blender are frequently used in the care of patients with ALS. The psychologic benefit to the patient and to those providing care is great when the patient's food is prepared at home. These psychologic factors may override the relative advantages of the commercial preparations. The person responsible for preparing the patient's meals should be counseled carefully by a dietitian. Frequently, such home diets contain an inadequate amount of fluid, and the nutrient content may vary. This inconsistency in composition occasionally may cause the patient to consume an excess solute load and lead to the syndrome well known with tube feedings: dehydration and azotemia. To avoid bacterial contamination, homemade diets should be made up daily and not stored. The blender should be cleaned thoroughly after each use to avoid a similar problem. If the patient receives his alimentation through tube feeding rather than gastrostomy or esophagostomy, particular care should be paid to the diameter of the tubing because particle size varies widely in homemade diets.

The routine use of tube feedings has become less frequent as more reliance has been placed on feeding esophagostomies and gastrostomies. Instructions should be given to the patient and to those directly responsible for monitoring the tube feedings as to the potential complications of this method, such as the tube being placed in the airway, the tube becoming coiled in the posterior pharynx, improper attachment of the tube to the face, too rapid a rate of food administration, or an inappropriate tube diameter. Several helpful publications are available that provide a detailed description of the method of tube feeding and the complications that may occur (17, 19, 25, 41).

Whether a patient receives a homemade diet, a commercially available preparation, or a combination of the two, there are certain commonly encountered mishaps that need to be anticipated and prevented. The following list is a summary of the major errors that may occur with these types of feeding regimens (17, 19, 25, 41).

1. Inadequate amounts of nutrients may be administered at a given feeding, and they may be either over- or underdiluted.

2. The composition of the diet may be inappropriate for a given individual, for example, a food item high in lactose may be fed to a lactase-deficient patient (3).

3. The food may be stored inappropriately or the utensils may be poorly cleaned, allowing growth of bacteria.

4. The temperature of the food may be too cold (below room temperature).

5. Patients may be placed directly on full strength feedings rather than undergoing a period of several days of diluted feedings.

6. The diet may contain excessively high protein and solute contents, which would predispose the patient to dehydration and life-threatening azotemia (17).

7. There is often failure to reevaluate the efficacy of the dietary regimen being employed.

8. Inadequate attention may be given to changes in the defecation pattern accompanying specific feeding regimens.

Patients with ALS frequently have complaints relating to gastrointestinal dysfunction, such as gastric distention, diarrhea, and constipation (Table 5) (11, 12). These problems are often related to an abnormal intake pattern in association with decreased physical activity. When they are not, these disturbances still affect intake patterns, nutrient absorption, or both. Diarrhea in ALS patients usually is not due to infection, infestation, inflammation, tumors, or metabolic disease (31). Table 5 lists the more frequent causes of this symptom in patients with ALS, and the treatment involves the removal of the causative stimulus. Several alternative diets may be needed to avoid diarrhea from solute overload. Increasing or decreasing the amount of fiber bulk in the diet may also be important in managing intestinal motility in patients with ALS (10, 14–16, 22, 38).

Constipation frequently results from inadequate water intake relative to the solute load the patient receives in the diet. Moreover, inactivity causes the patient to have decreased intestinal motility. Dietary

Table 5 Complaints and Possible Causes of Gastrointestinal Malfunction in Patients with ALS

Complaint	*Possible Causes*
Gastric distention	Excess solute in meal
	Severe bulbar symptoms
	Atropinelike medications
Diarrhea	Impaction
	Solute overload
	Lactose deficiency
	Laxative abuse
	Certain antacids (Mg^{++}, $PO_4^{=}$, $SO_4^{=}$)
Constipation	Impaction
	Dehydration
	Diet content and meal pattern
	Hypokalemia

alterations have an important therapeutic role in alleviating these symptoms in patients confined to a wheelchair or bed. Appropriate adjustment of dietary content to include adequate water and fiber, as well as the establishment of fixed meal patterns, will aid considerably in producing bowel regularity. Attention to water intake should significantly reduce the number of cases of impaction.

The overall management of constipation and diarrhea also requires obtaining a thorough diet history. This method allows the physician to estimate the solute load, total fluid intake, and bulk consumed in the diet when the patient developed the symptoms. Careful recording of mealtimes will aid in evaluating the timing of food intake on a day-to-day basis. This information is most helpful in treating irregular bowel-movement patterns. The use of various medications, particularly those that produce hypokalemia, may also predispose to decreased intestinal motility and constipation. Careful monitoring of serum potassium levels along with adequate potassium replacement may aid in preventing the development of constipation and bloating.

Various types of pancreatic abnormalities can develop in patients with ALS (4, 13, 20, 23, 29, 32, 34). Decreased exocrine pancreatic function occasionally predisposes these patients to the development of mild steatorrhea, decreased calcium absorption, and decreased absorption of fat-soluble vitamins (32). More often, patients develop abnormalities of endocrine pancreatic function. Glucose intolerance and insulin resistance are not uncommon, and for this reason occasional checks of oral glucose tolerance and fasting blood glucose levels may prove to be important in the overall nutritional management of patients with ALS. The etiology of the abnormal pancreatic function is unclear. The innervation of the pancreas may be altered in patients with ALS, and, as research in animals has demonstrated, abnormal pancreatic neural regulation may produce abnormal insulin release (8, 26, 35, 39). Decreased insulin release also occurs in atropinized subjects (21), and for this reason medications having atropinelike effects should be monitored carefully in patients with ALS.

SUMMARY

The overall nutritional management of patients with ALS presents major challenges to the physician and dietitian in view of the paucity of information available on the caloric needs of these patients and the efficiency of caloric utilization as the disease progresses. Serial evaluations of the patient's intake patterns with a three-day dietary history and a 24-hour dietary recall should aid in tailoring an effective nutritional approach to a specific patient. These serial dietary evaluations should help to avoid the development of obesity, nutritional deficiency states, and significant gastrointestinal dysfunction. Early detection of problems is possible through this approach and provides the physician and dietitian with a reasonable opportunity to manage successfully the problems affecting the nutritional status of patients with ALS as the disease progresses.

Acknowledgment

Our appreciation goes to Dr. David Goldblatt, Professor of Neurology at The University of Rochester School of Medicine and Dentistry, for his suggestions and counsel in preparing this manuscript.

REFERENCES

1. A daily food guide. In *Consumers All. Yearbook of Agriculture.* Washington, DC, USDA, 1965, p 394

2. Alleyne G, Hay R, Picou D, et al: *Protein-Energy Malnutrition.* London, Edward Arnold, 1977

3. Alpers DH, Isselbacher KJ: Disaccharidase deficiency. Adv Metab Disord 4:75–122, 1970

4. Astin KJ, Wilde LE, Davies-Jones GAB: Glucose metabolism and insulin response in the plasma and CSF in motor neuron disease. J Neurol Sci 25:205–210, 1975

5. Barac-Nieto M, Spurr G, Totero H, et al: Body composition in chronic undernutrition. Am J Clin Nutr 31:23–40, 1978

6. Benoit F, Martin R, Watten R: Changes in body composition during weight reduction in obesity. Ann Intern Med 63:604–612, 1965

7. Benoit FL, Martin RL, Watten RH: Changes in body composition during weight reduction in obesity: Balance studies comparing effects of fasting and a ketogenic diet. Ann Intern Med 63:604–612, 1965

8. Blackard WG, Andrews SS: Integration of the secretory control mechanism for insulin, glucagon, and growth hormone. Current Top Exp Endocrinol 2:130–154, 1974

9. Blackburn GL, Bistrian BR, Maini BS, et al: Nutritional and metabolic assessment of the hospitalized patient. J Parenteral Enteral Nutr 1:11–22, 1977

10. Bond J, Tevitt M: Effect of dietary fiber on intestinal gas production and small bowel transit time in man. Am J Clin Nutr 31:S169–S174, 1978

11. Boudin G, Barbizet J, Hillemand B, et al: Atonie et dilatation gastro-oesophagienne au cours de la sclerose laterale amyotrophique. Soc Med Hop Paris 70:641–648, 1954

12. Boudin G, Barbizet J, Hillemand B, et al: Le retentissement digestif de la sclerose laterale amyotrophique. Sem Hop Paris 31:7–14, 1965

13. Collis W, Engel W: Glucose metabolism in five neuromuscular disorders. Neurology 18:915–925, 1968

14. Connell A: The effects of dietary fiber on gastrointestinal motor function. Am J Clin Nutr 31:S152–S156, 1978

15. Devroede G: Dietary fiber, bowel habits, and colonic function. Am J Clin Nutr 31:S157–S160, 1978

16. Floch M, Fuchs H: Modification of stool content by increased bran intake. Am J Clin Nutr 31:S185–S189, 1978

17. Gault M, Dixon M, Doyle M, et al: Hypernatremia, azotemia, and dehydration due to high-protein tube feeding. Ann Intern Med 68:778–791, 1968

18. Goodhart RS, Shils ME: *Modern Nutrition in Health and Disease*, ed 5. Philadelphia, Lea & Febiger, 1973

19. Gormican A: Tube feeding—overview. Dietetic Currents (Ross) 2: 1–6, 1975

20. Gotoh F, Kitamura A, Koto A, et al: Abnormal insulin secretion in amyotrophic lateral sclerosis. J Neurol Sci 16:201–207, 1972

21. Hakanson R, Liedberg G, Lundquist I: Effect of vagal denervation on insulin release after oral and intravenous glucose. Experientia 27:460–461, 1971

22. Hunt J, Cash R, Newland P: Energy density of food, gastric emptying, and obesity. Am J Clin Nutr 31:S259–S260, 1978

23. Ionăsescu V, Luca N: Studies on carbohydrate metabolism in amyotrophic lateral sclerosis and hereditary proximal spinal muscular atrophy. Acta Neurol Scand 40:47, 1964

24. Jelliffe DB: *The Assessment of the Nutritional Status of the Community*. WHO Monograph Series, No. 53, Geneva, WHO, 1966

25. Kaminski MV: *Tube Feeding: Tips and Techniques*. Norwich, NY, Eaton Laboratory Publication, 1973

26. Lambert AE: The regulation of insulin secretion. Rev Physiol Biochem Pharmacol 75:98–140, 1976

27. Lewis SB, Wallin JD, Kane JP, et al: Effect of diet composition on metabolic adaptations to hypocaloric nutrition: Comparison of high carbohydrate and high fat isocaloric diets. Am J Clin Nutr 30:160–170, 1977

28. Mallette LE, Patten BM, Cook JD, Engel WK: Calcium metabolism in amyotrophic lateral sclerosis. Dis Nerv Syst 38:457–461, 1977

29. Mueller PS, Quick DT: Studies of glucose insulin and lipid metabolism in amyotrophic lateral sclerosis and other neuromuscular disorders. J Lab Clin Med 76:190–201, 1970

30. Patten BM, Mallette LE: Motor neuron disease: Retrospective study of associated abnormalities. Dis Nerv Syst 37:318–321, 1976

31. Phillips SF: Diarrhea—a broad perspective. View Dig Dis 7:1–6, 1975

32. Quick DT, Greer M: Pancreatic dysfunction in patients with amyotrophic lateral sclerosis. Neurology 17:112–116, 1967

33. *Recommended Dietary Allowances,* ed 8. Washington, DC, National Academy of Sciences, 1974

34. Steinke J, Tyler HR: The association of amyotrophic lateral sclerosis (motor neuron disease) and carbohydrate intolerance, a clinical study. Metabolism 13:1376–1381, 1964

35. Unger RH, Dobbs RE: Insulin, glucagon, and somatostatin secretion in the regulation of metabolism. Ann Rev Physiol 40:307–343, 1978

36. Van Itallie T, Yang M: Current concepts in nutrition, diet and weight loss. N Engl J Med 297:1158–1161, 1977

37. Webb P: *Bioastronautics Data Book.* Washington, DC, NASA, Scientific and Technical Information Division, SP-3006, 1964, pp 172–177

38. White P, Fletcher D: *Nutrients in Processed Foods.* Acton, MA, Publishing Sciences Group, 1974

39. Woods SC, Porte D: Neural control of the endocrine pancreas. Physiol Rev 54:596–619, 1974

40. Yang M, Van Itallie T: Composition of weight lost during short-term weight reduction. J Clin Invest 58:722–730, 1976

41. Ziegler E, Fomon S: Fluid intake, renal solute load, and water balance in infancy. J Pediatr 78:561–568, 1971

Commentary

Bernard M. Patten

As we see from Dr. Moxley's chapter, few data are available on nutrition in patients with ALS, but much has been published on nutrition in normal persons. Whether the facts obtained in studies of healthy subjects apply to patients with ALS needs to be worked out in the future. Obviously, weight standards that apply to healthy persons cannot be used for the patient with ALS because of the loss of muscle mass caused by the disease.

At our institution, once we determine whether the patient is too fat or too lean (by the formulas presented by Dr. Moxley in Table 2 of chapter 17) we apply the needed correction. In hopes that my system of management might help others with their patients, I describe it here.

If the patient is too fat, I tell him or her that reduction is necessary. After calculating the patient's ideal weight, I calculate the percentage overweight and then explain that weak muscles will function better when not required to move all that fat and that after weight reduction the patient will feel, look, and function better. Most patients need a clear statement of the problem and most need these assurances of improvement before they will cooperate in a weight reduction program.

Usually, I start by leaving the patient to his or her own devices. I give no diet and consult no dietitian; I just tell the patient to eat less. Patients who do not lose weight with this informal program require a formal diet. Those who still fail to lose require stronger measures. I ask such patients to deposit $1000 with me and weigh in every month. Those who reach a predetermined weight, agreed upon in advance by the patient and me, are refunded $200 and continue on to the next month's goal. Those who fail to reach the predetermined weight forfeit $200. This system, taught to me by a behavioral psychologist, puts the burden of weight reduction on the patient, where it belongs, and it works well. I have never had a patient not lose weight or fail to get the money back.

Undernutrition, the antipode of overnutrition, is more common in patients with ALS and is often associated with decreased ingestion of food secondary to a poor appetite, depression, difficulty in swallowing or chewing, or simple laziness in preparing the food. Some ALS patients, embarrassed by the long time needed to eat a meal, stop eating when the rest of the family stops despite their continued hunger. When choking, aspiration, etc., make adequate nutrition by mouth impossible, a nasal gastric tube comes to the rescue. In my experience, most patients manage well on nasal gastric tube feeding, and gastrostomy and left-sided esophagostomy are not needed.

Since commercially prepared tube feedings are expensive and because I believe they may not contain all the nutrients found in "real" food from the garden or grocery, my patients do not use commercial preparations for tube feeding. Instead, they purée their regular meal in a blender and flush that down the nasal gastric tube.

Dr. Moxley mentioned the complications of tube feeding but omitted one that can be quite strange and alarming: sometimes the tube slips out of the stomach into the duodenum. When food runs in there, the patient feels terrible, becomes hypotensive, sweats, and may develop diarrhea. Thus, malposition of the tube causes a true dumping syndrome, the remedy for which entails simply pulling the tube back a few inches so that the tip remains in the stomach.

When malnutrition is corrected in the ALS patient, he or she sometimes experiences an improvement in strength lasting a variable period of time, illustrating the rule Dr. Norris mentioned earlier that ALS patients do best when they are in an optimal state of health.

Before I talk about nutritional clues to what makes ALS progress rapidly or slowly, I want to mention something we all know but do not discuss. Dietitians know a lot more about nutrition than physicians do. The well-trained dietitian helps a great deal in managing patients with ALS. The dietitians know tricks like how to make food look good, how to change the color and taste for variety, how to prevent diarrhea or constipation by adjusting the fiber content, how to prevent splenic flexure syndrome (gas pains) by decreasing oligosaccharides, how to decrease thick saliva by avoiding milk and chocolate, and so forth. So, do your patients and yourselves a favor and get expert dietary consultation when your ALS patient appears to have a nutritional problem.

In a recent medical tape on motor neuron diseases, Dr. Bruce S. Schoenberg mentioned that some physicians in Africa and Asia report that ALS progresses slower there than it does in the United States. If this is true, we should know about it because it may provide a clue to environmental factors that control progression of ALS. Nutrition may be one of those factors that makes a difference, although what aspect of nutrition needs studying first remains unclear. We know that protein nutrition plays a major role in determining who gets cancer of the liver after hepatitis, and that poor protein nutrition in West Africa leads to a high incidence of liver cancer there. On the other hand, the high fiber content of the diet in the same region makes cancer of the colon rare. I have seen three patients who received intravenous amino acids in the form of Freeamine II undergo an apparent rapid progression of the disease. One thing seems clear: more work needs to be done to follow these leads to determine whether a high-protein diet accelerates the disease.

Another aspect of nutrition in ALS that needs additional study is calcium metabolism. A report by Dr. Mark Felmus and myself appraised the frequency of events that had previously been associated anecdotally with motor neuron disease (1). The study involved 25 patients with motor neuron disease, 25 age- and sex-matched healthy control persons, and 25 age- and sex-matched disease control patients. Our study revealed that a history of exposure to lead and mercury, participation in athletics, and consumption of large quantities of milk was found more often in patients with motor neuron disease than in controls. Karis questioned the statistical validity of the study (3), and Felmus replied that the differences in statistical results depended on how the expected frequency was determined in calculating chi square (2). We all agreed that a larger population was needed before firm conclusions could be drawn.

REFERENCES

1. Felmus MT, Patten BM, Swanke L: Antecedent events in amyotrophic lateral sclerosis. Neurology 26:167–172, 1976
2. Felmus M: Reply from author. Neurology 27:100, 1977
3. Karis R: Statistical data questioned in ALS. Neurology 27:100, 1977

Arthur J. Hudson

We attempt to maintain our patients with ALS who have bulbar symptoms on routine measures of nutrition for as long as possible. Accordingly, it becomes very important to consider the texture of food. For example, it has been mentioned that ALS patients have a propensity to drink excessive amounts of milk. We find, however, that milk should be avoided by ALS patients with bulbar symptoms, since it coagulates to form a sticky material in the throat and thus increases the bulbar difficulties. Some foods are desirable as they afford pleasure in eating, but their natural texture makes them difficult to swallow. However, this is often easily modified. For example, a patient with bulbar weakness may be unable to eat bran muffins, whereas the application of a little jam enables these to be swallowed fairly well.

Because a nasogastric tube creates problems of excessive salivation and sometimes gagging, we prefer to delay its use until it is necessary, although atropine or clonidine to reduce salivation does help. When nasogastric feeding is finally necessary, we believe it should be done with a small (pediatric size) tube of sufficient diameter to carry food that has been prepared in a home blender and should be as unobtrusive as possible. Being able to use food prepared at home is important, since the cost of commercially prepared foods and the more sophisticated supplements can be enormous, inasmuch as they are required every day.

H. Richard Tyler

Fifty-two percent of our last 75 patients had trouble swallowing. Only 35% of these 75 had lost weight, apparently secondary to their difficulty in swallowing, and 2% had gained weight by the time I saw them. More patients would have lost weight if they had not required fewer calories because of immobilization. If one asks such patients why they are losing weight, they will tell you, "I have difficulty chewing, I have difficulty with utensils, I get fatigued," and so forth. It is my impression that the commonest reasons for patients losing weight are that they have trouble asking their families to feed them and they have trouble just sitting the length of time it takes to eat. They often feel awkward about eating in the presence of other family members, so they just nibble. A simple solution to this problem, which I use often, is to encourage the families to sit at table longer with the patient and to encourage the patient to eat in more than one session.

The question of when to do a gastrostomy or esophagostomy relates to the following questions: Is the patient getting enough calories the way he or she is eating? Is the quality of his or her life in eating acceptable to patient and family? If early esophagostomy or gastrostomy is performed, the patient can still eat with the family and can use ordinary food put through a blender, if he or she wishes. This makes a distinct improvement in the quality of the patient's life. Most of my patients are initially reluctant to do it, but they are very pleased with the result afterward. It also helps with both fluid and caloric intake.

When patients are aspirating either saliva or food I encourage them to have a surgical procedure, either a gastrostomy or an esophagostomy, as soon as possible. Which procedure is preferable relies, I believe, on local expertise and the situation at the institution where the procedure will be done. We have had no trouble with gastrostomy. We usually administer local anesthesia and this works out well. The earlier we carry out the procedure, the less trouble we have. The only problem I have had with gastrostomies in the past few years is operating on patients who have had respiratory insufficiency. A gastrostomy can cause abdominal pain sufficient to immobilize the diaphragm and precipitate respiratory problems. Thus, when there is respiratory insufficiency, as defined by a rounded pulmonary flow curve, we usually prefer esophagostomy. Both procedures allow the patient to obtain adequate fluid and calories. Most patients prefer to sit and eat their meal with the family; we therefore usually encourage the use of a food blender.

W. King Engel

We very much prefer the higher opening—i.e., the esophagostomy—because, while the person is ambulatory, he or she can feed himself/herself without opening the clothes, and does not have to remain lying down after feeding. If the patient requires an abdominal respirator, that becomes easier to add. We had one ALS patient, a young man in his late twenties, who had a great deal of bulbar involvement while he was still ambulatory. We performed an esophagostomy, and the patient continued to go to cocktail parties in New York. At the parties, he would simply unbutton his collar, pour in his martini, and even pop in pieces of olive. Esophagostomy is socially much more convenient than the gastrostomy.

Forbes H. Norris, Jr

One patient of ours learned how to insert her own nasogastric tube. For 18 months she prepared the family dinner; they would sit down, and her husband would start to serve while she repaired to the bathroom and inserted the tube. Having blended some of the meal earlier, she would join the family and push in her portion with a syringe while the others ate. The meal over, she would again retreat and pull out the tube, wash it, put it aside, then return to clear the table and carry on with other kitchen duties.

This approach is obviously preferable to a surgical stoma, but few patients can manage as did that courageous lady. The group that I worked with had not done a gastrostomy in over nine years. We have been very pleased with cervical esophagostomy. The main problem is that many surgeons prefer to create the esophagostomy under general anesthesia, which involves certain other problems and risks (1).

REFERENCE

1. Lebo CP, Ü KS, Norris FH: Cricopharyngeal myotomy in amyotrophic lateral sclerosis. Laryngoscope 86:862–868, 1976

Richard T. Moxley III

Dr. Patten pointed out some of the problems one can encounter with tube feedings. I would like to recommend two excellent, simple-to-read articles on this subject. One describes an adaptation of the method of tube feeding developed at Walter Reed Army Hospital and is available as a handout for patients and doctors through Eaton Laboratories (2). The other is a practical guide to tube feeding that includes helpful details; this also could be used as a patient handout (1).

I suggest that we, as physicians responsible for the care of patients with ALS, are in a unique position to provide information that will be valuable in the development of dietary guidelines for these patients. If the clinical situation allows, a simple recording of basal oxygen consumption in such patients would be helpful. In some patients, it may also be possible to record oxygen consumption while they perform certain common daily activities. These oxygen consumption data would allow the physician to estimate a given patient's daily caloric needs much more accurately. If such measurements were made in a large number of patients, the results could help us to tailor diet recommendations to patients with ALS so that they could avoid becoming obese as their disease progresses. This is the only way I can foresee this important information ever getting into the literature. Such a study would allow us at some future time to talk very specifically about the real nutrient needs of patients with ALS.

REFERENCES

1. Gormican A: Tube feeding—overview. Dietetic Currents (Ross Laboratories) 2:1–6, 1975

2. Kaminski MV: *Tube Feeding: Tips and Techniques.* Norwich, NY, Eaton Laboratory Publication, 1973

18 Pulmonary Function Testing

Robert C. Griggs

Katharine M. Donohoe

Mark J. Utell

David Goldblatt

Pulmonary function tests are part of the initial evaluation of patients with amyotrophic lateral sclerosis and should be performed frequently thereafter. Patients with bulbar involvement should be studied most frequently. Although the following discussion focuses on laboratory testing, many important aspects of lung function can be approached best through history and examination. A history of smoking and symptoms such as aspiration, dyspnea, wheezing, and sputum production should be sought. Patients should be examined for impaired cough, for diaphragmatic excursion, and for inspiratory crackles at lung bases. The patient's weight should also be noted. At least 25% of patients with ALS have respiratory disease secondary to another cause such as obstructive airway disease, bronchitis, or congestive heart failure.

Pulmonary function testing in the patient with ALS helps to answer three major questions:

1. Are the respiratory muscles involved?

2. Is the impairment of respiratory muscles of such severity that respiratory failure is imminent or likely to occur with minor infections?

3. Is concomitant pulmonary disease present?

Early involvement of respiratory muscles can be detected best by measuring the pressure generated by these muscles. The maximum expiratory pressure (MEP) is the most sensitive indicator of muscle weakness in ALS, as in other neuromuscular diseases (1, 8). The MEP is useful for longitudinal follow-up of patients. It is, however, so greatly impaired in patients with marked weakness that it may be of little use as an indication of incipient respiratory compromise in such patients. It also requires that the patients have sufficient strength in their facial muscles to make a seal with the mouthpiece.

A mercury manometer for determining the MEP (Fig. 1) can be constructed for less than $200. It is particularly important to have a small-bore air escape to avoid measuring *buccal* pressures, which might give spuriously high readings in weak patients. The MEP is determined after the patient has taken a full inspiration. A substantial learning effect is seen with MEP determinations, and, if patients are to be followed sequentially, several observations should be made during the initial evaluation.

Maximum inspiratory pressure (MIP) can also be measured with the mercury manometer but, as shown in Figure 2, it is less impaired than MEP early in the course of ALS. The MEP is clearly abnormal in patients with neuromuscular disease before any reduction in spirometric studies is observed, such as forced vital capacity (FVC) or maximum mid-expiratory flow rate (MMEF), but whether this is true in all instances is not yet known (11).

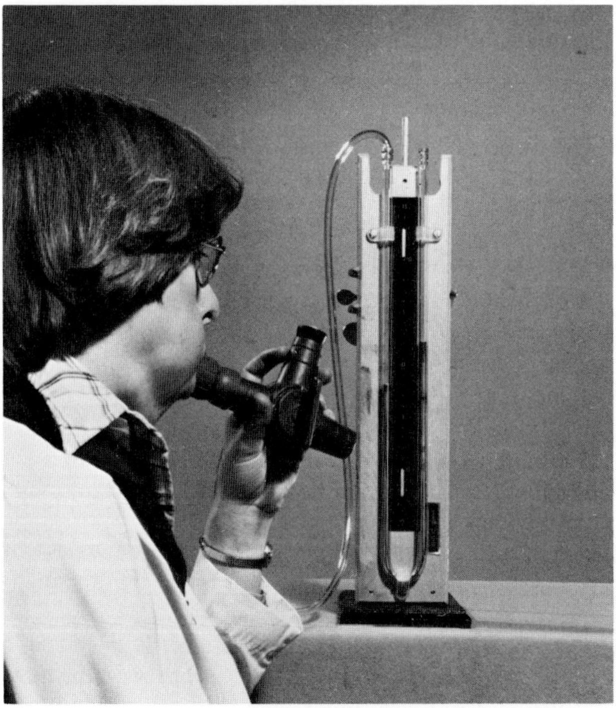

Figure 1 Apparatus for measuring maximum expiratory and inspiratory pressures. See reference (2).

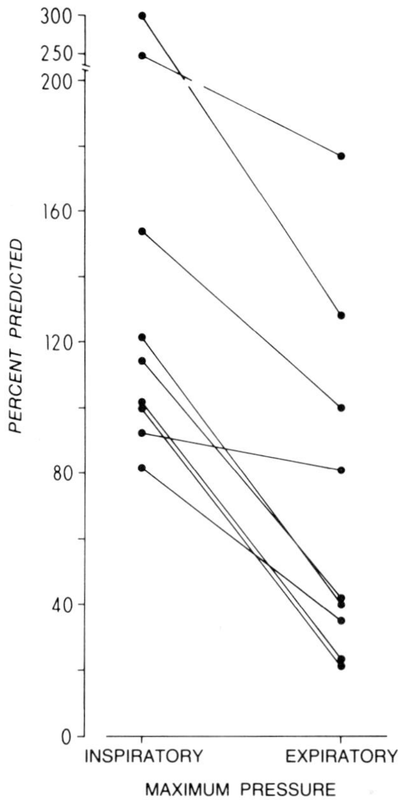

Figure 2 A comparison of maximum inspiratory pressure (MIP) and maximum expiratory pressure (MEP) in nine patients with ALS. MEP was abnormal in several patients who had normal MIP.

How does one decide which patient is at risk of respiratory compromise in ALS? Which patient will develop respiratory insufficiency with what would ordinarily be an inconsequential respiratory infection? When should one consider tracheostomy or make provision for respiratory support?

As yet, these questions have no definite answers. The best longitudinal data suggest that patients often have an FVC of over 50%, or even a normal determination, within weeks of sudden death from apparently respiratory causes (6). This abrupt deterioration from a vital capacity of over 2000 ml to severe respiratory insufficiency stands in striking contrast to patients with Duchenne or myotonic muscular dystrophy in whom an FVC of under 1000 ml is often compatible with years of life (3, 9). Such patients frequently develop CO_2 retention and hypoxemia of chronic restrictive pulmonary disease from muscle weakness. In ALS, by contrast, abnormal blood gases are seldom encountered (6).

It is our feeling, nonetheless, that all patients should have sequential follow-up measurements of FVC, one-second forced vital capacity (FEV_1), and MMEF. We believe that those with an FVC of less than 50% of the predicted value are at risk of respiratory compromise.

In addition, the maximum voluntary ventilation (MVV) is particularly useful in assessing the tendency to fatigue. Patients with myasthenia gravis or myasthenic features in their illness can develop an impairment of MVV long before FVC is impaired (7). Longitudinal observations of patients with ALS have not been published, but our preliminary studies suggest that the MVV is abnormal at times when the FVC is normal in this disorder as well.

Although we lack a clear indication of which patients are likely to develop respiratory insufficiency, we believe that patients with ALS should be managed with the following pulmonary function tests: FVC, FVC_1, MMEF, flow–volume loop, MEP, and MVV. Either the spirogram or the flow–volume loop should be used to detect obstructive airway disease, which often occurs concomitantly with ALS. Blood gas determinations are usually normal. In patients in whom the FVC or MVV falls below 50% of predicted, the possibility of subsequent respiratory compromise should be considered and, in appropriate circumstances, discussed with the patient.

A final factor to be considered in the evaluation of pulmonary function in patients with ALS concerns the selection of devices for outpatient measurements. Most data for evaluating the accuracy of spirometers have been generated in patients with normal muscle strength. We have compared pulmonary studies obtained from a Stead-Wells spirometer (formal laboratory testing) with those obtained from a portable electronic spirometer (Vanguard Model D-500) and from a widely utilized bellows spirometer (Vitalor) in patients with ALS.

Figures 3 and 4 demonstrate that the data from the electronic spirometer and the Stead-Wells spirometer correlate acceptably. On the other hand, the Vitalor values proved inaccurate for both FVC (Fig. 3) and FEV_1 (Fig. 4), as well as for MMEF. Previous studies have shown the inaccuracy of the Vitalor spirometer for the MMEF, but it has been considered satisfactory for determining FVC and FEV (13). It seems possible that patients with respiratory muscle weakness have greater difficulty generating the force necessary to move the bellows. The MVV determined by electronic spirometry and the Stead-Wells spirometer showed a close correlation. Our preliminary observations with a different bellows spirometer, the Vitalograph (14), suggest that it is comparable with the Stead-Wells.

More studies of pulmonary function in patients with ALS are needed to define the variables that predict respiratory compromise. Possible contributing factors include: upper airway obstruction during sleep such as has been shown to occur intermittently in many healthy individuals (2), a disturbance in ventilatory drive such as can occur in

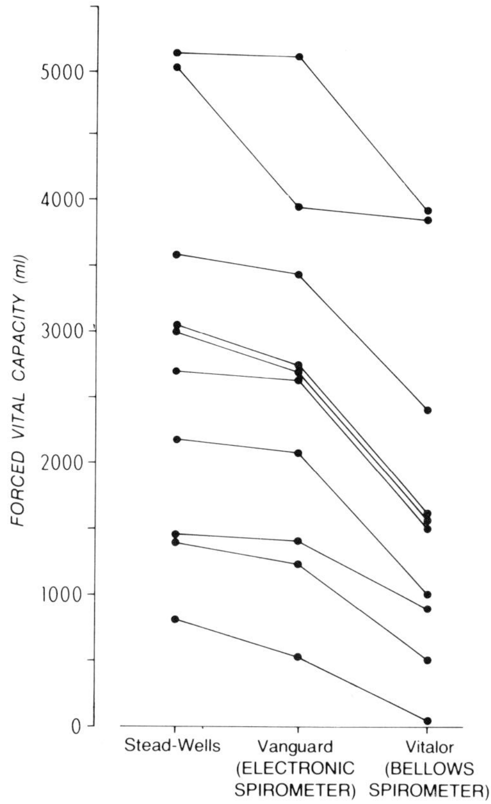

Figure 3 A comparison of forced vital capacity (FVC) determined by three types of spirometer in 10 patients with ALS. The FVC was consistently lower when measured with the Vitalor than with either of the other instruments.

patients with other neuromuscular diseases (4) or in normal individuals on a hereditary basis (5), myasthenic fatigue (10), and spasticity and bulbar or pseudobulbar impairment of glottic control.

Finally, studies of pulmonary compliance may prove to be important in evaluating the role of therapeutic intermittent positive-pressure breathing (IPPB). For example, in patients with respiratory compromise secondary to poliomyelitis, IPPB improved lung compliance in short-term studies (12). Whether normalization of compliance is of value to the patient remains uncertain.

SUMMARY

Respiratory function should be followed carefully in patients with ALS. A reduction in MEP is an early sign of respiratory muscle weakness.

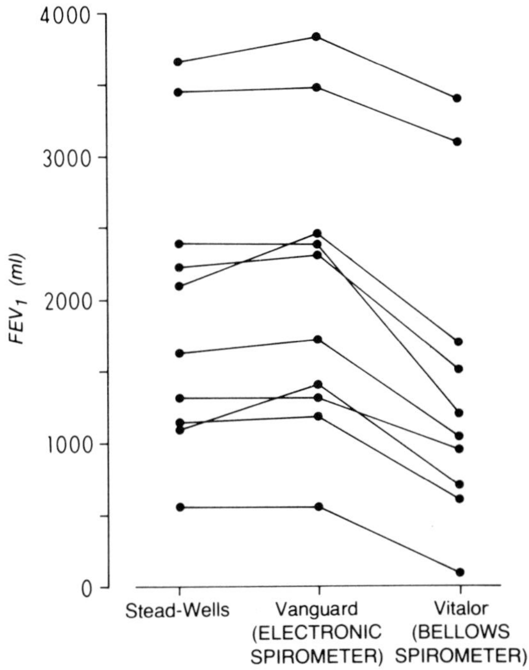

Figure 4 A comparison of the one-second forced expiratory volume (FEV_1) determined by three types of spirometer in 10 patients with ALS. The FEV_1 was consistently lower when measured with the Vitalor than with either of the other instruments.

In addition, FVC, MMEF, FEV_1, MVV, and flow–volume loop determinations will detect evidence of progressive restrictive or obstructive lung disease.

Respiratory failure becomes a concern when the FVC falls to below 50% of the predicted value, but, because the pulmonary function of patients whose FVC is nearly normal can deteriorate abruptly, more sensitive predictors of impending respiratory failure are needed.

Acknowledgments

We thank Ms. Donna Spears for technical aid in these studies. The studies reported were supported in part by grants from the Muscular Dystrophy Association to Dr. Griggs and Dr. Goldblatt and by US Public Health Service Grant RR00044 from the Division of Research Resources of the National Institutes of Health.

REFERENCES

1. Black LF, Hyatt RE: Maximal static respiratory pressures in generalized neuromuscular disease. Am Rev Respir Dis 103:641–650, 1971

2. Block AJ, Boysen PG, Wynne JW, et al: Oxygen desaturation in normal subjects. N Engl J Med 300:513–517, 1979

3. Buchsbaum HW, Martin WA, Turino GM, et al: Chronic alveolar hypoventilation due to muscular dystrophy. Neurology 18:319, 1968

4. Carroll JE, Zwillich C, Weil JV: A possible mechanism of respiratory failure in neuromuscular disorders. Neurology 7:360, 1977

5. Collins D, Scoggin CH, Zwillich CW, et al: Genetic factors in the control of breathing. Clin Res 25:132A, 1977

6. Fallat RJ, Jewitt B, Bass M, et al: Spirometry in amyotrophic lateral sclerosis. Arch Neurol 36:74–80, 1979

7. Florence JM, Brooke MH, Carroll JE: Evaluation of the child with muscular weakness. Orthop Clin North Am 9:409–430, 1978

8. Goldstein RL, Hyde RW, Lapham LW, et al: Peripheral neuropathy presenting with respiratory insufficiency as the primary complaint. Problem of recognizing alveolar hypoventilation due to neuromuscular disorders. Am J Med 56:443–449, 1974

9. Inkley SR, Oldenburg FC, Vignos PJ: Pulmonary function in Duchenne muscular dystrophy related to stage of disease. Am J Med 56: 297–305, 1974

10. Mulder DW, Lambert EH, Eaton LM: Myasthenic syndrome in patients with amyotrophic lateral sclerosis. Neurology 9:627, 1959

11. Nakano KK, Bass H, Tyler HR, et al: Amyotrophic lateral sclerosis: A study of pulmonary function. Dis Nerv Syst 37:32–35, 1976

12. Sinha R, Bergofsky EH: Prolonged alteration of lung mechanics in kyphoscoliosis by positive pressure hyperinflation. Am Rev Respir Dis 106:47–57, 1972

13. Wang CS, Boyington DG, Krumholz RA: Comparison of spirometry measurements using McKesson vitalor and Collins spirometer. Dis Chest 55:285–290, 1969

14. Wever AMJ, Britton MG, Hughes DDT: Evaluation of two spirometers. A comparative study of the Stead-Wells and the Vitalograph spirometers. Chest 70:244–250, 1976

Commentary

Robert J. Fallat

First, I agree fully with Dr. Griggs that one should pay attention to the type of spirometer one uses. Particularly when dealing with a patient with ALS, one should use a spirometer with a low resistance. A word of caution about electronic spirometers: they need to be calibrated carefully. They can be very erratic and should be calibrated against a standard displacement spirometer.

The very interesting data that Dr. Griggs included about the maximum expiratory pressure (MEP) being a good early finding should be reemphasized. It is even better, he says, than the maximum inspiratory pressure (MIP), and that is much better than the maximum breathing capacity (MBC), for detecting early disease. I think a complete battery of pulmonary function tests is useful. The final point made by Dr. Griggs is the most interesting part to me. It seems strange that we should see patients with ALS who have fairly severe reductions in respiratory function and yet so rarely see them with abnormal blood gases. I really think there is another factor present to explain their sudden death without a period of chronic respiratory failure.

W. King Engel

In regard to pulmonary function, we consider it a very important parameter to be measured. We use a simple bedside vital capacity measurement. It is quick and handy. In a study of several pulmonary function tests I conducted with Dr. Newball a few years ago, we found that the vital capacity gave us as much or more information useful in following the course of respiratory involvement in ALS as any of the other tests. I would allow that some of the types of studies Dr. Griggs mentioned might give more information on collateral disease, but I think that by simply following the vital capacity we can learn what is happening to the vital function of breathing. The precipitous death that Dr. Griggs described in some patients who had had a reasonably good vital capacity several weeks beforehand relates, in my view, to what several speakers have noted: that some patients exhibit a step-by-step decrease in strength. For example, an ALS patient can be clinically kept at a functional plateau for a period of time, and then suddenly over one day cannot get up off the toilet seat or begins falling. I think that in such cases a last few critical neurons may have ceased to function. In ALS patients there may also be insidious aspirations, of slight or moderate degree, but cumulative, as Dr. Griggs has mentioned and as demonstrated at autopsy in very elderly patients who died of causes other than ALS (U. Salamander, personal communication, 1979).

19 Respiratory Problems

Robert J. Fallat

Forbes H. Norris, Jr

Although respiratory problems and complications are frequent and are said to be the most common cause of death in patients with amyotrophic lateral sclerosis, little attention has been paid to the respiratory disease in these patients, at least in the general medical literature. Perhaps this neglect is caused by a presumption that ventilatory difficulties are not major clinical problems until the later stages of the disease, when a less-than-vigorous and sometimes even a nihilistic therapeutic approach is taken. Over the past several years, we have seen many pulmonary complications at an early stage of the disease. Recognition of these complications and appropriate interventions are a very important aspect of the management of patients with ALS.

This paper touches on several questions: What is the natural history of the respiratory illness in ALS? Is there a typical course, and what is the degree of variation? What is the best way to monitor the respiratory status of these patients? Are there clues to when the respiratory problems will become major or critical? What are the common respiratory complications that occur? Are there some guiding principles in the management of the respiratory problems?

In our experience, patients who have ALS are a stoic and highly optimistic group. Their subjective histories about respiratory problems are frequently misleading because of their optimism. These patients are very cooperative and perform pulmonary function tests of various complexities without difficulty. We have recently reported that relatively simple pulmonary function tests can be a most useful way to follow the natural history of the respiratory aspects of the disease (1).

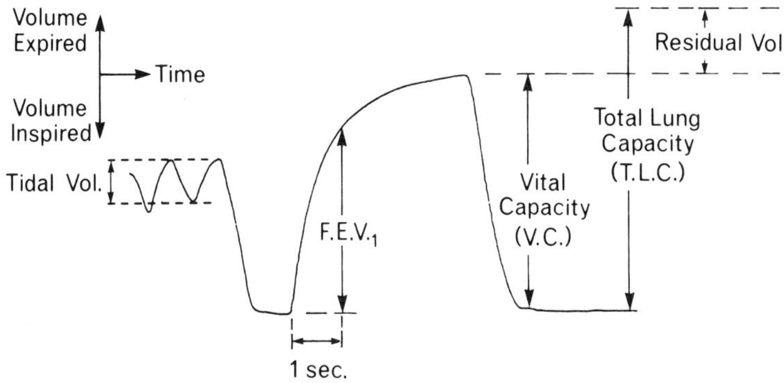

Figure 1 Volume-versus-time curves obtained during standard spirometry. Regular tidal volume breathing is followed by inhalation to total lung capacity, then by forced exhalation of the full vital capacity, leaving only the residual volume. Volume expired after 1 second (FEV_1) is measured to obtain an estimate of the rapidity of exhalation. This rate would be markedly reduced with airway obstruction. Residual volume must be measured by an independent maneuver such as by washout of lung nitrogen, equilibration with a small concentration of an inert gas (for example, helium), or by body plethysmography.

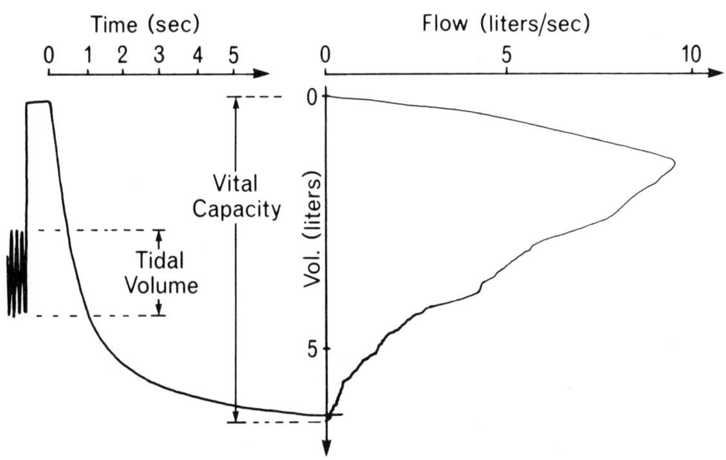

Figure 2 Electronic spirometers enable flow and volume to be measured simultaneously. A standard spirometric volume-time curve similar to that seen in Figure 1 is shown on the left. To the right, the time axis is replaced by a flow axis, while volume remains on the vertical axis. The forced exhalation maneuver produces a triangular-shaped flow-volume loop. Highest flows occur after approximately 20% of the vital capacity has been exhaled; and the flows then decline as residual volume is approached. The curve shown was obtained in a healthy 45-year-old male non-smoker with entirely normal pulmonary function.

METHODS OF ASSESSING LUNG FUNCTION

Various subdivisions of lung volume are shown in Figure 1, including tidal volume, vital capacity (VC), residual volume, and total lung capacity (TLC). Measurement of the forced expiratory volume in one second (FEV_1) during a forced vital capacity (FVC) maneuver is the simplest method to measure the neuromuscular capabilities of the chest muscles as well as the mechanics of the lungs themselves. Instead of using volume-time graphs of FVC, it has become more common to examine the flow-versus-volume curves, as shown in Figure 2. Patients with ALS generally show a restrictive pattern, although they can show any of the four patterns demonstrated in Figure 3. Other functional studies such as maximum voluntary ventilation (MVV), maximum inspiratory pressure (MIP), and maximum expiratory pressure (MEP) may be more useful as early indicators of neuromuscular involvement. The diffusing capacity is a useful measurement for defining lung parenchymal

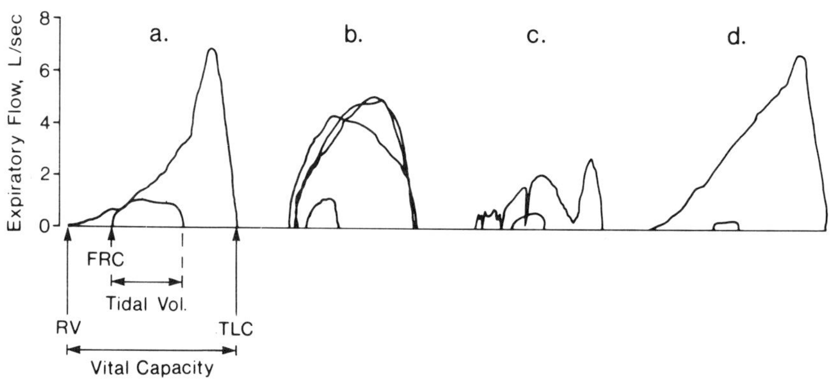

	a.	b.	c.	d.
VC, L	3.8 (91)	2.5 (52)	2.6 (61)	3.6 (79)
RV, L	2.9 (165)	3.7 (290)	2.1 (122)	3.1 (184)
TLC, L	6.7 (108)	6.3 (106)	4.7 (76)	6.7 (105)
FRC, L	4.2 (165)	4.0 (141)	3.5 (136)	4.2 (159)
FEV_1/FVC	65	96	62	85
MVV, L/min	86 (62)	92 (53)	49 (34)	150 (96)

Figure 3 Variations in characteristics of forced vital capacity (FVC) are shown as flow-versus-volume curves. **(A)** This subject has distinct airway obstruction. Note marked curvature compared with Figure 3D. Also note low FEV_1/FVC and high residual volume and total lung capacity. **(B)** Inability of this patient to exhale fully is shown by initiation of inspiration when expiratory flow is still quite high. Repeated efforts all result in the same early inspiration. **(C)** This patient with bulbar ALS shows an extremely erratic expiratory effort. The flow can decrease suddenly to zero, apparently because of occlusion of the glottis by discoordinated muscles. **(D)** The expiratory flow-volume curve appears normal, but the patient still has an unexplained high residual volume.

or vascular diseases, but it is not particularly applicable to patients with ALS. Arterial blood gases provide the most meaningful assessment of the integrity of pulmonary function, but generally these tests are not necessary until the later stages of the disease or until certain complications occur, as will be described later.

NATURAL HISTORY OF LUNG FUNCTION IN ALS

The FVC is probably the most common and useful measurement of respiratory function in patients with ALS. Figure 4 shows the progression of the FVC from 160 serial measurements in 28 patients during the three years before their death. Although there is considerable individual variation, one can see a distinct curvilinear trend in the data. During the early stages of disease, the FVC declines gradually, but a progressively more rapid loss occurs in the 12–15 months before death. This pattern is shown more precisely in a subgroup of 10 patients in Figure 5A and indicates that the rapid decline may begin at any time from one year to five years after the onset of symptoms. Figure 5B shows that in other patients the FVC can be quite stable for several years; a few patients had FVC values that were well below the normal range when they were first

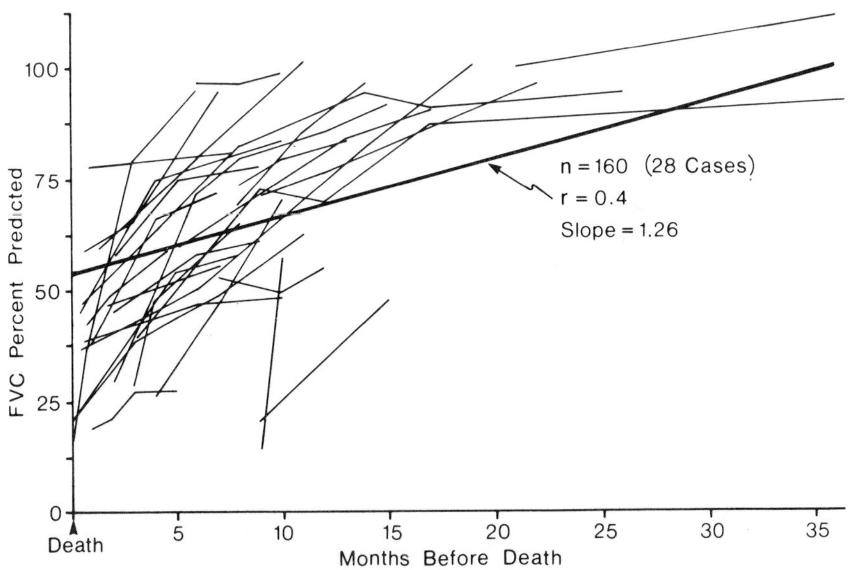

Figure 4 Longitudinal measurements of forced vital capacity (FVC) in 28 patients with ALS are shown. Each line represents a patient. The bold line indicates the mean regression for the group. This overall correlation does not reflect the curvilinearity seen in individual lines. The more rapid decline in FVC seen during the few months before death may have important prognostic value.

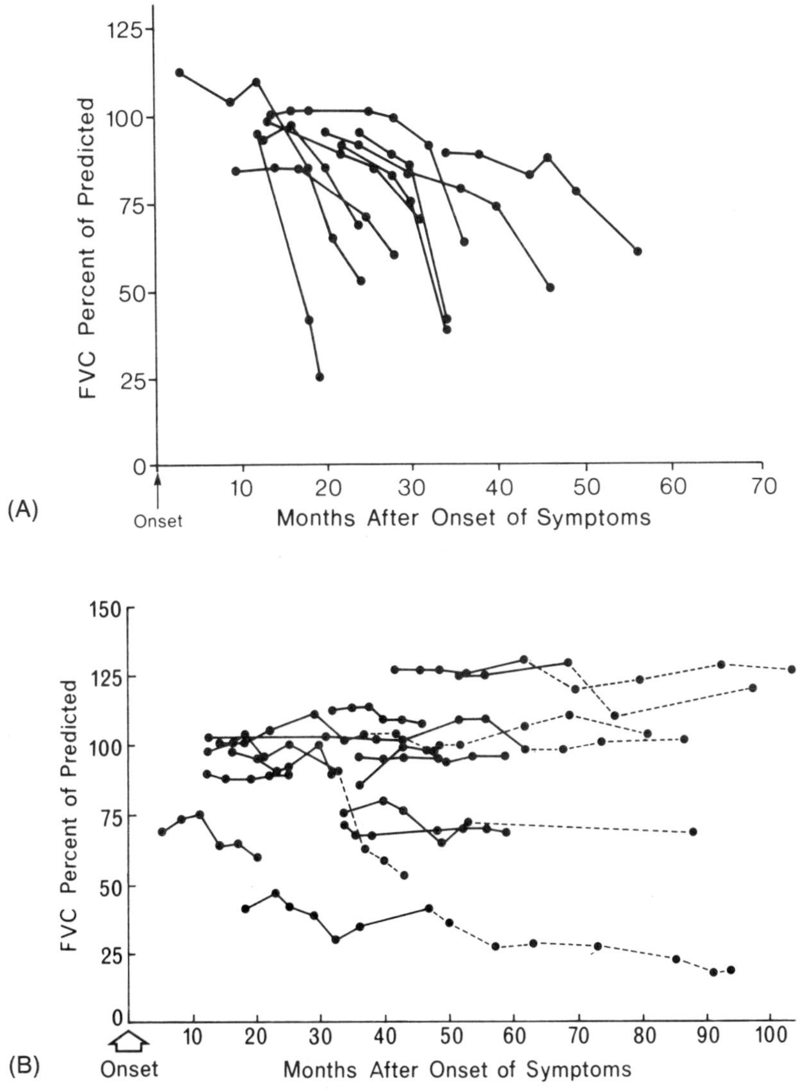

Figure 5 **(A)** Course of forced vital capacity (FVC) over five years after onset of weakness in selected patients with ALS. Note the variable latency before FVC began to decline in these 10 fatal cases and the tendency of the decline to accelerate late in the course of the disease. No patient had pneumonia, pulmonary embolus, or other pulmonary complication to account for the acceleration of pulmonary disability. **(B)** These 10 subjects, who showed stable lung function over a period of several years, were described in a previous publication (1). The dotted lines show their course since that publication. One patient entered the accelerated phase of the disease and died. The patient who had the lowest measurement of forced vital capacity shows the unusual response of a very gradual decline over a period of eight years, with no accelerated phase. This patient is now beginning to show some abnormality of gas exchange, as shown in Figure 6.

Table 1 Results of Four Pulmonary Function Tests in 136 Patients Studied in 1978[a]

Result	*Number of Patients*	*Percentage of Patients*
All studies normal	12	9
All studies abnormal	43	31
Only FVC abnormal	2	2
Only MVV abnormal	11	8
Only MIP abnormal	12	9
Only RV abnormal	15	11
MVV, MIP, or RV abnormal	43	31

[a] The tests were: forced vital capacity (FVC), maximum voluntary ventilation (MVV), maximum inspiratory pressure (MIP), and residual volume (RV).

evaluated and yet remained stable. Thus, the rate of change of the FVC is important to determine over a period of 3–6 months to give an objective assessment of the progression of the disease.

Our recent report indicates that MVV is reduced before the FVC and may decline at a more rapid rate than other indices of lung function (1). During the past year, we have started to measure the MIP as well, and have found this to be an even more sensitive indicator than the MVV. Table 1 indicates that, of 136 patients tested in 1978, all lung function tests were normal in only 12 (9%). On the other hand, FVC was abnormal in only 45 (33%). Thus, MVV, MIP, and residual volume measurements, or some combination of these three less common tests, were the only abnormalities in 81 (59%) of these patients, indicating the importance of these tests in the early evaluation of patients with ALS. The MEP may be an even more sensitive parameter, as indicated in chapter 18. This measurement may also be a better indicator of when to expect respiratory difficulties, since it may indicate more accurately the inability of these patients to cough and expel secretions.

The history and physical examination can be misleading in patients with ALS. Many of the patients whose ventilatory tests were under 50% of the predicted, which indicates severe restrictive disease, did not complain of respiratory symptoms and were given high respiratory scores by the physicians evaluating them. Perhaps this can be explained by the fact that, despite their poor lung volume and flow rate measurements, these patients are able to maintain quite good gas exchange. Figure 6 shows 54 measurements of arterial oxygen in 48 ambulatory patients, 38 of whom had a FVC of less than 60% of the predicted. Patients hospitalized with pulmonary complications were not included in the analysis. Only 6 patients had arterial oxygen below 70 torr, which

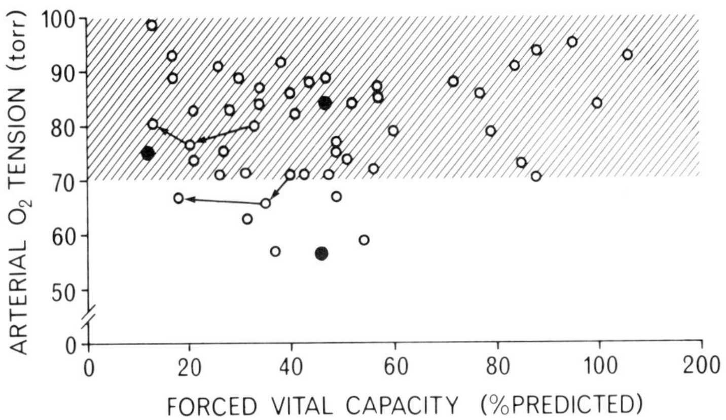

Figure 6 Arterial oxygen tension in a group of 48 ambulatory patients with ALS is shown. Because of the older age of these patients, the lower limit of normal is considered to be 70 torr. Six patients fall in the mildly hypoxic range, but all of these have values above 55 torr. The three solid symbols represent the three patients who also have mild CO_2 retention with arterial PCO_2 ranging from 50 to 52 torr. Note the lack of correlation of oxygen tension with decline in forced vital capacity seen in the three measurements made in two patients (arrows).

was considered normal for their age. Three of these 6 patients had obstructive airways disease in addition to ALS, and only one of these patients had an elevation in the arterial CO_2 of 51 torr. Of the 10 patients with a FVC of less than 25%, only one also had an increase in PCO_2 to 52 torr. It is of interest that this patient died "unexpectedly" at home the evening after the tests were performed. Note how serial measurements of P_aO_2 and FVC in 2 patients failed to show a correlation between these variables. It appears to be necessary to check arterial blood gases only when vital capacity is below 50% of the predicted. It is striking that we so seldom see chronic hypoxemia or hypercapnia in patients with ALS. The absence of such findings in the large number of patients followed during the past several years indicates that some more precipitous event than chronic respiratory failure must account for the death of these patients (Table 2).

In summary then, simple measurement of the FVC with a spirometer can be a useful way of objectively assessing the pulmonary status of patients with ALS. Although there is a characteristic decline that occurs in the last year or two before death, the onset and rate of that decline is quite variable. Measurement of FVC with each visit and perhaps also measurement of MIP and MEP are necessary to assess objectively the extent of respiratory muscle involvement; these tests are also very useful in making decisions about management.

When a patient with ALS has any pulmonary complaints or any new findings on examination, a chest x-ray may reveal some surprises.

sigh the lungs are distended with over 30 cmH_2O, so such pressures are not dangerous unless the patient is known to have had a pneumothorax or severe emphysema.

The use of IPPB devices generally should not be necessary until the vital capacity is less than 50% of the predicted. As pointed out earlier, this is usually a harbinger of the more rapid decline that occurs during the last year of life, when most patients have severe, diffuse neuromuscular involvement. Rarely, however, a patient may have marked progressive impairment of the respiratory muscles only, and this requires more frequent or prolonged use of IPPB. These patients may be candidates for tracheostomy and continuous ventilation if respiratory acidosis begins to develop. Portable systems are available. One ALS patient in Los Angeles has maintained an active business life for several years using such a portable system. A controlled leak around the tracheostomy tube makes speech possible while the ventilator is inflating the patient's lungs.

A common problem in these patients is difficulty in handling natural secretions. Due to weakness and discoordination of the glottis, aspiration is frequent when bulbar involvement develops. Use of a suction apparatus to clear the secretions from the mouth and oral pharynx may be sufficient. Sometimes transection of the cricopharyngeal muscle seems to alleviate aspiration problems, perhaps by facilitating the swallowing of saliva (2). Aspiration and dysphagia in general frequently stimulate new secretions which, in turn, aggravate the original problem. To this is added the even greater problem of aspiration of food and drink at mealtimes. Again, cricopharyngeal myotomy may alleviate these problems, but, in patients not helped by this procedure, major complications soon develop, and the quality of life declines rapidly.

Pneumonia has been called "the friend of the aged." When the patient with ALS is clearly near the terminal part of the disease, it may well be a friendly, quick mode of exodus. Frequently, however, it occurs as a complication early in the course of the disease. Treatment sometimes is not as specific as it might be because the sputum culture tends to become contaminated by the excessive oral secretions. A transtracheal needle aspiration of sputum for culture may help in the choice of an appropriate antibiotic. In addition to IPPB, one should also use postural drainage and percussion following the use of bronchodilator aerosols, particularly if airway obstruction is known to be present.

Another complication that can lead to respiratory failure is congestive heart failure with pulmonary edema, particularly in an older patient with associated cardiovascular disease. Routine measures with diuretics and digitalis preparations may be sufficient. However, because of the tendency toward atelectasis and subsequent respiratory failure, these patients may require transient intubation and artificial ventilatory support until the cardiac decompensation has been treated adequately.

Table 3 Lung Function in a 58-Year-Old Man with ALS

Date	FVC		FEV_1		MVV		MIP				
	Liters	% of predicted	Liters	% of predicted	Liters/ minute	% of predicted	cmH_2O	% of predicted	PaO_2 (torr)	PCO_2 (torr)	pH
7/10/78	3.4	70	2.0	53	68	48	66	64	—	—	—
After Bronchodilation	4.2	86	2.6	72	—		—		—	—	—
12/12/78	3.1	64	2.0	53	61	43	24	33	—	—	—
2/1/79	0.3	7	—		—		—		36	60	7.32
2/9/79	1.2	28	—		—		—		74[a]	49	7.38

[a] On 2 liters of oxygen per minute by nasal catheter.

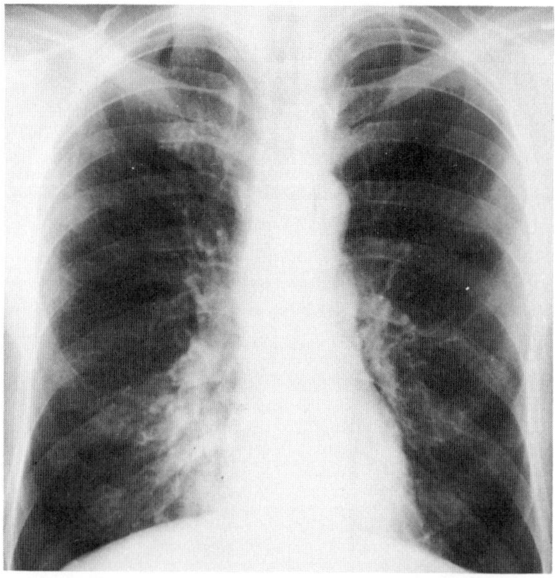

A

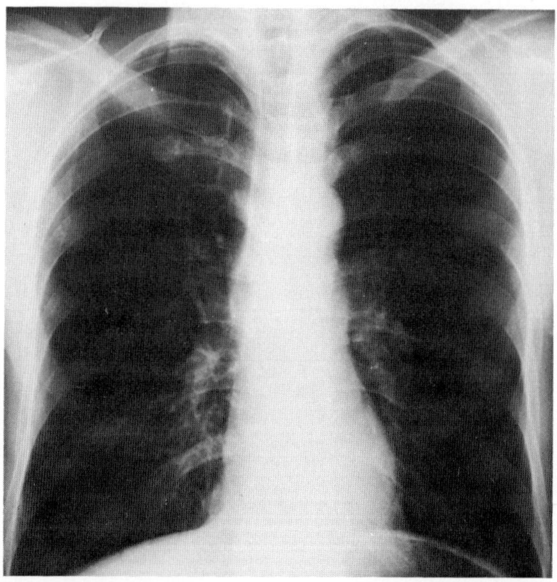

B

Figure 8 Serial x-rays obtained in a patient with ALS, as described in the text. **(A)** The initial x-ray, obtained 11/29/78, shows a right lower lobe infiltrate which was presumed to be aspiration pneumonia. **(B)**, obtained 12/8/78, shows complete clearing of the infiltrate and the absence of abnormalities in the lung fields. **(C)**, obtained 2/2/79, shows the same patient with a collapse of the right upper lobe and infiltrate in the left lower lobe and lingula. **(D)** shows complete reinflation of the right upper lobe and considerable clearing of the infiltrate in the left lung. This x-ray was obtained on the day the patient died.

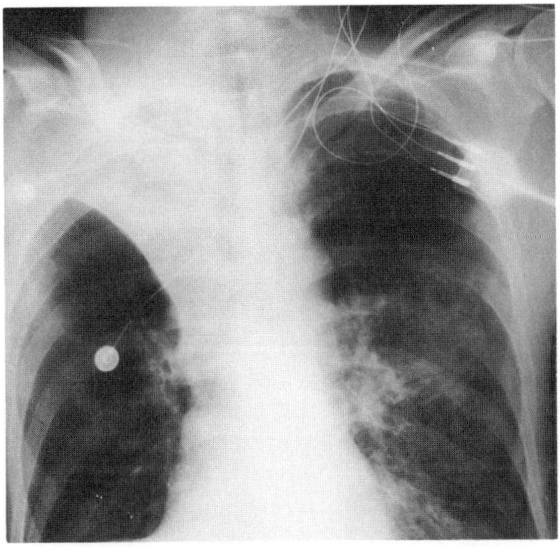

C

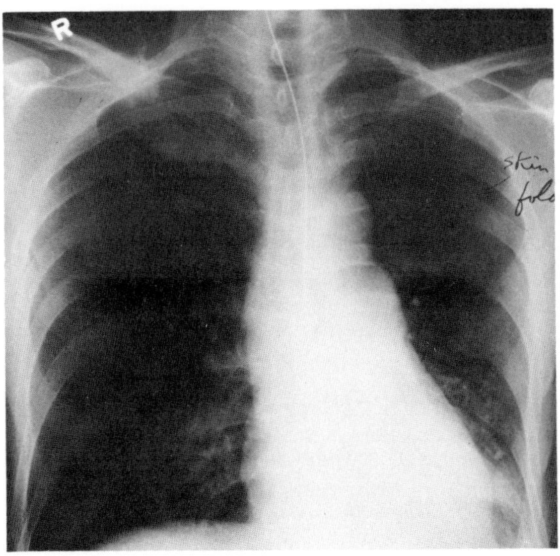

D

We have described a young adult patient with ALS and acute respiratory paralysis associated with the administration of guanidine (3). This patient subsequently had chronic cardiopulmonary failure which was managed at home using a cuirass at night. In addition to the cuirass, a rocking bed might be considered to help such patients maintain better ventilation during sleep, when further hypoxemia or respiratory acidosis may develop. We have used this successfully in only one patient, who had severe neuropathy rather than ALS. The absence of chronic respiratory acidosis in patients with ALS has limited the need for considering this mode of treatment.

When the course of the disease is complicated by severe atelectasis or infection, it may be necessary to intubate these patients and to use fiberoptic bronchoscopy to clear the mucous plugs and secretions. The decision to intervene with such invasive procedures is facilitated when recent serial measurements of FVC are available and indicate that the patient really is not in a rapid or terminal phase of the disease.

CASE HISTORY

A case history may help to exemplify some of these management problems. The patient was a 58-year-old, cigarette-smoking construction worker who noted his first symptoms of ALS, weakness of the upper extremities, in July 1977. By July 1978, the weakness had progressed only slightly, and the patient had his first respiratory evaluation, which showed the modest reductions in lung function typical of ALS and an associated moderate airways obstruction which responded well to bronchodilation, as shown in Table 3. Because of the airway obstruction, he was maintained on bronchodilators and did well until November 29, when he presented with dyspnea, fever, and a change in sputum. His lung fields were clear, but the chest x-ray showed pneumonia in the right lower lobe (Fig. 8A). Treatment included IPPB with bronchodilators, chest percussion, and postural drainage. Adequate sputum was not obtained for culture, but the patient responded to penicillin. He became afebrile and was discharged in three days. The diagnosis was presumed aspiration pneumonia.

His lung function showed only minimal deterioration on December 12 (Table 3), when the pneumonia had completely cleared (Fig. 8B). Note that the MIP had decreased considerably, probably indicating a loss of muscular force though not of volume. On February 1, 1979, he was hospitalized again with severe respiratory distress, severe hypoxia, and hypoventilation (Table 3). Chest x-ray showed collapse of the right upper lobe and pneumonia on the left (Figure 8C). Because his ventilatory function was known to be good just six weeks earlier, vigorous therapeutic efforts were instituted including nasotracheal intubation, bronchoscopy, vigorous bronchial toilet, and bronchodilators. By February 7, his FVC rose to 1.0 liter, and he maintained adequate arterial blood gases after extubation. He continued to improve, though mild hypoxemia and borderline CO_2 retention were present on February 9 (Table 3). On February 11, chest x-ray showed only minimal left lower lobe infiltration (Figure 8D). He died late that evening, less than an hour after he was seen by the nurse to be alert with no evidence of distress. Autopsy failed to show the cause of death. There was no airway occlusion or other evidence of acute respiratory collapse. Did the residual pulmonary motor neurons succumb suddenly?

Chronic respiratory difficulties extending over weeks or months might have been expected in this patient with combined airway obstruction and neuromuscular disease. Yet death occurred precipitously with no obvious cause. The question of why more of these patients do not have findings of chronic hypoxemia and chronic respiratory acidosis is puzzling. Is the acceleration of decomposition suggested in Figure 4 even more rapid in the last few days before death? Is some other acute respiratory event present such as glottic obstruction? Or is the mode of death related to something other than respiratory problems? These and many other challenging questions remain to be answered about the respiratory problems of these unfortunate patients.

REFERENCES

1. Fallat RJ, Jewitt B, Bass M, et al: Spirometry in amyotrophic lateral sclerosis. Arch Neurol 36:74–80, 1979

2. Lebo CP, Ü KS, Norris FH: Cricopharyngeal myotomy in amyotrophic lateral sclerosis. Laryngoscope 86:862–868, 1976

3. Norris FH, Fallat RJ, Calanchini PR: Increased paralysis induced by guanidine in motor neuron disease. Neurology 24:135–137, 1974

Commentary

Robert C. Griggs

Doctor Fallat's data on spirometry in ALS are the most extensive for this disease (3). Despite this large experience, as discussed previously (see chapter 18), the sudden demise of patients with apparently adequate vital capacities is not fully explained. It is noteworthy that neither he nor we have seen chronic hypercapnia in patients with ALS. In patients with muscular dystrophy, chronic restrictive pulmonary disease is routinely associated with hypercapnia. Possible reasons for the abrupt deterioration of patients with ALS include (*a*) impaired cough secondary to decreased expiratory flow rate, owing either to muscle weakness or to a coincident obstructive disease, (*b*) impaired cough coordination resulting from bulbar or pseudobulbar involvement, and (*c*) the potentially greater metabolic demand of muscles that are spastic rather than atrophic.

Patients with ALS appear to be at risk of respiratory insufficiency even at times when spirometric evaluation does not predict a need for respiratory support. Although we need better predictors for such patients, I feel that, at present, patients with dyspnea or those having difficulty handling secretions or who aspirate food should be considered for tracheostomy. At this point in their care, options such as tracheostomy and respiratory support should be discussed with the patient and his or her family.

When a tracheostomy is performed, even on an emergency basis, nasal or oral endotracheal intubation should be avoided, if possible. In the conscious patient with neuromuscular disease, such intubation is painful and frightening. In patients who require tracheostomy, a feeding procedure involving intubation is usually advisable to prevent aspiration.

Several outpatient needs of patients who have had a tracheostomy must be recognized, including:

1. Constant nursing care (often by family members) for suctioning, preventing tracheostomy dysfunction, etc.
2. Measures to prevent atelectasis.
3. Suctioning equipment (with manual back-up).
4. Respiratory support device.
5. Contingency plan in case sputum becomes infected.

Although the cause of death of the majority of ALS patients is respiratory insufficiency, a surprisingly small number of patients have been maintained at home for long periods with ventilatory support (1, 2, 4). Respiratory support devices have not changed much since the days of polio management, and I suspect there are many things to be learned concerning their use in patients with ALS. Table 1 lists some of these devices and notes some problems with each.

A combination of approaches might be useful in some patients. A positive-pressure device might be used during the day and coupled with a cuirass at night, or an abdominal pressure belt used during the day might be coupled with a positive-pressure system at night.

Patients with ALS and a respiratory support system usually need the following items:

1. A tracheostomy for suctioning.
2. A back-up respirator.
3. An AC/DC system.
4. An alternative power source (municipal power companies are often prepared to provide this service in emergencies).
5. An available manual system.

Table 1 Mechanical Devices Used for Home Respiratory Support

Type of Device	*Comments*
Positive Pressure	
IPPB (intermittent positive pressure breathing) device	Pressure regulated
Ventilator	Volume and pressure regulated
Negative Pressure	
Iron lung	Heavy, occupies a large area
Partial (wrap-around) lung[a]	Difficult with urinary and gastric catheters
Cuirass (encloses chest and abdomen)[b] or turtle shell (encloses chest)[b]	May not provide adequate gas exchange
Expiratory Assist	
Rocking bed	Heavy, may cause cardiovascular stress
Abdominal pressure (e.g., Pneumobelt)	Not effective in recumbent position, difficult to use with feeding gastrostomy

[a] Available through J. H. Emerson Co., 22 Cottage Park Ave., Cambridge, MA 02140.
[b] Available through Thompson Respiration Products, Inc., 1705 Range St., Boulder, CO 80301.

Unanswered questions on the management of respiratory failure in patients with ALS include:

1. What is the role of intermittent positive-pressure breathing (IPPB)? Is an increase in compliance beneficial?

2. What is the role of influenza virus or pneumococcal vaccines?

3. Are prophylactic antibiotics indicated during infections of the upper respiratory tract or for a change in sputum characteristics?

4. What are the relative long-term advantages of negative- or positive-pressure support systems?

Even without answers to these and other important questions, an increasing number of patients with ALS are electing to receive long-term respiratory support, and many have been maintained for many years.

REFERENCES

1. Adamson JP, Lewis L, Stein JD: Application of abdominal pressure for artificial respiration. JAMA 69:153–157, 1959

2. Alba A, Pilkington LA, Kaplan E, et al: Long-term pulmonary care in amyotrophic lateral sclerosis. Respiratory Therapy. December 1976

3. Fallat RJ, Jewitt B, Bass M, et al: Spirometry in amyotrophic lateral sclerosis. Arch Neurol 36:74–80, 1979

4. Norris FH, Fallat RJ, Calanchini PR: Increased paralysis induced by guanidine in motor neuron disease. Neurology 24:135–137, 1974

Richard A. Smith

The unexplained, relatively sudden death that Dr. Fallat cites might be analogous to sleep apnea. One might expect that weakness of the tongue and pharynx permits prolapse of the tongue so as to cause mechanical obstruction of the upper airway in patients with bulbar ALS. It would be of interest to determine whether sudden death occurs with equal frequency in males and females, since sleep apnea is primarily a disorder of males. Sleep studies might clarify these issues.

Robert J. Fallat

There might very well be a common mechanism involved in infant crib deaths, sleep apnea, and the enigma of sudden death in patients with ALS. Recently, the use of oxygen electrodes on the skin of infants has demonstrated marked decreases in arterial PO_2 during rather routine maneuvers. For example, when a premature infant has his or her diaper changed, the arterial PO_2 may fall to 30 mmHg, or below. Similarly, recent data published by Block et al., who used ear oximetry in normal adults, demonstrated that the arterial oxygen saturation can fall to below 72%, which is in the range of 30–40 mmHg PO_2 (1). If such hypoxemia can occur in normal adults, one can imagine that much more severe hypoxemic states can occur rather acutely in patients with ALS. The use of skin electrodes and ear oximetry might provide useful information on the cause of death in patients with ALS.

A second point concerns the vital capacity; 80% or higher is certainly not an indication that the patient has neuromuscular disease, much less a predictor of death. In our own series, all of the patients who were studied within three months of death had vital capacities below 60% of the predicted, which would be a distinctly abnormal level. Since many of the patients do decline very rapidly, it is conceivable that one could have a vital capacity of 80% six months before death. My guess would be that the vital capacity would decline to something under 60% before death, however.

REFERENCE

1. Block AJ, Boysen PG, Wynne JW, et al: Sleep apnea, hypopnea, oxygen desaturation in normal subjects. A strong male predominance. N Engl J Med 300:513, 1979

H. Richard Tyler

I would like to stress the importance to the clinician of recognizing pulmonary symptoms and to emphasize a few points. First, Dr. Fallat and Dr. Norris presented two curves, one a typical curve with a high peak, the other a curve with a rounded dome. The first is normal, and these patients are not likely to have respiratory trouble. The second, the rounded curve, shows a poor respiratory effort and indicates that the system is functioning so poorly that any resistance would seriously interfere with respiratory function. If the patient should aspirate, his or her resistance to respiratory function would go right up, and the vital capacity would close in. Often, in a matter of just minutes, a patient can develop hypoxia and cardiac arrhythmia, and sudden death may ensue. Thus, we do not lose patients from respiratory insufficiency alone, we lose them when a secondary factor, such as aspiration or chronic infection, is added. The life of the patient can usually be prolonged if we are very careful and meticulous in aiding respiratory function.

Of a series of patients studied recently at our institution, 35% (26 patients) had suffered loss of weight. Twenty-five of the 26 had experienced difficulty in swallowing or feeding, 10 had difficulty with both, and 12 had difficulty with swallowing only. Twenty-two of the patients were aspirating. If one has a patient who has respiratory insufficiency, one can probably help him or her by paying attention to the pulmonary toilet. I believe that attention to pulmonary toilet, early gastrostomy, and forbidding smoking are things that a physician can do to markedly lengthen the lives of these patients.

Victor M. Rivera

We are also impressed by the usefulness of pulmonary function data in the management of patients with ALS. Since we incorporated pulmonary function studies into our periodic objective measurements and assessments, and, of course, into the parameters for clinical trials, we have found that the arterial-alveolar gradient and the $PaCO_2$ are preserved fairly well until very late stages. When this parameter changes abruptly, it usually indicates that the patient is going into a catastrophic situation very soon. I do not know whether this finding can be used as a predictor of impending death. In contrast, the presence of a higher total lung capacity usually indicates an improved prognosis for the patient.

I would also point out that serial lung scans with ^{133}Xe clearance and wash-out curves are useful in some ALS patients. My consultant in the Nuclear Medicine Department reached a point where he could report these lung scans as "this is a typical lung scan in ALS." Actually, what we found was a typical pattern, characterized by trapping of the gas in the bases and hypoperfusion in the apices. Of course, as the ALS progressed, the trapping of the gas in the base increased, and the pattern became more and more spotty and disorganized (1).

REFERENCE

1. Alvarez A, Calderon M, Griffin BT, et al: Pulmonary function abnormalities in amyotrophic lateral sclerosis (abstract). In *Proceedings of the 11th World Congress of Neurology.* Excerpta Medica ICS #427:46, 1977

20 Ethical Issues

Theodore L. Munsat

The American medical community is in the midst of a radical change in the way it approaches and manages issues of death, life-support mechanisms, truth telling, quality versus duration of life, and other issues generally grouped under the rubric of bioethical considerations. We hope that the open discussion of these issues and the involvement of well-meaning and knowledgeable physicians, clergy, humanists, patients, and relatives will result in the kind of analysis that leads to more enlightened and humanistic patient care. The need for such discussion and analysis is particularly clear for the patient with ALS.

I would like to relate our own experiences in a rather large ALS Clinic at the Tufts–New England Medical Center and our particular philosophy in handling certain emotional and ethical aspects of patient care. The ALS Clinic is housed in a typical urban university teaching hospital. The staff meets weekly for three hours and consists of myself as the clinic director, two neuromuscular-disease fellows, a clinic nurse, a physiotherapist, and a secretary. Patient care is supported by third-party carriers and the Muscular Dystrophy Association. Part-time consultants include an Episcopal minister and a biomedical engineer working on communication devices. Patients are referred to us from a number of sources: private physicians (mainly neurologists), the Muscular Dystrophy Association, the ALS Societies, and other patients. All patients have a personal physician, either a generalist or internist. The ALS Clinic is structured and presented to the patient as a health care resource that will be available to him or her throughout the illness. The patient and the family are constantly assured that we will be available at all times in the future and will never abandon them.

We have found that fear of abandonment is the major concern of the patient and the family, although it is often unexpressed. This fear is enhanced when the patient is told he has an untreatable disease with a sharply defined life span—something we still hear over and over again. This sense of abandonment continues as the patient is shunted from physician to physician for frustrating consultations that are limited to one hour. Soon, the patient begins to perceive the physician's discomfort in managing a chronic illness that has no cure. The ALS Clinic and its personnel, with whom the patient and his or her family develop an increasingly trusting relationship, serves in great part as a constant reminder that people are concerned and always available.

A positive and enthusiastic therapeutic approach is both ethically and medically sound. Many of the therapies we use have already been discussed in detail. We have been particularly impressed with the use of baclofen to relieve upper motor neuron dysfunction, particularly pseudobulbar palsy, and the symptomatic benefit of antisialorrheics and the selective use of electronic communication devices.

Each of our patients and their families are told in great detail, often during several visits, of the many basic and clinical research projects being conducted throughout the world. They are assured that there is excellent communication among scientists and that when an important development occurs it will promptly be known to all. Volumes such as this are relayed to patients as quickly as possible. We believe it is important to keep patients well informed and up to date. Each of our patients is strongly encouraged to take part in one or more of our research projects. At present, these include peripheral nerve biopsy for study of morphology and axoplasmic transport, studies of gastrointestinal absorption, plasmapheresis, and the use of neurotransmitter precursors. Patients who are not directly involved are informed that if a particular approach proves to be effective they will be notified immediately. Conversely, they are assured that if a particular approach is not fruitful we are prepared to explore another. We are careful not to raise hopes falsely and have observed that most patients handle a negative drug trial remarkably well. It is the sense of participation in an effort that is the critical element. Patients do not want to sit by as observers while their motor function progressively fades.

Although one must generalize to communicate effectively, we have come to the conclusion that proper management of the psychologic turmoil and bioethical decisions that are part of the management of every ALS family must be highly individualized. Each patient is the unique product of his own psychosocial background, and each family has its own unique brand of interaction, prejudice, hostility, confusion, and fears. In order to advise the patient and family properly about such decisions as tracheostomy, feeding gastrostomy, and life-support procedures, a broad understanding of the patient as an individual is important. This takes time, many visits, and is not cost effective. There is no easy or fast road to arriving at this information. The wishes of the well informed patient are paramount in the making of any decision, and should not be overshadowed by a well-meaning, more dominant relative. This is particularly a problem with dysarthric patients; it is much easier and faster to get information from a relative rather than directly from the patient.

In general, we counsel against tracheostomy, except in those patients with early bulbar involvement and sparing of the trunk and limbs. Orders not to resuscitate are written only after it is clear that these are the wishes of the patient and his family. If the patient develops an acute respiratory problem at home, the family is advised to bring the patient to an emergency room as quickly as possible.

The management of a hospitalized patient in the terminal state of ALS requires all the skill, compassion, and emotional strength the physician can muster. Families seemingly prepared for the end may suddenly decompensate. Nurses, medical students, and house staff who may be more intimately involved with terminal care often require their own support. After death occurs, many problems and questions remain unresolved and require attention. Many families wish to continue to contribute to the fight against ALS, and these opportunities should be made available.

Our concerns can be summarized as follows:

1. Emotional and ethical issues constitute a major element in the management of the patient with ALS. It is an element that can be mismanaged or handled effectively.

2. The major fear of the patient and family is that they will be abandoned by loved ones and by the medical profession. We try to allay this fear.

3. We favor a multidisciplinary approach in a setting that provides an opportunity for the patient to take an active role in clinical research.

4. Bioethical decision making must be highly individualized, and the final decisions may vary greatly depending on individual circumstances.

21 Patient Autonomy as Therapy

Christine Cassel

Ethics is as integral a part of the practice of medicine as differential diagnosis. Physicians have probably always been confronted with ethical dilemmas, so medical ethics is not a new field. But the complexity of modern medicine and the impersonal alienating forces of modern society have combined to present ever more perplexing problems to which solutions cannot be reached by intuition alone. The discipline of medical ethics draws on the philosophic methods of systematic and analytic thinking in the hope that these methods are more adequate to the dilemmas we face.

Many of the problems encountered by physicians caring for patients who have amyotrophic lateral sclerosis are similar to those engendered by other maladies afflicting human beings. Yet ALS is also unique in certain ways that pose a special challenge to the ethicist as well as to the physician. It is a disease of mysterious etiology, insidious onset, and relentless—if variable—progression toward death. Patients with ALS lose the motor function of their nervous system but generally maintain intelligence and awareness. They do not usually have intense pain requiring narcotics that cloud consciousness. No curative therapy is known to exist, and the horizon is not brimming with hopeful experimental procedures or drugs. Even cancer, the most dreaded disease in our culture, has greater statistical chances of medically or surgically induced cure or remission. Consideration of the ethical aspects in the care of persons with ALS is inextricably intertwined with the medical. We must confront the limits of our own power, and perhaps thereby gain greater power of a different sort.

Many of the ethical issues in the care of patients with ALS derive from a psychologic phenomenon that is present in any relationship between physician and patient. The physician is healthy, knowledgeable, powerful, respected by society, and has access to medical technology. The patient is sick, ignorant, vulnerable, pitied—if not rejected—by society, and a supplicant to professionals for access to help. The person as patient has lost many of the characteristics that give people power in the world. I will refer to this power as *autonomy*, which I believe to be a very important element in living a meaningful life in our culture.

Although there is a movement toward greater personal responsibility for health, the basic underlying truth to this conception of the physician/patient relationship remains unchanged. A person who is ill or in pain goes to a physician for help and relief. If that person has an acute, reversible condition, this relationship may be satisfactory, because the physician provides treatment or advice and the patient gets better. The patient gets back on his or her feet with autonomy reinstated. In the face of any incurable or chronic disease, however, the dynamic changes. It does not work as neatly for many reasons, not the least of which is our own anxiety in dealing with the limits of our curative powers. The patient in such a situation is in danger of being permanently stripped of his or her autonomy and thereby losing a crucial element of personhood.

Patients with ALS are also in danger of outright abandonment occurring under the guise of professionalism. The physician may make the diagnosis, which is his or her "job," and then send the patient away claiming there is "nothing else I can do." Physicians who respond in this way undoubtedly believe that they have nothing more to offer. One reason for this is that medical school curricula devote a far greater amount of time to the study of mechanisms of disease than to mechanisms of supportive relationships. Another is that physicians are all too aware of the fragility of human life. It may be less painful to work within the arena of control offered by science than to face one's own mortality in the form of a person with an incurable or disabling disease.

I am pleased to see that we health professionals are beginning to discuss the sources of help and support that we need in dealing with this disease as it affects our patients. If we can be strong, we can help the patients to be strong. Their inner strength enhances their autonomy and our respect for them as persons. If our verbal and nonverbal messages contain only anxiety and avoidance, our ability to give meaningful help through the difficult times ahead is severely limited. Many health professionals have reported learning how to tap their own sources of strength and hope from patients, thus making them partners in the therapeutic relationship.

The notion of autonomy for critically ill patients was recently addressed by Imbus and Zawecki in a report from their burn unit (4).

In this unit, patients who are so badly burned that survival is unprecedented are asked to decide whether they want aggressive or palliative therapy. This is a kind of all-or-nothing autonomy, for the patients rapidly become obtunded, and death is swift. Maintaining autonomy for a person who has ALS is a day-to-day activity. It involves not one decision but many. It involves an ongoing relationship that changes over time, presenting new problems and new demands. It involves the patient's family and friends and many different health professionals. In this setting, the patient's autonomy can be fostered in many ways. These include sharing of information, sharing of decision making, participation in research, and respect for the values of each individual.

Knowledge is an avenue to power. Therefore, full disclosure of the nature of the disease and its prognosis must be made whenever possible. This does not mean "dropping it like a bomb" (in the words of one ALS patient) and beating a hasty retreat. It means that a persistent and supportive effort should be made to get the information across and to help the patient deal with it. Cicely Saunders stated:

> The fact that a patient does not ask does not mean that he has no questions. One visit or talk is rarely enough. It is only by waiting and listening that we can gain an idea of what we should be saying. Silences and gaps are often more revealing than words as we try to learn what a patient is facing as he travels along the constantly changing journey of his illness and his thoughts about it. . . . The main argument against a policy of deliberate, invariable denial of unpleasant facts is that it makes such communication extremely difficult, if not impossible. Once the possibility of talking frankly with a patient has been admitted, it does not mean that this will always take place, but the whole atmosphere is changed. We are then free to wait quietly for clues from each patient, seeing them as individuals from whom we can expect intelligence, courage, and individual decisions. They will feel secure enough to give us these clues when they wish. (6)

Many physicians worry that disclosure of a poor prognosis will cause a person to give up hope and become depressed or even suicidal. It is equally likely, however, that uncertainty causes more anxiety and despair, as well as preventing the patient from realistically confronting the situation. Doubt renders him or her helpless, whereas information given in the right way offers a measure of autonomy. Hope can be sustained by an honest, supportive relationship, and is damaged more by abandonment than by the telling of an unpleasant truth.

In her discussion of lies to the sick and dying, Sissela Bok mentions psychologic risks of disclosure:

> Physicians know only too well how uncertain a diagnosis or prognosis can be. They know how hard it is to give meaningful and correct answers regarding health and illness. They also know that disclosing their own uncertainty or fears can reduce those benefits that depend upon faith in recovery. (3)

I would argue that sharing our uncertainty with patients enhances trust as well as allowing room for hopefulness. Ironically, it is exactly the limitations of the physician's knowledge that can help to sustain hope, and so it is also important that we never rule out the possibility of a long survival and productive life for ALS patients.

In disclosing the limitations of our understanding of the etiology of the disease and our ignorance of any possible cure or reversal, we need also to emphasize that we do have skills in methods of care and technologies of assistance. Help is available. There *is* something we can do. Care and attention can be an essential buttress to the autonomy of the patient with ALS. Health professionals have an obligation to any person who is sick. Sick persons have the same rights as any other persons, and our help can be directed toward maintaining those rights for the most vulnerable. Therefore, it is crucial to respect patients as persons, which means "... they have the same right to their judgements as we have to our own ... [for the reason] that the other is a person and therefore rightfully a rational determiner of his or her destiny" (2). Respect leads us to set limits to our paternalism, but this does not mean setting limits to our caring. With the knowledge and consent of the patient, medical care for those with ALS can be as energetic and meticulous as it is for patients with any other disease.

Great progress has been made in the development of technologies to assist patients with ALS, including refinements of esophagostomy, gastrostomy and tracheostomy, as well as elaborate devices for assisted respiration, communication, and other functions. These techniques can do a great deal to enhance the patient's autonomy, if he or she feels free to choose the forms of therapy desired, as well as to set limits to it. Some patients do not want to be the primary decision makers. There are those who want to hand their fate over completely to their physicians. In such a case we cannot force information, nor should we ask them to make decisions for which they are not emotionally prepared. But we should always be aware that these attitudes are not irreversible. They may change as the physician's relationship with the person progresses and as the person's relationship with the disease progresses. We owe it to all patients to make an offer of partnership in decision making, to make the offer vigorously and genuinely, and to stay open to changes in the patient's attitudes. For example, there are many patients for whom the idea of a tracheostomy may initially be abhorrent. They may say, "No, I draw the line at that," but they may change their minds as they learn to cope with their limitations and reevaluate their criteria for acceptable quality of life.

Attention to patients' values is as important in developing new forms of assistance as it is in determining the extent of assistance. In the design of communications devices, for example, professionals place much importance on the speed of communication. This is not always of real concern to the patient, however, since he or she is in no great rush. Often the patient is not so frustrated as the physician at the slowness of the communication process, for the physician is the one with the busy schedule who is always in a hurry. We must remember to ask, *whose* values are we responding to?

Another aspect of the problem of setting limits to therapeutic intervention can be seen in terms of cost-benefit analysis: how much, and for whom? The cost considerations occur on two levels: the cost (financial and otherwise) to the patient and family, and the cost to society at large. The second level is particularly troublesome, especially in the current climate of concern over burgeoning medical spending, some of which is attributable to high-technology care for patients who are unlikely to recover their premorbid functional condition (7). How should a physician take this issue into account when dealing with an individual patient? I believe it is not the physician's role to limit a patient's access to high-cost technology in order to limit overall medical spending. As especially knowledgeable citizens, health professionals should certainly exhibit concern for societal issues, but rationing decisions must be made on a policy level that applies equally to everyone, if such decisions are to be ethically sound. It is quite impossible to make a convincing moral argument based on computing how much something is costing society against how much benefit a single person is getting from it. Such a calculation erodes the specificity of the individualized caring relationship that is the central obligation of the medical profession. If reimbursement for a given treatment modality is available, then the decision to use it should be based on its appropriateness in the care of a particular patient, not on considerations of harm or benefit to society as a whole.

In the area of personal and family cost, I think we have to make a sort of cost-benefit calculation in a manner that furthers patient autonomy. Cost-effectiveness has to be judged by the real benefit to the patient and family in terms of what *they* want and what benefits *them*. This is not the same thing as efficiency. If something requires a great outlay of energy, time, and resources on the part of health professionals but really does benefit the patient, not just in terms of prolongation of life but also in terms of improving the quality of life, then it is justified. We could consider it cost-effective, even though it may not appear to be efficient.

A distinction between ordinary and extraordinary means may be helpful in this context. This concept was first clarified when philosophers and religious leaders began to address the problems faced by the medical profession with the advent of life-extending technology. Most of the problems in those early days concerned irreversibly comatose patients or patients with terminal disease for whom someone other than the patient had to make the decision whether to continue or to stop artificial life support. The distinction that was made was intended to be helpful in clarifying which methods of therapy were morally obligatory and which were morally optional or conditional on other factors. Confusion arose when physicians began to use these terms in a way that equated ordinary means with customary or accepted therapeutic modalities and extraordinary means with heroic or experimental modalities. With the inflationary technology of modern medicine, the reference points for these concepts are never fixed or stable. Things that were extraordinary last year are quite ordinary this year.

In *The Patient as Person,* Ramsey quotes Father Kelly's quite different interpretation of these terms:

> Ordinary means of preserving life are all medicines, treatments, and operations which offer a reasonable hope of benefit for the patient and which can be obtained and used without excessive expense, pain, or other inconvenience. Extraordinary means of preserving life mean all medicines, treatments, and operations which cannot be obtained without excessive expense, pain, or inconvenience, or which, if used, would not offer a reasonable hope of benefit. (5)

This statement contains several significantly ambiguous terms: ordinary, extraordinary, reasonable, benefit, and excessive. How are we to judge what is a *reasonable* benefit? How are we to judge what is an *excessive* cost, *excessive* pain, or *excessive* inconvenience? Ramsey claims, and I think that this makes the most sense for our purposes, that these words must not be defined in terms of current medical values, or in terms of a particular physician's values, or even in terms of the values of a well-meaning family member, but strictly in terms of the patient's own values. The range of what is considered excessive or not excessive may vary widely from patient to patient. Reasonable benefits should be seen in terms of the quality of life acceptable to that patient. This evaluation will be based on self-image, on spiritual resources and orientation, on the patient's own moral values, and on his or her concept of a useful life and a good death. For some people, the "fighters," this can mean that they are willing to endure a great deal of disability and still conduct a useful and fulfilling life. For others, not being able to move or speak inflicts intolerable suffering. We may not initially be able to accept these decisions at face value, but after exploring values and reasons with the patient we are obligated to accept what his or her value system dictates and to provide all possible supportive therapy up to the point where the patient draws the line.

One interesting option we have to offer that may enhance patient autonomy is the ability to participate in research. This is especially true for those patients who are "fighters." The chance to participate in research can offer dignity and a means of sustaining autonomy and hope because the patient becomes a coadventurer with the physician. A note of caution is necessary, however. In this setting, the researcher has to realize that he or she is filling two roles that are not always easily compatible (8). Many patients who choose to be research subjects derive satisfaction from the idea that they may be helping future victims of the disease. This attitude is authentic and can be very precious as a source of strength. Other motives that are more dangerous to patient autonomy may coexist, however, such as a desire to please the caregivers, or a fear of abandonment if one does not participate. It is the responsibility of the researcher to give priority to the welfare of the individual patient to avoid taking unfair advantage of his or her altruistic motives. The physician/patient relationship always morally precedes the researcher/subject relationship. The patient may fear that the physician's interest will decrease if he or she drops out of a research project, or that he or she has failed personally if the research trial is unsuccessful. Clinical researchers must take great care not to let their ego involvement in therapeutic trials influence their attitude toward patients. There are some very fine lines to tread in this area, but participation in research remains a significant option that can offer a source of autonomy to patients with ALS.

A person with ALS is truly unique as a potential partner in decision making. He or she usually maintains intelligence and awareness throughout the illness. This is not true for many other medical and surgical patients, especially in situations of life-threatening illness. Patients with ALS have time to deal with the emotional aspects of their disease, unlike patients with myocardial infarctions, for example, who are in a state of fear and disbelief in the face of a very real risk of sudden death at any moment. The role played by time is crucial and unavoidable. The patient with ALS has time to work through various reactions to what is happening to him or her and has time to develop a supportive relationship with medical professionals as well as with family members and friends. The professional also has time to get to know the patient and to make this therapeutic relationship a real partnership.

Medieval Christian philosophy considered the best death to be one that was foreseen, for which a person had ample time to prepare (1). I think most people in our culture feel that the best death is a sudden and unexpected one, so one does not have to think about it too much. We vigorously deny death as we deny other realities such as aging, suffering, and poverty. In medieval times ALS patients would have been considered especially blessed because they have a long period of time in which to confront their mortality and confront the meaning of life as well as the meaning of death. Patients with a strong spiritual orientation bear witness to this value. In ALS, most significant decisions can be made ahead of time. Events can be anticipated, alternatives can be discussed. There is time to think things over, time to reconsider grievances and to correct misunderstandings. There is time to make and change decisions about acceptable or desirable forms of medical help. These opportunities are not present in many other serious diseases; usually there is neither time nor a conscious partner, and the health care professionals have to proceed without really knowing what the patient would have wanted.

In summary, it seems clear that medical professionals can offer a great deal to the patient with ALS. It is *not* true that there is nothing we can do. Through the means I have discussed, and probably through many others as well, we can offer respect and a degree of autonomy consistent with meaningful living and dying.

Acknowledgments

I am indebted to Albert R. Jonsen, PhD, Professor of Bioethics, University of California at San Francisco, and the Reverend John Dame for critical assistance and shared insight.

REFERENCES

1. Aries P: *Western Attitudes towards Death: From the Middle Ages to the Present.* Translated by M Ranum. Baltimore, Johns Hopkins University Press, 1974

2. Beauchamp TL, Childress JF: *Principles of Biomedical Ethics.* New York, Oxford University Press, 1979, p 59

3. Bok S: *Lying: Moral Choice in Public and Private Life.* New York, Random House, 1978, p 237

4. Imbus S, Zawecki B: Autonomy for burned patients when survival is unprecedented. N Engl J Med 297:308–311, 1977

5. Ramsey P: *The Patient as Person.* New Haven, Yale University Press, 1970, p 122

6. Saunders CMS: Telling patients. In *Ethics in Medicine.* Edited by SJ Reiser, AJ Dyck, WJ Curran. Cambridge, MIT Press, 1977, pp 238–240

7. Shroeder SA, Showstack JA, Roberts HE: High cost patients in 17 acute-care hospitals. N Engl J Med 300:1306–1309, 1979

8. Spiro HM: Constraint and consent—on being a patient and subject. N Engl J Med 293:1134–1137, 1975

Commentary

H. Richard Tyler

I would like to raise some questions that I cannot answer. In my view, many of the subjects mentioned here do raise ethical problems. If we believe that it is justifiable to try new things and to call such trials "research," does it follow that we should not charge the patients who participate in these efforts? Or, do we have a right to charge these patients because we are really treating them with "research"? We have to be careful of these words.

In order to conduct a true research trial, one has to obtain informed consent from the patients, a requirement that brings up other considerations. We have to provide full information, yet in so doing we usually will be telling the patients that there is no evidence to support our trials. The patients cannot give truly informed consent unless they know the truth as we see it. Some of their ideas, hopes, and beliefs concerning getting better, which we can understand and accept, are not appropriate in a research setting.

Another thing that troubles me is that this type of trial is being supported by third-party payments. Is it the responsibility of the physician to inform Blue Cross and Blue Shield that he or she has had a patient admitted to the hospital for research purposes? If hospitalization is paid by third parties, what provision shall we make to ensure that the individual without insurance has equal access to the same research projects that a well-to-do patient has?

These problems all relate to caring for patients and therefore require some sort of sanction by society, or at least an acceptance that these things are being done in a morally responsible manner. The hospital should not have to pay for these studies. The physician can wait for his or her fee, but who is going to pay for the tests required by the research protocol? Certainly, it is not clear to me that government or voluntary agencies want to support informal studies. The time it takes to mobilize support from these sources is often one to three years. Our snake venom study cost over $500,000. That money had to be found and did not come from any of the usual sources. I think that these considerations are important. Society, if it asks such things of the physician, must assume responsibility. It must pay for its expectations and must face up to such issues. Physicians do not have the answers. Perhaps societies like the ALSSOA can encourage systems like the government to face up to such consequences and make it easier for physicians to seek the answers they expect us to produce.

The definition of "treatment" in ALS is not the definition of treatment in any other disease. Blue Cross, Blue Shield, and other insurance companies have to understand what we are doing, where we are doing it, and why we are doing it. No one wants to be deceptive about it, yet many of us do not always put down a full explanation in response to their requests for information. This point is very important to me, at least in terms of the things that we are expected to do and wish to do to help these patients in the future.

Brian S. Gould

I think that a rather simple notion is tripping up many of us. Treatment means taking care of a patient, it does not mean curing him or her and does not depend on the efficacy of any specific agent. The best treatment for a patient with a chronic, progressive, irreversible illness may be to participate in a clinical research trial. The idea that it is improper to charge for such treatment, I think, is going to cause great difficulties and is an unnecessary restriction.

H. Richard Tyler

The physician charges for his or her time, I think, not his or her effectiveness. I do not think there is any ethical or medical problem with this whatsoever. We can treat patients with various agents on a prototype basis more or less indefinitely, and it could still constitute good treatment. So far as the point about informed consent is concerned, you raise a vexing problem. However, on the psychologic level, the studies that have examined informed consent seem to indicate that it is impossible to obtain truly informed consent from any patient with any disease. The patients do not remember accurately what you have told them, and they do not understand the implications of the decisions they are making. It is a legalistic view that sounds good in bioethical discussions, but in the clinical practice of medicine it seems to have very little relevance. I think it is important to inform patients to the best of one's ability about the choices that confront them, but one has to keep in mind that this is imperfect at best and ultimately inadequate. We see patients making contradictory decisions all the time. They will not admit there is anything wrong but, yes, they will take the medications we prefer. Is that informed consent?

Christine Cassel

I am familiar with the studies showing that patients do not remember anything the physician has said after they sign the consent form. I do not think that this is because they are lacking in intelligence or are unable to remember what they are told. I think it is because the information is not transmitted properly and persistently. They may be too upset to retain complex information the first time they are told, but one must keep the dialogue going. It is not an impossible task.

Brian S. Gould

I am a physician, and I had the unfortunate experience a few years ago of being with my father when he received the terrible diagnosis of malignant melanoma. We were at his oncologist's office together, and I found myself doing the very same thing all patients and their families do. I was nodding "yes" before I had even heard what he had to say. I could not think of questions; we were just overcome with anxiety, and I know more about that illness than most people do. It is not a question of informing, it is a question of handling one's own psychologic need. A few months later, I could not have told you anything that the physician had said except "malignant melanoma," and my response: "Yes, Dad, I think you should take whatever treatment he prescribes."

22 Therapeutic Trials in Amyotrophic Lateral Sclerosis: A Review

Barry W. Festoff

Nancy Jones Crigger

Since the formal description and pathologic characterization of amyotrophic lateral sclerosis by Charcot in 1865, several causes of the disease have been proposed and various treatments attempted to cure or substantially halt the progressive deterioration it causes. However, the cause of ALS is still unknown, and clearly no treatment, whether drug, replacement, or physical therapy, has proved to be more useful than any other in altering its course. We decided that a review of previous reports might close the chapter on a particular theory or treatment and, perhaps more important, reopen some chapters to modern investigation for a closer look.

At the outset, several assumptions had to be made. First, selection of an empirical treatment should be guided by some notion as to cause. Second, treatment might involve efforts not only to cure, but also to improve specific abnormalities in the motor system or to halt the progression of wasting and weakness. Last, symptomatic therapies agreed upon by those involved in planning this conference as essential in the management of ALS patients would be excluded in the present discussion. To be sure, evaluation of previous trials with such a disease, which was described by Cooper as "one of the cruelest, most demeaning, most unbearable of the neurologic disorders" (26), is fraught with inherent problems. For example, many authors have discussed the ethical and moral issues surrounding single- or double-blind trials in ALS. These discussions have established the notion that withholding of possibly ameliorative medication is not warranted in attempts to evaluate the clinical usefulness of some treatment. Recently, Tyler has addressed this point in a particularly humanistic, as well as scientific, way (100).

For the purpose of this review, we have attempted to identify a previous study as being adequate or inadequate. Our means for determining this are themselves quite limited. However, despite these limitations, it can safely be said that almost all studies have been inadequate, according to the criteria outlined in Table 1.

We have organized the subject matter, as much as possible, in a chronologic fashion within each etiologic category. Table 2 lists the various theories regarding etiology of ALS and serves as the point of reference in the material which follows.

VITAMIN OR SPECIFIC NUTRIENT DEFICIENCY

During the 1940s, several conflicting reports were published concerning the use of tocopherol (vitamin E) as a treatment for ALS. The rationale for these drug trials was based on reports of development of muscular and neurologic signs in rats fed diets deficient in tocopherol (Table 2) (38). Several authors noted improvement of ALS patients after treatment with vitamin E (Table 3) (69, 91, 102). A larger group of researchers concluded that the therapy was ineffective (32, 33, 36, 63, 105). Interestingly, the rats did not improve either.

Ask-Upmark (3) and, later, Ask-Upmark and Muerling (4) reported that the so-called deficiency factor was related to gastric dysfunction. They examined 111 patients with a history of gastric resection. Of those examined, they reported two cases of clinically undetected ALS. From another perspective, of 20 individuals with ALS, 5 had a previous history of gastric surgery. Some years later, Stiel found that none of 125 ALS patients had had gastric surgery before onset of the disease (96). Gastric secretion was normal in all of the 5 patients studied.

Two other drug trials of vitamin supplements are worthy of note. Pieper and Fields reported a trial of intrathecal administration of vitamin

Table 1 Criteria for Evaluating Clinical Trials of ALS

Diagnosis made by clinical examination plus EMG and/or muscle biopsy
Randomized drug therapy
Inclusion of control group taking placebo
Double-blind study
Standardized treatment for both groups
Objective measurement of follow-up evaluation and analysis of results

B_{12} and hydrocortisone in 21 patients (87). Dorman et al. evaluated the effect of vitamin E and pancreatic extract on patients with ALS; both clinical drug trials were ineffective in alteration of the disease (35). Although we feel that these studies were inadequate, our impression is that further investigation into use of vitamin E as specific therapy for ALS is unwarranted. However, since there has been no documentation of untoward effects of vitamin E in moderately high dosages, we do not feel it should be totally rejected either.

HEAVY METALS AND OTHER TOXINS

Heavy metals, particularly lead, have long been considered of possible etiologic significance in ALS. For our purposes, we will examine only some of the more recent reports of possible lead toxicity.

Campbell et al. found an increased incidence of history of lead exposure in ALS patients as compared with controls (15). Bone biopsies did not reveal a greater amount of lead in ALS patients. More recently, Conradi et al. compared blood of 16 ALS patients and 18 controls by means of atomic absorption spectrophotometry (23–25). Blood levels of lead were reported as being in the normal range; however, as compared with control patients, levels were significantly higher. Several authors have reported unsuccessful results of trials with chelating agents (15, 31). Table 4 lists some of these reports. Boothby et al. report a case of severe lead exposure that improved after treatment with penicillamine (8).

In 1954, Brown published an article reporting 6 patients who exhibited an ALS-like picture and who had mercurial intoxication (11). Kantarjian observed 11 farmers with ALS-like symptoms and signs who were exposed to mercury (53). In both reports, individuals with the disease developed other systemic signs and symptoms of acute intoxication (i.e., nausea, vomiting, lines on gums). In both groups of patients, treatment with dimercaprol did not alleviate the symptoms. It seems reasonable that lead or mercury exposure may induce a motor neuron disease syndrome in some patients. However, whether such exposure alone can account for all cases of classic ALS remains to be determined.

Manganese has also been implicated by Yase as a possible agent in ALS (106, 107). The high amount of manganese in soil and the higher incidence of ALS developing in individuals on the Kii Peninsula of Japan and on Guam who have a history of manganese mining lend suspicion to the metal as a possible etiologic factor. A further discussion of manganese is included in the section on *Mineral Metabolism*, below.

More recently, selenium has been associated with development of ALS. Reports by Kilness and Hochberg have resulted in a flurry of letters for and against this idea and have even led to discussion of the possible dangers of selenium-based shampoo (55). Their original

Table 2 Theories Concerning the Etiology of ALS

Theory	*Explanation*
Deficiency factor	
Evans and Burr (38) Ask-Upmark (3) Ask-Upmark and Muerling (4) Stiel (96)	Laboratory study with rats; Ask-Upmark reports a relation between gastric surgery and ALS. Stiel did not support an increased incidence of ALS in patients with gastric surgery.
Heavy metals, toxins	
Mercury	
Brown (11) Kantarjian (53)	Relation between mercury intoxication and ALS-like symptoms. Not classic ALS picture.
Lead	
Campbell et al. (15) Boothby et al. (8) Felmus et al. (40) Conradi et al. (24, 25)	Higher incidence of exposure to lead. Case report of improvement of ALS-like symptoms with chelating agent. Lead levels greater in ALS patient than in control.
Selenium	
Kilness and Hochberg (55) Schwartz (94) Kurland (59) Norris and Ü (76)	High selenium and increased incidence of ALS. ALS is as common in selenium-deficient areas. Selenium excretion not greater in ALS patients.
Cycad	
Kurland (59)	Possible etiologic factor. No greater ingestion of cycad in Guamanians.
Metabolic dysfunction	
Impaired glucose metabolism/ endocrine dysfunction	
Tom and Richardson (98) Barris (6) Cumings (30) Ionasescu and Luca (51) Steinke and Tyler (95) Quick and Greer (88) Collis and Engel (21) Friedman et al. (41) Mueller and Quick (70) Gotoh et al. (46) Astin et al. (5) Koerner (56) Saffer et al. (92)	Relation between pancreatic tumor and ALS symptoms. High incidence of abnormal GTT[a] and ALS. Site of dysfunction disputed: pancreatic dysfunction, decreased receptor space, or both. Normal CSF glucose.

Table 2 Theories Concerning the Etiology of ALS (*continued*)

Theory	*Explanation*
Metabolic dysfunction (*continued*)	
Exocrine pancreatic dysfunction	
Quick and Greer (88)	Conflicting reports of abnormal pancreatic exocrine function. Dysfunction of indirect mechanism speculated.
Brown et al. (12)	
Friedman et al. (41)	
McEwan-Alvarado et al. (66)	
Charchaflie et al. (19)	
Homovanillic acid (HVA)	
Brody et al. (10)	Increased HVA and 5-HIAA[b] (steady state) in CSF of ALS patients.
Chase et al. (20)	
Mendell (68)	
Abnormal mineral metabolism	
Yase (106)	Disturbance in Ca++ metabolism.
Yase et al. (107)	Relation between manganese exposure and ALS. Increased Ca++ content in CNS tissue. Mechanism speculated to be soft tissue calcification with interaction of divalent and trivalent cations (manganese and aluminum). Patten et al. concluded that hyperparathyroid persons may have treatable motor neuron disease. Speculation on relation between vitamin D deficiency and malabsorption of Ca++.
Patten et al. (83)	
Nakagawa et al. (71)	
Mallette et al. (67)	
Increased age	
Fullmer et al. (42, 43)	Collagenolytic factor.
Hirano et al. (47) Carpenter (18)	Axoplasmic transport blocking of neurofilaments; axostasis.
Störtebecker et al. (97)	Decreased number of functioning muscle units in elderly.
McComas et al. (65)	Increased incidence of disease in elderly; neuropathic changes in senile muscle.
Viral factors	
Zil'ber et al. (109)	Reported transmission to monkeys. Increased HLA-3 in ALS patients; virus-like particles seen on EMG[c] with immunosuppression cellular response to myelin protein and poliovirus; viral antigens in jejunal tissue. Relation between polio and later progression of motor neuron disease. Defective lymphocytes. Conflicting reports of elevated antibodies and immune deposits; deposits of IgG and C3 in glomeruli.
Nathanson and Goldblatt (72)	
Norris et al. (77)	
Antel et al. (2)	
Oshiro et al. (81)	
Kott et al. (57)	

Table 2 Theories Concerning the Etiology of ALS (*continued*)

Theory	*Explanation*
Remote effects of cancer	
Norris and Engel (75) Norris et al. (79)	Reported 10% incidence of major neoplasms in ALS patients. Few pathologic differences between primary motor neuron disease and carcinomatous neuropathy.
Circulating neurotoxins	
Wolfgram and Myers (104) Horwich et al. (50) Conradi et al. (23)	Cytotoxic effects of ALS sera on spinal cord extracts in animal and human. Circulating protein binding of lead in ALS patients.

[a] GTT = glucose tolerance test.
[b] 5-HIAA = 5-hydroxyindoleacetic acid.
[c] EMG = electromyogram.

observations concerned an apparent cluster of four cases in a small town of 1000 in South Dakota known to have seleniferous soil. However, to date no increase in body burden for selenium has been specifically found to be associated with ALS. Various letters refuting the suggestion of selenium as a factor in ALS may be referred to (58, 94).

Other possible noninfectious exogenous agents, such as aluminum and cycad, have also been suggested as etiologic agents of ALS, but neither enough interest nor enough data are available for intelligent comment at this point (59, 107). Our feeling is that exogenous factors should be sought in individual patients and vigorously treated if found.

METABOLIC DYSFUNCTION

Impaired Glucose Metabolism/Endocrine Dysfunction

Observations of ALS-like syndromes associated with pancreatic islet-cell tumors by at least two sources in the early 1950s gave some credence to the possible connection between hypoglycemia and ALS (6, 98). Cumings reported an abnormal oral glucose tolerance test (OGTT) in 16 of 41 patients with ALS (30). Ionasescu and Luca speculated, after studying 10 patients with motor neuron disease, that there was "defective glucose assimilation and consumption" (51). An article with great impact by Steinke and Tyler concluded that abnormality of glucose metabolism existed in patients with ALS was most likely related to pancreatic dysfunction (95). However, Collis and Engel reviewed this suggestion and concluded that a reduction of glucose receptor space was the most likely mechanism behind the abnormal OGTT (21). Numerous other reports on the topic followed (see Table 5) (41, 46, 56, 70). Recently, Saffer et al. studied 8 patients matched for degree of wasting with

8 controls and arrived at the conclusion that an abnormality in carbohydrate metabolism does exist in ALS (92). Astin examined CSF insulin and glucose and found no difference in the values of ALS patients as compared with those of a control population (5). The most outstanding problem with many of the studies concerning glucose metabolism is the numerous variables involved (i.e., age, history of diabetes mellitus, diet, exercise, muscle mass, family history, other diseases that may be associated with abnormal glucose tolerance). An additional problem is the definition of what is "normal" in studies that did not use matched controls.

Results of a clinical trial with amitriptyline reported by Brown and Mueller suggested that this drug might improve glucose utilization and relieve underlying depression in persons with ALS (13). Anecdotally, amitriptyline is used by several clinicians for symptomatic treatment of ALS patients. The issue of carbohydrate metabolism is not yet resolved. We are hopeful that our own preliminary results, which show an increase in the hemoglobin A_{1c} (HbA_{1c}), will reopen this problem (14). If HbA_{1c} levels, which reflect the total glucose metabolism in the 120-day life span of a red blood cell, are consistently elevated, a treatment trial will be initiated.

Abnormal Exocrine Pancreatic Function

The possibility of abnormal exocrine function as a factor in ALS has also had support. Quick and Greer described both abnormal endocrine and exocrine pancreatic function (88). However, Brown et al. (12), Friedman et al. (41), and McEwan-Alvarado et al. (66) reported normal exocrine function in patients with ALS. Seventeen ALS patients studied by Charchaflie et al. were evaluated for parotid and pancreas function (19). These studies suggested impaired flow rate and bicarbonate levels with indirect stimulation as compared with these measurements in control patients, while direct stimulation was normal.

Clinical drug trials using a pancreatic extract have been conducted by several groups. Quick and Greer reported no alteration in the disease process of their patient populations with use of this drug (88).

Homovanillic Acid

In the early 1970s, several investigators analyzed the CSF of ALS patients with regard to levels of homovanillic acid (HVA) and 5-hydroxyindoleacetic acid (5-HIAA) (9, 20, 68). All three groups concluded that a decreased steady state for HVA existed in the respective samples studied. On the basis of both this observation and the striking response of patients with Parkinson's disease to L-dopa, a clinical drug trial was conducted by Mendell et al (68). Levels of HVA in CSF increased with

(Text continues on page 350.)

Table 3 Clinical Trials of Vitamin or Specific Nutrient Deficiency as a Factor in ALS

Study	*No. of Patients*	*No. of Controls*	*Duration*	*Vitamin and Dosage*	*Patient Response*	*Evaluation of Therapy*
Bicknell[a]	4 ALS	0	?–18 mos	Wheat germ	"Not enough patients were used for a trial, however, results are promising."	Inadequate
Doyle and Merritt (36)	8 ALS	0	6–12 mos	Wheat germ oil; Vitamin E, 60 mg/day	". . . unable to produce improvement or to arrest the course of the disease with vitamin therapy."	Inadequate
Worster-Drought and Shafar (105)	25 ALS	0	5–10 mos	Oral Vitamin E, 30 mg/day	". . . general result of vitamin E has been disappointing." (3 of 25 patients had some improvement)	Inadequate
Weschler (102)	2 ALS	0	1–4 mos	Vitamin E, 60 mg tid	". . . the prompt response to vitamin E seemed to me to be of unusual significance."	Inadequate
Rosenberger (91)	9 ALS	0	Several mos to 1 yr	Vitamin E and Vitamin B, 100–300 mg combined, 3 times a day	"Improvement was noted in 8 of 9 patients."	Inadequate

DeJong (32)	35 "mixed"[b] 19 ALS	0	1 yr?	Wheat germ oil, 240 mg/day	No objective evidence of improvement.	Inadequate
Denker and Scheinman (33)	11 ALS	0	21–91 days	Vitamin E, 100 mg (total) po and im	"No therapeutic effects of any kind were observed."	Inadequate
Merwarth (69)	5 ALS	0	Variable	Vitamin E, 20–50 mg/day	Temporary improvement: ". . . drug is not without effect."	Inadequate
Lubin (63)	35 "mixed"[a] 7 ALS	0	3 days to 11 mos	Vitamin E, 300–?500 mg/day (variable)	"No patient with ALS . . . showed any definite improvement."	Inadequate
Zech and Telford[c]	3 ALS	0	23–120 days	Vitamin E, 23–90 g over total trial period	". . . results were negative and discouraging . . ."	Inadequate
Dorman et al. (35)	12 ALS	0	Minimum of 7 mos; followed up to 6 yrs on trial of both drugs.	Pancreatic extract, 6.3 g/day; vitamin E, 1500 U/day, iv	Negative	Inadequate

[a] Data taken from Bicknell F: Vitamin E in the treatment of muscular dystrophies and nervous diseases. Lancet 1:10–13, 1940.
[b] "Mixed" indicates that patients had mixed neurologic disease.
[c] Data taken from Zech V, Telford IR: Negative therapeutic effects of massive doses of vitamin E on amyotrophic lateral sclerosis. Arch Neurol Psychiatry 50:190–192, 1943.

Table 4 Clinical Trials of Heavy-Metal Toxicity as a Factor in ALS

Study	*No. of ALS Patients*	*No. of Controls*	*Duration*	*Dosage*	*Patient Response*	*Evaluation of Therapy*
Mercury						
Brown (11)	1	0	2 wks or until patient died	Dimercaprol, 1.5 cc q 4 hr for 2 weeks	No response to therapy	Inadequate
Kantarjian (53)	11	0	4 patients followed up for 6 mos	Dimercaprol, 300 mg/day for 2 days; 200 mg/day for 2 days; 100 mg/day for 8 days; vitamin B complex; vitamin B_{12}, 100–300 mg/day; vita-	Disease progressed in all 4 followed up; no immediate response with initial therapy.	Inadequate

Currier and Haerer (31)	31 (13 treated)	0	Variable	4 patients given Ca-disodium edetate; 1 given 2 g/day for 4–10 days; 3 given thioctic acid, 2–4 cc for 9 days; 1 given thioctic acid plus disodium edetate; 4 given penicillamine, 1 g/day for 10–14 days	"In none of the patients did the therapy appear to change the course of the disease."	Inadequate
Campbell et al. (15)	7	0	Up to 16 yrs	Varying courses of EDTA, penicillamine; some courses repeated	5 of 7 are reported to have an "altered" course.	Inadequate
Boothby et al. (8)	1	0	1 yr	Penicillamine, 1–2 g/day for 4 1-mo periods (1 mo on, 1 mo off)	Symptoms improved; EMG[a] and strength improved slightly.	Inadequate

[a] EMG = electromyogram.

Table 5 Clinical Trials of Metabolic Dysfunction as a Factor in ALS

Study	*No. of Patients*	*No. of Controls*	*Duration*	*Dosage*	*Patient Response*	*Evaluation of Therapy*
Impaired glucose metabolism/endocrine dysfunction						
Brown and Mueller, 1968	9 ALS	None stated	?1yr	Amitriptyline, 100–150 mg/day	Initial observation suggests alleviation of motor neuron symptoms; improved function in 3 patients.	Inadequate
Abnormal exocrine pancreatic function						
Quick and Greer (88)	Unknown	Unknown	Unknown	Vitamin E, pancreatic enzymes	Clinical improvement with treatment	Unknown
Brown et al. (12)	4 ALS	0	3–7 mos	Pancreozymin, 12 g/day at mealtime	No alteration of disease	Inadequate

Dorman et al. (35)	12 ALS	0	?3 yrs	Pancreatic extract, 6.3 g/day; Vitamin E, 1500 U/day	No alteration of disease	Inadequate
Homovanillic acid (HVA)						
Mendell et al. (68)	10 ALS	Comparison with pre-treatment pace of deterioration	1.5–9 mos (5.5 mos average)	L-dopa, average max. dose of 6.4 g/day	HVA increased 30-fold during trial, but motor performance did not improve.	Inadequate
Mineral metabolism						
Mallette et al. (67)	2 ALS (with previous findings of hypocalcemia and hypoparathyroidism)	0	Several wks	Vitamin D analogue, 0.25–0.5 mg/day	"Neurological disease continued to progress."	Inadequate

L-dopa treatment, but clinical weakness did not improve as compared with the pretreatment period.

Mineral Metabolism

Manganese mining takes place both on Guam and on the Kii Peninsula (15, 106). During the aging process, calcium metabolism is disturbed, with a decalcification of most body organs except for muscle and the central nervous system (CNS). A hypercalcemic state apparently may influence the absorption of manganese (106). Later reports by Yase et al. postulated a mechanism of soft-tissue calcification with an interaction of divalent (manganese) and trivalent (aluminum) cations (107). Patten et al. examined several patients with hyperparathyroidism (83). Fourteen of 16 individuals studied had electromyographic changes suggesting denervation. The authors concluded that many patients with hyperparathyroidism may have a treatable neuromuscular disease. Subsequently, Mallette et al. studied 12 ALS patients and found mild hypocalcemia in 2 (67). The investigators concluded that the abnormality in calcium metabolism was unclear, and they speculated on an "inborn defect in cellular metabolism" that may react to metabolic or toxic stimuli. The authors treated the 2 mildly hypocalcemic patients with vitamin D for several weeks and noted no alteration in disease progression. However, the topic of divalent- and trivalent-cation metabolism deserves more intensive evaluation and clinical trials. Of particular interest is both our own finding of elevated parathormone levels in more than half of our ALS patients (BW Festoff, CR Hartman, unpublished data) and the evidence of enhanced intestinal absorption and neural deposition of aluminum in rats given parathyroid hormone.

INCREASED AGE

Older persons in general have decreased muscle mass, and the incidence of ALS is higher in this population. McComas et al. speculated that motor neuron disease may be an example of an accelerated aging process (65). Fullmer et al. found a disorder of connective tissue that was associated with a collagenolytic factor. This is a very intriguing result whose impact was somewhat diminished by similar findings in patients with muscular atrophy and parkinsonism (42–44). Both Carpenter (18) and Hirano et al. (47) reported an accumulation of neurofilaments that was presumed to block axoplasmic transport. Because proliferation of neurofilaments is seen in aged nervous systems, the accumulation of neurofilaments in ALS patients suggests accelerated aging. In a study by Störtebecker, 9 of 15 patients with ALS had focal degenerative, nonarteriosclerotic changes in arterial biopsy samples (97).

Other findings that seem to fit into the theory of accelerated aging are studies by Deshmukh and Taylor (34), Hirano et al. (47, 48), and McClain (64). Neurolathyrism induces aginglike changes in the nervous system, with proliferation of neurofilaments. Lathyritic collagen has been characterized as having a decrease in cross-linking (64). It is intriguing to speculate whether similar compounds, which are concentrated in the chickpea (*Lathyrus sativas*), have effects on motor neuron or motor unit function or on collagenous or fibrous proteins. In this regard, an active ingredient, β-aminopropionitrile (BAPN), is used to induce the formation of lathyritic soluble (non-cross-linked) collagen. Another analogue, β,β-iminodipropionitrile (IDPN), induces spasticity, motor neuron alterations, and neurofilament accumulation in rats (34). It has also been reported recently that IDPN causes impaired slow transport of neurofilament proteins. Clinical observations in healthy aged persons have shown that there is a decrease in functioning motor units in persons older than 60 years; in addition, neuropathic changes similar to those seen in progressive muscular atrophy have been found in senile muscle (17).

Aside from several studies with isoprinosine (see section on *Viral Etiology*), drug trials concerned with the possibility of accelerated aging have not been reported. Isoprinosine was initially evaluated for use with senile dementia because the drug was thought to stimulate RNA synthesis. However, no effect of this drug on the course of ALS has been found. The concept of accelerated aging of the motor system tends to support the concept of abiotrophy found in the older literature. However, even so-called degenerative diseases may become treatable once the underlying defect is recognized and understood.

VIRAL FACTORS

In 1963, Zil'ber et al. reported the transmission of ALS in monkeys by administration of extracts from the medulla and spinal cord of persons who presumably had died from the disease (109). The monkeys were stricken with the disease after a long latent period (up to five years). However, this study has not been reproduced outside the Soviet Union.

Motor neuron disease following poliomyelitis has been observed by some authors since the phenomenon was first postulated by Charcot in 1875. Campbell et al. extensively reviewed 88 cases of poliomyelitis that were followed by development of a motor neuron syndrome in limbs initially unaffected by the acute polio infection (16). In 1973, Cremer et al. were unable to transmit poliovirus to cell cultures of various tissues from ALS patients and found no difference in antibody titers to poliovirus in these patients as compared with titers found in control patients (29). Lehrich et al. also studied neutralizing antibody titers of polio and mumps virus and reported no difference between titers in 27 ALS patients and those of 18 controls (60). In an uncontrolled study of 33 ALS patients, Oldstone et al. observed circulating immune complexes and moderate deposits of IgG and C3 in renal glomeruli (80). They also observed some degree of correlation between circulating immune complexes and rapidity of disease progression.

Other data supporting the theory of viral etiology include the presence of viruslike particles in muscle tissue of one ALS patient and an increased number of viral antigens in biopsy specimens of jejunal mucosa (81, 86). More recently, Jokelainen et al. concluded that an association of HLA-BW40 with ALS was possible; they also said that the lymphocytes observed in ALS patients seemed defective (52). Different conclusions regarding HLA antigens have been reached by four other groups. Kascak et al. examined 23 ALS patients and reported negative complement-fixing and hemagglutinin-inhibiting activity to 76 arboviruses (54).

Several clinical drug trials have been conducted on the possibility of viral etiology of ALS (see Table 6). Liversedge reported a trial of idoxuridine, which had no effect on the disease process (62). Isoprinosine was given clinical trials but proved to be of no efficacy on an objective basis (10, 39, 85). Engel and Munsat are reported to have tried amantadine, which also was unsuccessful (45). To our knowledge, a controlled study regarding the effect of amantadine in ALS has not been reported.

IMMUNOLOGIC FACTORS

Urbánek and Jansa studied cellular response in ALS patients by means of the skin-window technique and found a delayed migration and decreased number of macrophages as compared with controls (101). Pederson et al. found no significant deviation in HLA antigens of 25 ALS patients from those of control patients (84). In 1978, Barron and Heffner examined samples of muscle tissue from 20 ALS patients and found no immune deposits (7). Palo et al. reported the presence of immune complexes in muscle but stated that these complexes were thought to be a "generalized, immunological reaction" of secondary origin (82). Hoffman et al. evaluated cellular immunity in patients with Guamanian ALS and in those with parkinsonism-dementia and concluded that a defect existed; however, they did not find this defect in patients with classic ALS (49).

Two studies have reported on the use of corticosteroid therapy for ALS. Pieper and Fields evaluated the effects of intrathecal administration of 50 mg of hydrocortisone alone (87) (Table 6), and Norris has reported on a trial of oral azathioprine and prednisone. Both groups felt

Table 6 Clinical Trials of a Viral or Immunologic Etiology for ALS

Study	*No. of Patients*	*No. of Controls*	*Duration*	*Dosage*	*Patient Response*	*Evaluation of Therapy*
Pieper and Fields (87)	21 ALS	0	9–10 mos	Vitamin B_{12}, 1000 mg; hydrocortisone, 50 mg; 16 intrathecal injections of each, 4 per mo	"This investigation project is reported to show the failure of another therapy for ALS . . ."	Inadequate
Liversedge (62)	10 ALS (unselected, successive)	0	2 mos follow-up	Idoxuridine, 1.5 g iv, in 50 cc D5W on 5 successive days	"The treatment had absolutely no influence on the course of the disease . . ."	Inadequate
Percy et al. (85)	9 ALS (double-blind)	5	6 mos	Isoprinosine, 6 g/day (2 wks off out of 8 wks)	". . . no statistical difference between the 2 groups."	Inadequate
Fareed and Tyler (39)	13 ALS	12	3 mos	Isoprinosine, 300 g/day	Ineffective by subjective and objective criteria.	Inadequate
Brody et al. (10)	8 ALS	8	2 yrs	Isoprinosine, 4 g/day	Ineffective; subjectively, patients were "helped."	Inadequate
Engel and Munsat (45)	Unknown	?	?	Amantadine (dosage unknown)	Unsuccessful	Unknown
Olson et al.[a]	16 ALS	Double-blind, placebo controlled	48 wks	Tilorone, 1 g/wk	Treatment did not alter course of disease.	Adequate

[a] Data taken from Olson WH, Simons JA, Halaas GW: Therapeutic trial of tilorone in ALS: lack of benefit in a double-blind, placebo-controlled study. Neurology 28:1293–1295, 1978.

the therapies were ineffective. To our knowledge, a controlled study of immunosuppressive therapy for ALS has not been reported.

REMOTE EFFECTS OF CANCER

Reports of carcinoma and ALS in the literature prompted a study by Norris and Engel (75). Of 130 ALS patients evaluated, 10% were found to have major neoplasms. Later, Norris et al. compared 8 cases of "carcinomatous neuropathy" with 12 cases of primary motor neuron disease (79). The authors concluded that "There are few pathological differences to separate the various types of primary and secondary motor neuron disease." However, most clinicians have not confirmed the 10% incidence of carcinoma.

Two case reports of insulinoma were associated with ALS (1 patient reportedly improved after removal of the tumor). Norris and Engel commented that 7 of 13 patients with major neoplasms were "cured" of the tumor by radiation therapy, surgery, and/or chemotherapy (75). However, none of the 7 had remission of ALS-like symptoms.

CIRCULATING NEUROTOXINS

Recently, interest has developed in the circulating-factor theory. In 1973, Wolfgram and Myers demonstrated a specific cytotoxic effect of 70% of ALS sera on mouse embryonic motor neurons in culture (104). This factor was nondialyzable and was speculated to be a protein. Horwich et al. found a specific toxic effect of sera from 8 control patients and from 14 ALS patients on motor neurons, suggesting that there was no unique effect of ALS sera on motor neurons (50).

A blind study conducted by Wolfgram was reported in the proceedings of a recent symposium on research trends in ALS (104). In that study, the author found a high incidence of specific cytotoxic effects of ALS sera on motor neurons. He concluded that technical factors may have precluded specificity in the study by Horwich et al. (50). Recently, positive results were reported by Bartfeld's group, giving credence to the earlier reports (90). Whatever the toxic factor is, it seems to possess two features—its specificity for motor neurons and its nondialyzability—that require it to be characterized and purified as soon as its biologic effect is confirmed. The latter feature may have relevance to studies reported by Conradi et al. (23), who hypothesize that a retrograde axonal transport of lead is pathogenetic in ALS. In ALS patients, the lead may be bound to serum proteins in increased concentration (25).

Drug studies that are related to the circulating-factor theory have involved therapy with trypan red (dye) and modified neurotoxin (see Table 7). In 1948, Aird's rationale for the trial of trypan red was his

Table 7 Clinical Trials of Circulating Neurotoxin as a Factor in ALS

Study	*No. of Patients*	*No. of Controls*	*Duration*	*Dosage*	*Patient Response*	*Evaluation of Therapy*
Aird (1)	12 ALS (double-blind)	0	12–57 mos	Trypan red, 25 mg/kg; Vitamin A, 25,000 U/day	"Course of ALS appears to be modified in half of patients . . ." (lowers permeability to CSF barrier).	Inadequate
Sanders and Fellowes (93)	Unknown	0	6 wks	Modified neurotoxin, 1.0–1.7 ml, qod im	"Partial treatment"; 10% "functional improvement"; 15%–42% stabilized with im injection of modified neurotoxin.	Inadequate
Norris ([45] and personal communication)	50 ALS	0	Unknown	Neurotoxin (dosage unknown)	No effect	Inadequate
Tyler (100)	74 ALS	Double-blind	6 mos	Modified neurotoxin or placebo, 1.0–1.7 ml, qod im	Modified neurotoxin had no objective meaningful improvement in course of ALS.	Adequate

Table 8 Empirical Trials of Drugs for the Treatment of ALS

Study	*No. of Patients*	*No. of Controls*	*Duration*	*Drug and Dosage*	*Patient Response*	*Evaluation of Therapy*
Copperman et al. (28)	1 ALS	0	?~ 1 yr	Securinine, 1.2 mg bid po, increased to 4 mg bid; then 2 mg subcutaneously, increased to 16 mg bid po	Symptomatic improvement	Inadequate
Norris (73)	84 ALS	0	5 yrs	?Guanidine in combination with or as alternative to other medications	". . . in the presence of disease that is often fatal, the major side effects are low enough to justify a controlled trial in ALS."	Inadequate
Copperman (27)	8 ALS	0	Unknown	Securinine (dosage not stated)	No significant effect on progression of disease. Significant ameliorating effects.	Inadequate

Norris et al. (78)	30 ALS; 11 received "adequate dosages"	6 patients given EDTA; only 13 given low-dose guanidine	6 to 9–10 mos	Guanidine, 1.5–2.5 mg/kg/day or 25 mg/kg/day (dosages randomly assigned)	No significance after 3 mos, but after 6 mos the group on 25 mg/kg/day was considered to have "better status" as measured by objective testing.	Inadequate
Erfahrungen (37)	Unknown; patients had combinations of ALS, spinocerebellar degeneration, dystrophic muscle disease, peripheral nervous system disease		Not stated	Guanidine, 20–40 mg/kg/day	Supports the assumption that guanidine slows progress of the disease.	Inadequate

study, which demonstrated a "lowered permeability of the CSF barrier" to various drugs (e.g., cocaine) in combination with supravital dyes (1). He studied 12 patients with ALS and concluded that the disease course was modified in 50% of the patients. We were unsuccessful in locating other references to this treatment of ALS.

Sanders and Fellowes reported 10% improvement and 15%–42% stabilization in ALS patients treated with injections of modified neurotoxin (93). This study stimulated enthusiasm in a large number of ALS patients. More recently, Tyler evaluated modified neurotoxin in a double-blind trial but did not observe improvement in the course of the disease with this treatment (100). Tyler conducted his study with 48 patients over six months. It is a vitally important study from two perspectives. First, it represents the first carefully controlled, double-blind clinical trial (fulfilling most of the criteria in Table 1); second, it documents variations not previously stressed in the clinical course of ALS. The latter point represents an important foundation for a prospective two-phase study of the natural history of ALS, while the former should serve as a model for future clinical trials. A double-blind study by Rivera evaluating the efficacy of modified neurotoxin showed similar results.

EMPIRICAL TRIALS

Copperman described an ALS patient who responded symptomatically to securinine, a CNS stimulant used in the Soviet Union and China (28). A later publication based on a study of eight individuals reported no significant effect of the drug on disease progression but noted "significant ameliorating effects" (27).

Guanidine was studied by Norris et al., who concluded that the group of patients on therapeutic doses were considered to have a "better status" as measured objectively (73, 78). Erfahrungen reported a "slowing down" of diseases (ALS, spinocerebellar degeneration, dystrophic muscle disease, peripheral nervous system disease) after treatment with guanidine (37). (See Table 8 for summary of empirical drug trials.)

CONCLUSION

After reviewing the vast numbers of published reports that deal with suggested etiologies and therapeutic trials, we were struck by the recurring stories of success and failure. It is interesting that, although the earlier treatment trials were enthusiastic, the positive results were clearly not strong enough to stand the test of time. We had hoped that this review would reveal a particular area of investigation that could be pursued on the basis of previous treatment trials. Although we did not realize that goal, certain clues may be uncovered in the areas of metabolic failure or deficiency.

Two threads can be found in the fabric of the various reports described in this review. First, the etiology of ALS may be multifactorial. Amyotrophic lateral sclerosis may be a syndrome that has diverse causes leading to motor neuronal or nerve–muscle failure either that is irreversible or whose reversibility has not yet been identified. The role of the concept of abiotrophy in this context, as discussed by early neurologists, is not yet known. If abiotrophy does represent an etiology of ALS, then the disease may have no more nosologic meaning than congestive heart failure, seizure, or syncope. However, we are not firmly led in this direction, primarily because of the specificity of ALS for the motor system.

Second, clinical therapeutic trials have demonstrated increasing application of problem-solving techniques to the study of ALS (22). Application of the scientific method has been difficult in general, but even more so with regard to understanding motor neuron disease. The latter point encourages us that the puzzle of ALS can be put together, with both the pieces that constitute this review and future definitive studies. In this regard, we feel it pertinent to include the comments of Liversedge.

> Whatever information emerges from current experiments and theories on the biochemistry of neural function, the true assessment of the efficacy of treatment in motor-neurone disease will come from clinical trials; hence one is justified in carrying on empirical clinical experiments even in the absence of definitive scientific justification (61).

Acknowledgments

The authors gratefully acknowledge the assistance of Ms. Patsy Rush and Ms. Sherry Rampani in the preparation of this manuscript. Partial support for this project came from the Veterans Administration Medical Center, Kansas City, MO, and the Endowment Fund, University of Kansas Medical Center, Kansas City, KS.

REFERENCES

1. Aird RB: Trypan red therapy of amyotrophic lateral sclerosis. Arch Neurol Psychiatry 59:779–789, 1948

2. Antel JP, Arnason GW, Fuller TC, et al: Histocompatibility typing in amyotrophic lateral sclerosis. Arch Neurol 33:423–425, 1976

3. Ask-Upmark E: Amyotrophic lateral sclerosis observed in 5 persons after gastric resection. Gastroenterology 15:257–259, 1950

4. Ask-Upmark E, Muerling S: On the presence of a deficiency factor in the pathogenesis of amyotrophic lateral sclerosis. Acta Med Scand 152: 217–221, 1955

5. Astin KJ, Wilde CE, Davies-Jones AB: Glucose metabolism and insulin response in the plasma and CSF in motor neuron disease. J Neurol Sci 25:205–210, 1975

6. Barris RW: Pancreatic adenoma (hyperinsulinism) associated with neuromuscular disorders. Ann Intern Med 38:124–129, 1953

7. Barron SA, Hoffner RR: Immune complexes in amyotrophic lateral sclerosis (letter). Lancet 1:1040, 1978

8. Boothby JA, DeJesus PV, Rowland LP: Reversible forms of motor neuron disease. Arch Neurol 31:18–23, 1974

9. Brody J, Chase TN, Gordon EK: Depressed monoamine catabolite levels in CSF of patients with Parkinson dementia of Guam. N Engl J Med 282:947–950, 1970

10. Brody JA, Chen K-M, Yase Y, et al: Inosiplex and amyotrophic lateral sclerosis. Therapeutic trial in patients on Guam. Arch Neurol 30: 322–323, 1974

11. Brown IA: Chronic mercurialism. Arch Neurol Psychiatry 72:674–681, 1954

12. Brown J, Colin R, Kater MH: Pancreatic function in patients with amyotrophic lateral sclerosis. Neurology 19:185–189, 1969

13. Brown WA, Mueller PS: Psychological function in individuals with amyotrophic lateral sclerosis. Psychosom Med 32:141–152, 1970

14. Bunn HF, Gabbay KH, Gallop PM: The glycosylation of hemoglobin: relevance to diabetes mellitus. Science 200:21–27, 1978

15. Campbell AMG, Williams ER, Barltrop D: Motor neuron disease and exposure to lead. J Neurol Neurosurg Psychiatry 33:877–885, 1970

16. Campbell AMG, Williams ER, Pearce J: Late motor neuron degeneration following poliomyelitis. Neurology 19:1101–1106, 1969

17. Campbell MJ, McComas AJ, Petito F: Physiological changes in aging muscles. J Neurol Neurosurg Psychiatry 36:174–182, 1973

18. Carpenter S: Proximal axonal enlargement in motor neuron disease. Neurology 18:841–851, 1968

19. Charchaflie RJ, Fernandez LB, Perec CJ, et al: Functional studies of the parotid and pancreas glands in amyotrophic lateral sclerosis. J Neurol Neurosurg Psychiatry 37:863–867, 1974

20. Chase TN, Schnur JA, Brody JA, et al: Parkinson-dementia and amyotrophic lateral sclerosis of Guam. Arch Neurol 25:9–13, 1971

21. Collis WJ, Engel WK: Glucose metabolism in 5 neuromuscular disorders. Neurology 18:915–925, 1968

22. Colton T: *Statistics in Medicine.* Boston, Little, Brown & Company, 1974, pp 254–271

23. Conradi S, Ronnevi LO, Stibler H: Serum protein binding of lead in vitro in amyotrophic lateral sclerosis patients and controls. J Neurol Sci 37:95–105, 1978

24. Conradi S, Ronnevi LO, Vesterberg O: Abnormal tissue distribution of lead in amyotrophic lateral sclerosis. J Neurol Sci 29:259–265, 1976

25. Conradi S, Ronnevi LO, Vesterberg O: Increased plasma levels of lead in patients with amyotrophic lateral sclerosis compared with control subjects as determined by flameless atomic absorption spectrophotometry. J Neurol Neurosurg Psychiatry 41:389–393, 1978

26. Cooper IS: *Living with Chronic Neurologic Disease—A Handbook for Patient and Family.* New York, WW Norton Co, 1976

27. Copperman R: Securinine (letter). JAMA 228:288, 1974

28. Copperman R, Copperman G, Ara-Den M: Securinine—a central nervous system stimulant as used in treatment of amyotrophic lateral sclerosis. Pa Med 76:36–41, 1973

29. Cremer NE, Oshiro LS, Norris FH, et al: Cultures from tissue from patients with amyotrophic lateral sclerosis. Arch Neurol 29:331–333, 1973

30. Cumings JN: Motor neurone disease. Proceedings of the Royal Society of Medicine 55:1023–1024, 1962

31. Currier RD, Haerer AF: ALS and metallic toxins. Arch Environ Health 17:712–719, 1968

32. DeJong RN: Vitamin E and alpha tocopherol therapy of neuromuscular and muscular disorders. Arch Neurol Psychiatry 46:1068–1075, 1941

33. Denker PG, Scheinman L: Treatment of amyotrophic lateral sclerosis with vitamin E. JAMA 116:1893–1895, 1941

34. Deshmukh P, Taylor JJ: Neurofibrillary tangles in experimental neurolathyrism in rats induced by iminodipropionitrile. Acta Neuropathol (Berl) 41:17–22, 1978

35. Dorman JD, Engel WK, Fried DM: Therapeutic trial in amyotrophic lateral sclerosis. JAMA 209:257–258, 1969

36. Doyle AM, Merritt HH: Vitamin therapy of diseases of the neuromuscular apparatus. Arch Neurol Psychiatry 45:672–679, 1941

37. Erfahrungen I: Use of guanidine (summary). Wien Klin Wochenschr 2:43, 1978

38. Evans HM, Burr GO: Development of paralysis in the suckling young of mothers deprived of vitamin E. J Biol Chem 76:273–293, 1928

39. Fareed GC, Tyler RH: The use of isoprinosine in patients with amyotrophic lateral sclerosis. Neurology 21:937–940, 1971

40. Felmus CT, Patten BM, Swanke L: Antecedent events in ALS. Neurology 26:167–172, 1976

41. Friedman HM, Tzagournis M, Ruppert RD: Pancreatic exocrine and endocrine function in ALS. Neurology 19:283–284, 1969

42. Fullmer HM, Lazarus G, Gibson AW, et al: Collagenolytic activity of the skin associated with neuromuscular diseases including ALS. Lancet 1:1007–1009, 1966

43. Fullmer H, Lazarus GS, Stam AC, et al: Collagenase in neuromuscular diseases. In: *Motor Neuron Diseases. Research on Amyotrophic Lateral Sclerosis and Related Disorders.* Edited by FH Norris Jr, LT Kurland. New York, Grune and Stratton, 1969, pp 242–244

44. Fullmer HM, Siedler HD, Krooth RS, et al: A cutaneous disorder of connective tissue in amyotrophic lateral sclerosis. Neurology 10:717–724, 1960

45. Goldblatt D: Treatment of ALS. Adv Neurol 17:786–796, 1977

46. Gotoh F, Koto KA, Kataoka K, et al: Abnormal insulin secretion in ALS. J Neurol Sci 16:201–207, 1972

47. Hirano A, Kurland LT, Sayre GP: Familial amyotrophic lateral sclerosis. Arch Neurol 16:232, 1967

48. Hirano A, Llena J, Streifler M, et al: Anterior horn cell changes in a case of neurolathyrism. Acta Neuropathol (Berl) 35:277–283, 1976

49. Hoffman PM, Robbins DS, Gibbs CJ, et al: Histocompatibility antigens in amyotrophic lateral sclerosis and parkinsonism-dementia on Guam. Lancet 2:717–718, 1977

50. Horwich MS, Engel WK, Chauvin PB: ALS sera applied to cultured motor neurons. Arch Neurol 30:332–333, 1974

51. Ionasescu V, Luca N: Studies on carbohydrate metabolism in amyotrophic lateral sclerosis and hereditary proximal spinal muscular atrophy. Acta Neurol Scand 40:47–57, 1964

52. Jokelainen M, Tiilikainen A, Lapinleimu K: Polio antibodies and HLA antigens in ALS. Tissue Antigens 10:259–266, 1977

53. Kantarjian A: A syndrome resembling ALS following chronic mercurialism. Neurology 11:639–644, 1961

54. Kascak RJ, Shope R, Donnefeld H, et al: Antibody response to arboviruses. Absence of increased response in amyotrophic lateral sclerosis and multiple sclerosis. Arch Neurol 35:440–442, 1978

55. Kilness AW, Hochberg FH: ALS in a high selenium environment. JAMA 237:2843–2844, 1977

56. Koerner DR: Abnormal carbohydrate metabolism in amyotrophic lateral sclerosis and parkinson dementia on Guam. Diabetes 25:1055–1065, 1976

57. Kott E, Livni E, Zamer R, et al: ALS: cell mediated immunity to poliovirus and basic myelin protein in patients with high frequency of HLA-BW 35 (abstract). Neurology 26:378, 1976

58. Kurland LT: Amyotrophic lateral sclerosis and selenium. JAMA 238:2365–2366, 1977

59. Kurland LT: An appraisal of the neurotoxicity of cycad and the etiology of ALS on Guam. Fed Proc 31:1540–1542, 1972

60. Lehrich JR, Oger J, Arnason BGW: Neutralizing antibodies to poliovirus and mumps in amyotrophic lateral sclerosis. J Neurol Sci 23:537–540, 1974

61. Liversedge LA: Glycocyamine and betaine in motor neuron disease. Lancet 2:1136–1139, 1956

62. Liversedge LA, Swinburn WR, Yuill GM: Idoxuridine and motor neuron disease (communication). Br Med J 755:749–750, 1970

63. Lubin AJ: Use of alpha tocopherol in the treatment of neuromuscular disorders. Arch Intern Med 69:836–855, 1942

64. McClain PE: In vitro aging-like changes in the cross-linking characteristics of collagen from intramuscular connective tissue. Gerontology 17:139–147, 1971

65. McComas AJ, Upton ARM, Sica REP: Motor neuron disease and aging. Lancet 2:1477–1480, 1977

66. McEwan-Alvarado G, Hightower N, Carney LR, et al: Exocrine pancreatic function in patients with amyotrophic lateral sclerosis. Am J Dig Dis 16:107–110, 1971

67. Mallette LE, Patten B, Cook JD, et al: Calcium metabolism in amyotrophic lateral sclerosis. Diseases of the Nervous System 38:457–461, 1977

68. Mendell JR, Chase TN, Engel WK: Amyotrophic lateral sclerosis: a study of central monoamine metabolism and therapeutic trial of levodopa. Arch Neurol 25:320–325, 1971

69. Merwarth HR: Synthetic vitamin E in the treatment of amyotrophic lateral sclerosis and related disorders. Diseases of the Nervous System 2:325–329, 1941

70. Mueller PS, Quick DT: Studies of glucose, insulin and lipid metabolism in amyotrophic lateral sclerosis and other neuromuscular diseases. Journal of Latin American Medicine 76:190–201, 1970

71. Nakagawa S, Suematsu C, Kumamato T, et al: Calcium and magnesium deficiency-induced atrophy of muscle and calcium accumulation in the spinal cord. Experientia 32:915–917, 1976

72. Nathanson N, Goldblatt D: Spinal ganglion involvement in experimental poliomyelitis. Neurology 14:1132–1148, 1964

73. Norris FH: Guanidine in ALS (letter). N Engl J Med 288:690–691, 1973

74. Norris FH: Discussion. Trans Am Neurol Assoc 97:22–23, 1972

75. Norris FH, Engel WK: Carcinomatous myelopathy. In: *The Remote Effects of Cancer on the Nervous System.* Edited by Lord Brain and FH Norris. New York, Grune and Stratton, 1964, pp 24–34

76. Norris FH, Ü KS: Amyotrophic lateral sclerosis and low urinary selenium levels. JAMA 239:404, 1978

77. Norris FH, Aguilar MJ, Colton RP, et al: Tubular particles in a case of recurrent lymphocytic meningitis followed by amyotrophic lateral sclerosis. J Neuropathol Exp Neurol 34:133–147, 1975

78. Norris FH, Calanchini PR, Fallat RJ, et al: The administration of guanidine in ALS. Neurology 24:721–728, 1974

79. Norris FH, McMenemey WH, Barnard RO: Anterior horn pathology in carcinomatous neuromyopathy compared with other forms of motor neuron disease. In *Motor Neuron Diseases. Research on Amyotrophic Lateral Sclerosis and Related Disorders.* Edited by FH Norris, LT Kurland. New York, Grune and Stratton, 1969, pp 100–111

80. Oldstone MBA, Perrin LH, Wilson CB, et al: Evidence for immunocomplex formation in patients with amyotrophic lateral sclerosis. Lancet 2:169–172, 1976

81. Oshiro L, Cremer NE, Norris FH, et al: Virus-like particles in muscle from a patient with amyotrophic lateral sclerosis. Neurology 26:57–60, 1976

82. Palo JA, Rissanen E, Jokinen J, et al: Kidney and skin biopsy in ALS (letter). Lancet 1:1270, 1978

83. Patten BM, Harati H, Acost L, et al: Free amino acid levels in amyotrophic lateral sclerosis. Neurology 3:305–309, 1978

84. Pederson I, Platz P, Jersild C, et al: HLA (SD and LD) in patients with amyotrophic lateral sclerosis. J Neurol Sci 31:313–318, 1977

85. Percy AK, Davis LE, Johnston D, et al: Failure of isoprinosine in ALS (letter). N Engl J Med 285:689, 1971

86. Pertschuk LP, Cook AW, Gupta JK, et al: Jejunal immunopathology in ALS and multiple sclerosis identification of viral antigens by immunofluorescence. Lancet 1:1119–1123, 1977

87. Pieper SJL, Fields WS: Failure of ALS to respond to intrathecal steroid and vitamin B_{12}. Arch Neurol 19:522–526, 1957

88. Quick DT, Greer M: Pancreatic dysfunction in patients with amyotrophic lateral sclerosis. Neurology 17:112–116, 1967

89. Quick DT, Mueller PS: Glucose, fatty acid, insulin and growth hormone abnormalities in amyotrophic lateral sclerosis (abstract). Neurology 19:283, 1969

90. Roisen FJ, Baxter J, Bartfeld H, et al: Amyotrophic lateral sclerosis: *in vitro* neuron-specific cytotoxicity of human sera. In *Proceedings of the 4th International Congress on Neuromuscular Diseases* 114a, 1978

91. Rosenberger AI: Observations on the treatment of amyotrophic lateral sclerosis with vitamin E. Medical Record (New York), 1941, pp 97–100

92. Saffer D, Morley J, Bell PLA: Carbohydrate metabolism in motor neuron disease. J Neurol Neurosurg Psychiatry 40:533, 1977

93. Sanders M, Fellowes J: Use of detoxified snake neurotoxin and the partial treatment for ALS. J Cancer Cytol 15:26–30, 1975

94. Schwartz K: Amyotrophic lateral sclerosis and selenium. JAMA 238:2365, 1977

95. Steinke J, Tyler HR: The association of amyotrophic lateral sclerosis (motor neuron disease) and carbohydrate intolerance, a clinical study. Metabolism 13:1376–1381, 1964

96. Stiel JN: The incidence of gastrectomy and gastric secretion in motor neuron disease. Australas Ann Med 16:176–177, 1967

97. Störtebaker P, Pap de Pesteny M, Seeman T, et al: Vascular and metabolic studies of amyotrophic lateral sclerosis. Neurology 20:1157–1160, 1970

98. Tom MI, Richardson JC: Hypoglycemia from islet cell tumor of pancreas with amyotrophy and cerebrospinal nerve cell changes. J Neuropathol Exp Neurol 10:57–66, 1951

99. Tomanaga M: Histochemical and ultrastructural changes in senile human skeletal muscle. J Am Geriatr Soc 25:125–131, 1977

100. Tyler HR: Double-blind study of modified neurotoxin in motor neuron disease. Neurology 29:77–81, 1979

101. Urbánek K, Jansa P: Amyotrophic lateral sclerosis—abnormal cellular inflammatory response. Arch Neurol 30:186–187, 1974

102. Weschler IS: Recovery in amyotrophic lateral sclerosis. JAMA 114: 948–950, 1940

103. Wilson SAK: *Neurology*, 2nd ed. Edited by AN Bruce. Baltimore, Williams & Wilkins, 1955, pp 1164–1165

104. Wolfgram F, Myers L: ALS: effect of serum on anterior horn cells in tissue culture. Science 179:579–580, 1973

105. Worster-Drought C, Shafar J: Motor neurone degeneration treated with vitamin E. Lancet 2:209–212, 1941

106. Yase Y: The pathogenesis of amyotrophic lateral sclerosis. Lancet 2:292–295, 1972

107. Yase Y, Fumio Y, Vebaystti Y, et al: ALS, interaction of divalent metals in CNS tissue and soft tissue calcification. Proc Jap Acad 50:401–406, 1974

108. Zech V, Telford IR: Negative therapeutic effects of massive doses of vitamin E on amyotrophic lateral sclerosis. Arch Neurol Psychiatry 50:190–192, 1943

109. Zil'ber LA, Bajdakova ZL, Angardaus J, et al: Study of the etiology of amyotrophic lateral sclerosis. Bull WHO 29:449–456, 1963

Commentary

H. Richard Tyler

Dr. Festoff and Dr. Crigger's review of previous therapeutic trials demonstrates that our present system of carrying out and reporting clinical trials in ALS is unsatisfactory. I would like to discuss some of the problems and suggest a system that might be of help.

This chapter reviews all previously published studies on agents used to treat ALS and rejects most of them as being inadequate, yet all were published in responsible journals. The best aspect of this review is that it describes nearly 50 possible therapies for ALS patients that have not been adequately studied and for which tests have not disproved the initial claims. One problem is that we have no journal of negative results. Thus, many of us have tried some of the items reported here and can guarantee that they do not work, but what can we do? Do we submit papers stating that the therapy did not work on 15 patients? As I see it, this lack of a forum for such failures is one of the problems with the literature.

Although this chapter rejects most previous trials as being inadequate, I do not think that a double-blind study is necessary for any treatment that proves to be a cure for ALS. If one were to inform me of five patients who were cured of this disease by a responsible investigator, I would accept it and I would be delighted to prescribe the treatment for my patients. I would not need a double-blind study. Thus, there will be no problem when we find a cure. I think the problem arises when someone says that he or she has been able to demonstrate stabilization of the disease or claims to have found a partial treatment. Then we get into the problem of what these terms might mean. Thus, I believe that double-blind studies, which are terribly expensive and difficult to do right, should not be done initially. For instance, the study we carried out using cobra venom did not answer many of our questions; it did not show the effect of the drug on the young person or the effects of administration over a period longer than six months. It really only answered a few limited questions.

There are a few specific problems that are inherent in the diagnosis of ALS; these problems are related to communication among neurologists and to governmental control. First, neurologists do not always agree on diagnosis or prognosis. An investigator who claims to have demonstrated partial treatment or partial cure must have a comparable control series. Whatever the therapist is talking about has to be spelled out clearly; a control series that conforms to his criteria will solve that problem. If an investigator wants to define ALS narrowly, I can understand and accept that. But, in a therapeutic trial, I want the control series to be identical to the treated cases; we must avoid mixed series.

Second, the neurologist must be in a position to counsel his or her patients or to supervise trial of the drug in question directly. The solution is building a better communication system than that currently provided by our system of meetings and journals. Such a system would allow neurologists to know who is experimenting with what therapies and with what results.

The third problem involves governmental licensure, which is required for any experimental use of a drug. Although this is a complicated situation, it poses problems only with unique medicines. The government limits use of these drugs to a small number of investigators and thus forces dislocation of patients to where the medicine is. I think that, if a physician is in possession of a medicine that requires governmental control, the government should either insist that the physician using the medicine be responsible for the claims he or she makes for it, or withdraw the physician's license to use the medicine. I also think that the government should guarantee availability of that medicine to other investigators.

It is my belief, therefore, that our present system of dealing wth ALS has failed. Thus, I would like to make the following suggestions with an aim toward improving the situation.

I think that a cadre of neurologists or physicians should be established who see about 20–25 ALS patients a year, who remain responsible for them, and who are willing to treat them with experimental medications. The cadre should be open to all physicians. The only requirement would be submission of a quarterly report on what they are doing and the results. The Medical Advisory Board of the Amyotrophic Lateral Sclerosis Society of America or of another medical society would make comments and recommendations on only those reports that look promising. These reports would be published and sent to all neurologists and physicians who are interested and, about two weeks later, sent to patients and to the press so that everyone would learn what is going on and who is doing what. Members of the cadre could also test drugs or treatments suggested by physicians who are not members. This system would guide people who are not a part of the establishment into approved channels.

In addition, a Board of Experts would decide, on the basis of these reports, whether a full double-blind study should be performed. The double-blind studies would be set up with appropriate questions asked (the questions are critical). Funded studies would be carried out in two to three places with the originator of the idea of the trial having priority. It would be possible, however, for anyone who found the money and had the drug available to carry out such a study. It would be best to have two or three studies that are clearly centrally funded and conducted only after a central committee has indicated a need for them. Once the drug has been studied, the report would go back to this panel, and the members would express an opinion on it and encourage publication. If necessary, there would be minority and majority statements.

What benefits would this system offer? It would keep physicians who are treating patients with ALS informed of progress with various therapies. Physicians would be able to use any medication they wished, or could send a patient to an investigator for a particular treatment. The physician not only would receive a quarterly report on what investigators are willing to say publicly, but would also know that patients would be receiving the same information. Patients would also be better equipped to decide whether or not to start or discontinue a particular treatment. In short, the system would ensure that investigators, physicians, and patients would be working together toward the same ends.

23 Research Strategies

Richard T. Johnson

Cure for the greatest part of human misery is not radical but palliative.
Samuel Johnson, *Rambler No. 32,* 1750

The cause of amyotrophic lateral sclerosis is unknown, and we have no definitive method to prevent, arrest, or reverse its tragic course. It seems appropriate, therefore, that this conference has focused on the mitigation or alleviation of symptoms, i.e., on summarizing the information now available on the optimal management of the physiologic and psychologic symptoms of our patients. One supportive treatment is to share with our patients the hope that a cause and cure for ALS will be found, if not for them, at least for the next generation. Such research is still in its formative stage, but the horizon is broadening.

Amyotrophic lateral sclerosis is one of several degenerative diseases that gave neurology the unhappy reputation of being "the specialty for the diagnosis of untreatable disease." The neuropathologic concept of abiotrophy, popularized by Gowers at the turn of the century, did not help this grim image of inevitable nerve cell death. The concept of abiotrophy assumed that under proper circumstances cells were immortal, and that death of specific cells in particular diseases occurred as a "consequence of a defect of vital endurance" (14). Studies of cell biology have disproved the immortality of normal cells and have provided understanding of normal cell function and maintenance and the intrinsic and extrinsic factors that interfere with cellular integrity. As this knowledge is applied to neural cells, degenerative processes of the central nervous system are becoming promising targets of research.

BASIC NEUROBIOLOGY

During the past two decades the field of neurobiology has burgeoned, but interest has focused primarily on development. Most studies have dealt with cell differentiation, cell migration, and the development of cell-to-cell contact and interaction. Little attention has been directed toward the maintenance of function in the mature, differentiated, neural cell. For example, how can a motor neuron, maintaining an axon over a meter in length, survive and function for over 70 years? Even if one disregards the wear and tear of daily use and the potential for damage from background radiation, trauma, or environmental toxins, the laws of chemical kinetics mandate that the simple maintenance of normal body temperature must cause a certain denaturation of proteins and nucleic acids (11). Proteins and RNA can, of course, be replaced over the lifetime of the motor neuron, but what of the DNA itself in this static cell population? One possibility is that the motor neurons contain sufficient copies of the genetic information that the injuries caused by thermal noise and other insults can be incurred without loss of function. A more likely explanation is that the enzymes that excise and repair damaged DNA are active in neural cells. Fibroblast cultures from patients with xeroderma pigmentosum, a disease in which DNA repair mechanisms have been shown to be defective, exhibit varying defects in DNA repair when exposed to ultraviolet radiation. Patients with the least effective DNA repair have the greatest incidence of chronic neurologic disease, including upper and lower motor neuron involvement (1). Nevertheless, the majority of research on DNA repair has been directed toward the pathogenesis of neoplasia, the consequence of DNA damage to replicating cell populations, rather than toward cell death, which would be the natural consequence of a failure of DNA repair in a static cell population.

Maintenance of neural integrity over many years may also depend on trophic factors. A protein, nerve growth factor, has been isolated from sympathetic and certain sensory neurons and characterized. It not only stimulates enzymes and promotes growth but also maintains cell survival. Indeed, the administration of exogenous nerve growth factor prevents cell death after the surgical or chemical induction of lesions in the neurites of sympathetic neurons (17). Similar trophic factors probably exist for other neuronal populations. A nerve growth factor specific for motor neurons may well exist, and failure of its production, blocking of its action, or failure of its transport to the soma might well lead to premature motor neuron death.

Both anatomic and physiologic studies suggest that motor neurons of the spinal cord are normally lost with age. This loss becomes prominent at approximately 60 years of age (16, 22). McComas et al. noted the similarity of this age to the average age of onset of ALS and postulated that ALS might represent an acceleration of normal aging (16). However, if this were the case, the incidence of ALS would increase progressively with age. Instead, the disease has a unimodal age-distribution curve with a peak incidence at about age 60. The incidence does not continue to increase with age as it does for osteoarthritis, prostatic malignancy, or gray hair. The correlation of mean onset with the time of initial, significant loss of motor neurons does suggest that some compensatory mechanism may be lacking in individuals who develop ALS.

Recently, neural plasticity has been demonstrated in the brains of aging animals. Studies in aging rats have shown a loss of olfactory bulb mitral cells beginning abruptly at 24 months of age, but coincident with this loss is a dramatic increase in the volume and length of dendritic projections of the remaining mitral cells, which presumably compensates for this loss (10).

Maintenance and repair of neurons and compensation for neuronal loss are not well understood. Basic neurobiologic studies aimed not at development but at long-term maintenance of normal neural integrity may provide clues to the sites of failures that lead to selective degeneration of the motor system.

EPIDEMIOLOGIC CONSIDERATIONS

In general, epidemiologic studies show a monotonously uniform incidence of ALS throughout the world. These studies provide no evidence that the incidence has been increasing or decreasing over recent decades, as might be expected if the disease were related to environmental pollutants, dietary inadequacies or excesses, or other environmental factors that have undergone regional or worldwide changes. Conversely, these epidemiologic studies do not rule out some widespread toxin, nutritional abnormality, or infectious agent.

Exceptions to this uniform incidence do exist, specifically among the Chamorros of Guam or the population of the Kii Peninsula of Japan, where the incidence of ALS is 100 times higher than in other areas (3). There is also a motor neuron disease of high incidence in a remote area of New Guinea, but the disease has not been characterized pathologically (6). Furthermore, throughout the world approximately 5%–10% of cases are familial with a pattern of autosomal dominant inheritance (3).

These isolated geographic foci and familial aggregates may represent diseases of the motor system due to other causes, but intensive study of these exotic foci or familial cases might provide the critical clue to the etiology of ALS. For example, if a specific inherited biochemical defect were found in familial cases, we could investigate mechanisms of induction of such a defect by environmental factors. Similarly, the high incidences in Guam and the Kii Peninsula may represent a greater concentration of the causative factor among these populations, or they might represent a genetic or environmental factor that predisposes those populations to the causative agent or agents of ALS.

We have no evidence that familial or focal cases have the same cause as the widespread sporadic disease, that the sporadic disease is due to a single etiologic agent, or that the disease in an individual patient is not of multifactorial causation. Studies of the familial cases and high-incidence foci could provide the entree to a new direction for research.

ANIMAL MODELS

Spontaneous neurologic diseases of the motor system have been observed in a variety of animals, including monkeys, dogs, cats, mice, rabbits, and zebras (2, 5, 9, 20, 23). These diseases have varying degrees of clinical and pathologic similarity to ALS in humans. Some are genetically determined, some are produced by viruses, and some are of unknown etiology.

Of the inherited motor neuron diseases of animals, the Wobbler mouse model has been the most extensively investigated. This disease is due to an autosomal recessive gene. Heterozygous animals are normal clinically and pathologically. The homozygous animals show early growth retardation and during the third week of life show abnormalities of gait with progressive weakness that leads to death after two or three months. Widespread abnormalities are present in motor neurons as well as other cell populations. Histologically, the major finding is neuronal vacuolization, a finding unlike any seen in motor neuron diseases of humans (2, 5).

A slowly progressive motor neuron disease that was identified recently in Brittany spaniels has both clinical and pathologic similarities to progressive spinal muscular atrophy in humans. This disorder also appears to have an autosomal recessive mode of inheritance. A striking feature of the pathology is the early presence of neurofilamentous swelling in the proximal axons of motor neurons (4) which resembles the argenophilic neurofilamentous swellings seen in both the sporadic and familial forms of ALS (19).

Intoxication with lead, mercury, magnesium, or selenium; dietary deficiencies; or occult malignancy have all been implicated clinically in motor neuron diseases, but none has been substantiated as a cause by experimental studies. Intoxication with β,β-iminodipropionitrile causes axonal swellings with accumulations of neurofilaments resembling those seen in patients with ALS and in the spaniels with spinal muscular atrophy. Studies of this intoxication in rats have shown an impairment of slow axoplasmic flow without alteration of fast anterograde or retrograde transport (8). Although this experimental disease has not yet been shown to cause anterior horn cell death resembling that in motor neuron diseases, it may clarify the abnormalities of axoplasmic flow that have been postulated in these diseases.

Although viral infections have been postulated as a cause of ALS for over 100 years, the evidence is not convincing. The recent demonstration of the transmissibility of kuru and Creutzfeldt-Jakob disease and the recovery of viruses from subacute sclerosing panencephalitis and progressive multifocal leukoencephalopathy have certainly heightened expectations that viral etiologies will be uncovered for other chronic neurologic diseases of humans. However, thus far, claims of virus recovery or serologic evidence of viral infections in patients with ALS have not been independently confirmed (12).

Viruses can selectively infect motor neurons, as in acute poliomyelitis, but the allegation that patients with sequelae of paralytic poliomyelitis are predisposed to the development of ALS is not generally accepted (18). Furthermore, we have no evidence indicating persistence of polioviruses, presence of poliovirus genome in the tissues of patients with ALS (25), or abnormal serologic responses to polioviruses in patients with ALS (13).

Recently, a spontaneous motor system disease of mature mice has been associated with a retrovirus (type C) infection (7). This disease resembles ALS in that it occurs in middle life, presents with both upper and lower motor neuron signs, and has a progressive course to paralysis and death. The pathologic features, however, are characterized during the early phase of the disease by the vacuolization of neurons and glial cells (2, 21). Furthermore, recent sequential electron microscopic studies have shown that neuronal disease develops when virus infection can be demonstrated only in histologically normal vascular endothelial cells and pericytes (21). Focusing research solely on the affected neurons in ALS may be a mistake, not only as judged from this viral model, but also in view of another classic degenerative disease, subacute combined degeneration, in which the primary lesion occurs in the gastrointestinal tract.

Recognition of retrovirus-induced motor neuron disease in mice led to studies of possible endogenous retrovirus infections in patients with ALS. Although initial studies suggested viral reverse-transcriptase activity in the neural tissue of patients from Guam (24), this enzyme activity has proven to be due to a brain terminal deoxynucleotidyl transferase rather than to a viral polymerase (MV Viola, GJ Gibbs Jr, P Norton, unpublished data). An immunologic disease involving the anterior horn cells of mice has also been reported, but a recent study indicates that this disease is also due to a viral infection (15).

CONCLUSIONS

Questioning of patients regarding life events, analysis of environmental factors, chemical analyses of trace metals, and attempts to isolate viruses have been unsuccessful in uncovering the etiology of ALS. However, none of these studies can be called truly negative. It may be that the patients were never asked the proper questions, that the correct chemical was not analyzed, or that the right method was not employed to recover an infectious agent. A crucial place still remains for critical clinical observation of individual patients, since serendipity is often the greatest ally of scientific advancement.

Although I am a virologist, I have tried not to overemphasize virologic studies. In my laboratory we have investigated virus-induced animal models of motor neuron disease and will continue to carry out virologic and immunologic studies of patients with the disease. However, this is not because of a deep conviction that ALS has a viral etiology, but because virology is our area of competence. We know too little about the cause of motor system diseases to press forward in a single direction. We know too little about the normal maintenance of motor neurons and too little about the intrinsic as well as the environmental factors that may cause their premature death. We know too little to abandon any lead.

REFERENCES

1. Andrews AD, Barrett SF, Robbins JH: Relation of DNA repair processes to pathological ageing of the nervous system in xeroderma pigmentosum. Lancet 1:1318–1320, 1976

2. Andrews JM, Andrews RL: The comparative neuropathology of motor neuron disease. In *Amyotrophic Lateral Sclerosis, Recent Research Trends, UCLA Forum in Medical Diseases.* Edited by JM Andrews, RT Johnson, MAB Brazier. New York, Academic Press, 1976, pp 181–216

3. Bobowick AR, Brody JA: Epidemiology of motor neuron diseases. N Engl J Med 288:1047–1055, 1973

4. Cork LC, Griffin JW, Munnell JF, et al: Hereditary canine spinal muscular atrophy. J Neuropathol Exp Neurol, in press

5. Duchen LW: Motor neuron disease in man and animals. Invest Cell Pathol 1:249–262, 1978

6. Gajdusek DC: Motor neuron disease in natives of New Guinea. N Engl J Med 286:474–476, 1963

7. Gardner MB, Henderson BE, Officer JE, et al: A spontaneous lower motor neuron disease apparently caused by indigenous type-C RNA virus in wild mice. J Natl Cancer Inst 51:1243–1254, 1973

8. Griffin JW, Hoffman PN, Clark AW, et al: Slow axonal transport of neurofilamental proteins: Impairment by β,β-iminodipropionitrile intoxication. Science 202:663–665, 1978

9. Higgins RJ, Vandevelde M, Hoff EJ, et al: Neurofibrillary accumulation in the zebra (Equus burchelli). Acta Neuropathol 37:1–5, 1977

10. Hinds JW, McNelly NA: Aging of the rat olfactory bulb: Growth and atrophy of constituent layers and changes in size and number of mitral cells. J Comp Neurol 171:345–368, 1977

11. Johnson HA, Pavelec M: Thermal noise in cells. Am J Pathol 69: 119–129, 1972

12. Johnson RT: Virological studies of amyotrophic lateral sclerosis: An overview. In *Amyotrophic Lateral Sclerosis, Recent Research Trends, UCLA Forum in Medical Diseases.* Edited by JM Andrews, RT Johnson, MAB Brazier. New York, Academic Press, 1976, pp 173–180

13. Kurent JE, Brooks BR, Madden DL, et al: Cerebrospinal fluid viral antibody titers in amyotrophic lateral sclerosis and late onset post-poliomyelitis progressive muscular atrophy. Arch Neurol, in press

14. Lewis PD: Abiotrophy revisited. In *Motor Neurone Disease.* Edited by F Clifford Rose. Kent, England, Pitman Medical Publishing Co., 1977, pp 30–35

15. Martinez D, Wolanski B, Tytell AA, et al: Viral etiology of age-dependent polioencephalomyelitis in C58 mice. Infect Immun 23:133–139, 1979

16. McComas AJ, Upton ARM, Sica REP: Motor neurone disease and ageing. Lancet 2:1477–1480, 1973

17. Mobley WC, Server AC, Ishii DN, et al: Nerve growth factor. N Engl J Med 297:1096–1104, 1149–1158, 1211–1218, 1977

18. Mulder DW, Rosenbaum RA, Layton DD: Late progression of poliomyelitis or forme fruste amyotrophic lateral sclerosis. Mayo Clin Proc 47:756–761, 1972

19. Schochet SS, Hardman JM, Ladewig PP, et al: Intraneuronal conglomerates in sporadic motor neurone disease. Arch Neurol 20:548–553, 1969

to know more about concordance in twins and about HL-A typing in familial and sporadic cases. What we need most is information about the biochemical abnormalities in ALS. However, there are no clues. The only feasible approach would be what scientists disdainfully call a "fishing expedition"—screening blood, urine, and CSF for common and exotic constituents. In a sense, this brings us back to unanswered basic questions. What is the difference between genetically dominant and recessive diseases? Why has it been so difficult to identify the biochemical abnormalities of autosomal dominant diseases? Why are dominant diseases, including motor neuron disease, so much more variable in clinical expression?

Biochemical genetics is not a neglected field, and we can anticipate progress—but when? Biochemical information about genetic ALS would surely influence our concepts about the more common idiopathic forms.

Finally, Dr. Johnson discussed animal models. Here, I respectfully part company with him, at least in relation to spontaneous diseases. Enormous amounts of money, effort, and intelligence have been devoted to the study of animals with "muscular dystrophy"; but we still do not understand the fundamental biochemical abnormality in any of these diseases, and we do not know which animal diseases, if any, are related to which human diseases. Unfortunately, there is no indication that study of animal motor neuron diseases is going to be any more productive. I do not look on these animal models as models of anything.

Experimental diseases, however, are another matter, and it is a measure of the corruption of our language that they have to be called "animal models," or that the study of viral diseases is put together with the study of the animal model in Brittany spaniels. In contrast to my skepticism about spaniels or Wobbler mice, Dr. Johnson and his colleagues in virology have provided an overwhelming amount of data suggesting that a virus may cause the idiopathic human disease. If this is so, then animal models are of little help. We have to know the limits of attempts to isolate, transmit, or identify viruses in humans with ALS. If present techniques fail, new approaches will be devised, and the search for a virus is likely to continue unless some other cause is found. The rest of us, including funding agencies, will have to be patient. Slow virus research is painfully slow.

Again, we return to the problem of basic science. What is the nature of the scrapie agent and of the transmissible agents that cause human diseases but elicit no detectable immunologic responses? What host factors affect the clinical expression of these chronic infections? We have a long way to go in these areas.

There is another kind of experimental disease that should not be neglected. If lead, mercury, and x-rays can cause human motor neuron diseases, it would be valuable to determine what exactly these substances do to the motor neuron. This question can be studied experimentally.

One additional category of research does not fit neatly into Dr. Johnson's three major divisions: study of the human patient. For instance, we have very little information about the humoral and cell-mediated immune status of patients with ALS, and there has been no prospective study of the ultrastructure of motor neurons in this disease. I would not neglect controlled therapeutic trials. The recent flurry of reports has not indicated objective benefit from any agent, but the trials themselves have been psychologically important for patients and physicians. This activity should continue, because there are effective treatments for other diseases of unknown pathogenesis. Although any agent with reasonable promise and low hazard can be used, I believe it is crucial to use double-blind trials. Although such trials are expensive, tiring for the investigator, and unacceptable to many patients, they are the only way to avoid fiascos such as the snake-venom test experience.

I would conclude with two hopes: first, that our larger society, not the Amyotrophic Lateral Sclerosis Society of America alone, can support adequate funding for basic biomedical research, since those of us who are interested in ALS cannot predict how or when the crucial information is going to appear; and second, that our larger society can provide adequate funding for the training of young investigators who will bring us new ideas, funding to make a career in clinical investigation sufficiently attractive to bright young men and women.

Index